Advances on Scoliogeny, Diagnosis and Management of Scoliosis and Spinal Disorders

Advances on Scoliogeny, Diagnosis and Management of Scoliosis and Spinal Disorders

Editor

Theodoros B. Grivas

MDPI • Basel • Beijing • Wuhan • Barcelona • Belgrade • Manchester • Tokyo • Cluj • Tianjin

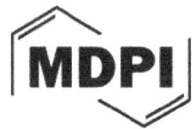

Editor
Theodoros B. Grivas
Tzanion General Hospital
Greece

Editorial Office
MDPI
St. Alban-Anlage 66
4052 Basel, Switzerland

This is a reprint of articles from the Special Issue published online in the open access journal *Journal of Clinical Medicine* (ISSN 2077-0383) (available at: https://www.mdpi.com/journal/jcm/special_issues/scoliosis_spinal_disorders).

For citation purposes, cite each article independently as indicated on the article page online and as indicated below:

LastName, A.A.; LastName, B.B.; LastName, C.C. Article Title. *Journal Name* **Year**, *Volume Number*, Page Range.

ISBN 978-3-0365-6005-2 (Hbk)
ISBN 978-3-0365-6006-9 (PDF)

© 2022 by the authors. Articles in this book are Open Access and distributed under the Creative Commons Attribution (CC BY) license, which allows users to download, copy and build upon published articles, as long as the author and publisher are properly credited, which ensures maximum dissemination and a wider impact of our publications.

The book as a whole is distributed by MDPI under the terms and conditions of the Creative Commons license CC BY-NC-ND.

Contents

About the Editor ix

Preface to "Advances on Scoliogeny, Diagnosis and Management of Scoliosis and Spinal Disorders" xi

Edyta Kinel, Krzysztof Korbel, Piotr Janusz, Mateusz Kozinoga, Dariusz Czaprowski and Tomasz Kotwicki
Polish Adaptation of the Italian Spine Youth Quality of Life Questionnaire
Reprinted from: *J. Clin. Med.* **2021**, *10*, 2081, doi:10.3390/jcm10102081 1

Lorenzo Costa, Tom P. C. Schlosser, Hanad Jimale, Jelle F. Homans, Moyo C. Kruyt and René M. Castelein
The Effectiveness of Different Concepts of Bracing in Adolescent Idiopathic Scoliosis (AIS): A Systematic Review and Meta-Analysis
Reprinted from: *J. Clin. Med.* **2021**, *10*, 2145, doi:10.3390/jcm10102145 9

Hans-Rudolf Weiss
Comment on Costa et al. The Effectiveness of Different Concepts of Bracing in Adolescent Idiopathic Scoliosis (AIS): A Systematic Review and Meta-Analysis. J. Clin. Med. 2021, 10, 2145
Reprinted from: *J. Clin. Med.* **2022**, *11*, 752, doi:10.3390/jcm11030752 25

Lorenzo Costa, Tom P. C. Schlösser, Moyo C. Kruyt and René M. Castelein
Reply to Weiss, H.-R. Comment on "Costa et al. The Effectiveness of Different Concepts of Bracing in Adolescent Idiopathic Scoliosis (AIS): A Systematic Review and Meta-Analysis. *J. Clin. Med.* 2021, *10*, 2145"
Reprinted from: *J. Clin. Med.* **2022**, *11*, 918, doi:10.3390/jcm11040918 29

Lorenzo Costa, Steven de Reuver, Luc Kan, Peter Seevinck, Moyo C. Kruyt, Tom P. C. Schlosser and René M. Castelein
Ossification and Fusion of the Vertebral Ring Apophysis as an Important Part of Spinal Maturation
Reprinted from: *J. Clin. Med.* **2021**, *10*, 3217, doi:10.3390/jcm10153217 33

Luis González Vicente, María Jiménez Barrios, Josefa González-Santos, Mirian Santamaría-Peláez, Raúl Soto-Cámara, Juan Mielgo-Ayuso, Diego Fernández-Lázaro and Jerónimo J. González-Bernal
The ISJ 3D Brace, a Providence Brace Evolution, as a Surgery Prevention Method in Idiopathic Scoliosis
Reprinted from: *J. Clin. Med.* **2021**, *10*, 3915, doi:10.3390/jcm10173915 43

Hong Jin Kim, Jae Hyuk Yang, Dong-Gune Chang, Se-Il Suk, Seung Woo Suh, Yunjin Nam, Sang-Il Kim and Kwang-Sup Song
Long-Term Influence of Paraspinal Muscle Quantity in Adolescent Idiopathic Scoliosis Following Deformity Correction by Posterior Approach
Reprinted from: *J. Clin. Med.* **2021**, *10*, 4790, doi:10.3390/jcm10204790 55

Edyta Kinel, Krzysztof Korbel, Mateusz Kozinoga, Dariusz Czaprowski, Łukasz Stepniak and Tomasz Kotwicki
The Measurement of Health-Related Quality of Life of Girls with Mild to Moderate Idiopathic Scoliosis—Comparison of ISYQOL versus SRS-22 Questionnaire
Reprinted from: *J. Clin. Med.* **2021**, *10*, 4806, doi:10.3390/jcm10214806 65

Steven de Reuver, Jelle F. Homans, Tom P. C. Schlösser, Michiel L. Houben, Vincent F. X. Deeney, Terrence B. Crowley, Ralf Stücker, Saba Pasha, Moyo C. Kruyt, Donna M. McDonald-McGinn and René M. Castelein
22q11.2 Deletion Syndrome as a Human Model for Idiopathic Scoliosis
Reprinted from: *J. Clin. Med.* **2021**, *10*, 4823, doi:10.3390/jcm10214823 75

Katarzyna Politarczyk, Mateusz Kozinoga, Łukasz Stepniak, Paweł Panieński and Tomasz Kotwicki
Spirometry Examination of Adolescents with Thoracic Idiopathic Scoliosis: Is Correction for Height Loss Useful?
Reprinted from: *J. Clin. Med.* **2021**, *10*, 4877, doi:10.3390/jcm10214877 87

Yujia Wang, Huanxiong Chen, Jiajun Zhang, Tsz-ping Lam, A.L.H. Hung, J.C.Y. Cheng and W.Y.W. Lee
Potential Muscle-Related Biomarkers in Predicting Curve Progression to the Surgical Threshold in Adolescent Idiopathic Scoliosis—A Pilot Proteomic Study Comparing Four Non-Progressive vs. Four Progressive Patients vs. A Control Cohort
Reprinted from: *J. Clin. Med.* **2021**, *10*, 4927, doi:10.3390/jcm10214927 101

Marlene Dufvenberg, Elias Diarbakerli, Anastasios Charalampidis, Birgitta Öberg, Hans Tropp, Anna Aspberg Ahl, Hans Möller, Paul Gerdhem and Allan Abbott
Six-Month Results on Treatment Adherence, Physical Activity, Spinal Appearance, Spinal Deformity, and Quality of Life in an Ongoing Randomised Trial on Conservative Treatment for Adolescent Idiopathic Scoliosis (CONTRAIS)
Reprinted from: *J. Clin. Med.* **2021**, *10*, 4967, doi:10.3390/jcm10214967 115

Stefano Negrini, Sabrina Donzelli, Francesco Negrini, Chiara Arienti, Fabio Zaina and Koen Peers
A Pragmatic Benchmarking Study of an Evidence-Based Personalised Approach in 1938 Adolescents with High-Risk Idiopathic Scoliosis
Reprinted from: *J. Clin. Med.* **2021**, *10*, 5020, doi:10.3390/jcm10215020 133

Elias S. Vasiliadis, Dimitrios Stergios Evangelopoulos, Angelos Kaspiris, Christos Vlachos and Spyros G. Pneumaticos
Sclerostin and Its Involvement in the Pathogenesis of Idiopathic Scoliosis
Reprinted from: *J. Clin. Med.* **2021**, *10*, 5286, doi:10.3390/jcm10225286 155

Theodoros B. Grivas, George Vynichakis, Michail Chandrinos, Christina Mazioti, Despina Papagianni, Aristea Mamzeri and Constantinos Mihas
Morphology, Development and Deformation of the Spine in Mild and Moderate Scoliosis: Are Changes in the Spine Primary or Secondary?
Reprinted from: *J. Clin. Med.* **2021**, *10*, 5901, doi:10.3390/jcm10245901 165

Steven de Reuver, Tom P. C. Schlösser, Moyo C. Kruyt, Keita Ito and René M. Castelein
Comment on Grivas et al. Morphology, Development and Deformation of the Spine in Mild and Moderate Scoliosis: Are Changes in the Spine Primary or Secondary? *J. Clin. Med.* 2021, *10*, 5901
Reprinted from: *J. Clin. Med.* **2022**, *11*, 1160, doi:10.3390/jcm11051160 173

Theodoros B. Grivas, George Vynichakis, Michail Chandrinos, Christina Mazioti, Despina Papagianni, Aristea Mamzeri and Constantinos Mihas
Reply to de Reuver et al. Comment on "Grivas et al. Morphology, Development and Deformation of the Spine in Mild and Moderate Scoliosis: Are Changes in the Spine Primary or Secondary? *J. Clin. Med.* 2021, *10*, 5901"
Reprinted from: *J. Clin. Med.* **2022**, *11*, 2049, doi:10.3390/jcm11072049 177

Christian Wong and Thomas B. Andersen
Evaluation of Brace Treatment Using the Soft Brace Spinaposture: A Four-Years Follow-Up
Reprinted from: *J. Clin. Med.* **2022**, *11*, 264, doi:10.3390/jcm11010264 . . . . **183**

Alberto Romano, Elena Ippolito, Camilla Risoli, Edoardo Malerba, Martina Favetta, Andrea Sancesario, Meir Lotan and Daniel Sender Moran
Intensive Postural and Motor Activity Program Reduces Scoliosis Progression in People with Rett Syndrome
Reprinted from: *J. Clin. Med.* **2022**, *11*, 559, doi:10.3390/jcm11030559 . . . . **195**

Agnieszka Stepień and Beata Pałdyna
Neurodynamic Functions and Their Correlations with Postural Parameters in Adolescents with Idiopathic Scoliosis
Reprinted from: *J. Clin. Med.* **2022**, *11*, 1115, doi:10.3390/jcm11041115 . . . . **209**

Rebecca Sauvagnac and Manuel Rigo
Evolution of Early Onset Scoliosis under Treatment with a 3D-Brace Concept
Reprinted from: *J. Clin. Med.* **2022**, *11*, 1186, doi:10.3390/jcm11051186 . . . . **227**

Mateusz Kozinoga, Łukasz Stoliński, Krzysztof Korbel, Katarzyna Politarczyk, Piotr Janusz and Tomasz Kotwicki
Regular School Sport versus Dedicated Physical Activities for Body Posture—A Prospective Controlled Study Assessing the Sagittal Plane in 7–10-Year-Old Children
Reprinted from: *J. Clin. Med.* **2022**, *11*, 1255, doi:10.3390/jcm11051255 . . . . **243**

About the Editor

Theodoros B. Grivas

Dr Theodoros B. Grivas, MD, PhD. Dr Theodoros is an orthopaedic and spinal surgeon who graduated from the Medical School at the "Aristotle" University of Thessaloniki (1978), Central Macedonia, Greece. He completed his training in General Surgery, in paediatric and adult orthopaedics and traumatology in Greece and received an MD Diploma. He also received a PhD from the National and Kapodistrian University of Athens, Greece. He worked at the "University Hospital", Queen's Medical Centre, Nottingham, "Harlow Wood" Orthopaedic Hospital, Mansfield, UK, under Mr. JK Webb, and under Professor RG Burwell. Subsequently he worked at at "Evangelismos" and "Thriasio" Hospital in Athens, Greece. At "Thriasio" Hospital, he served as Director of the department of Orthopaedics and Traumatology for 5 years. He is a member of the Hellenic Association of Orthopaedic Surgery and Traumatology, in addition to his membership of numerous other scientific societies. He is a member and Traveling Fellow of both AOA and SRS. He served as an IRSSD, SOSORT (of which he was also a founder) and Hellenic (Greek) Spine Society president. He completed several research projects, studied and implemented the School Screening program, established a National Training Center for school-screening examiners (www.schoolscreening.gr), published numerous peer-review articles and chapters in books and was invited to lecture on various general orthopaedic and spinal topics. He has written or edited 9 books, as well as numerous scientific Medline-indexed papers, (see http://www.ncbi.nlm.nih.gov/pubmed/?term=grivas+t) publications and presentations. He was scientific responsible/principal investigator or collaborator of 20 research projects, financed by Greek national or European sources (see also at https://www.researchgate.net/profile/Theodoros_Grivas/contributions). He served as the Chief Editor of BMC open access Scoliosis and Spinal Deformities, former editor of the Scoliosis journal and is member of editorial board or reader for several peer-review journals. During 2019–20, he served as a member of the National Examination Committee for the specialty of Orthopaedics and Traumatology and as a member (2020-2021) of the Crisis and Selection Council of Hellenic National Health System, the competent authority for the appointment of Orthopaedic Surgeons in State Hospital Positions, in the 2nd Health District of Piraeus and the Aegean. His department was invited to provide the "Trialect platform" Fellowship—Traineeship in Orthopaedics and Traumatology. He retired (2021) from the Orthopaedic and Traumatology Department at "Tzaneio" General Hospital of Piraeus, Greece, where he has served as Director for 12 years. He served the Hellenic National Health System for 35 years as an Orthopaedic and Spinal Surgeon. Currently he is working to establish the Hellenic Scoliosis Foundation.

Preface to "Advances on Scoliogeny, Diagnosis and Management of Scoliosis and Spinal Disorders"

Scoliosis, a 3-D deformity of the spine and the thorax, mainly affects children, who are the future of any society. The medical societies that specialize in this ailment have recently focused intensely on the study of the epidemiology, etiology, pathobiomechanics and laboratory work, in addition to clinical and imaging documentation and treatment, either non-operative or operative. The advent of new technologies is key in the study and advancement of our insight into these diseases, with the aim of improving the quality of life of those who live with the condition. Our ultimate goal is to diminish or even eliminate the disease.

It is interesting to note the impressive developments in the implementation of growth modulation for the surgical treatment of early-onset scoliosis. These developments have led to better patient quality of life compared to what was experienced in the past. However, this topic is still under development and new instrumentation systems are being introduced.

When proper management is not implemented, spinal disorders may lead to significant social problems and enormous economic burdens. Therefore, treatment decisions based on the recent evidence-based literature will result in the optimum outcomes. Proper management, including prevention and treament, whether operative or not, must be tailored and implemented.

Therefore, it is very important to increase awareness and advocacy for a social mission regarding the early detection of scoliosis and prevention of progressive spinal deformity. It is imperative to raise awareness about scoliosis and to inform the public, as well as the healthcare and policy-making communities, about the individual, familial and societal burdens of spinal deformity, as well as the benefits of proper detection, diagnosis and optimal care for all patients.

This Special Issue and its papers aim to serve the above-mentioned objectives.

Theodoros B. Grivas
Editor

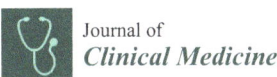

Article

Polish Adaptation of the Italian Spine Youth Quality of Life Questionnaire

Edyta Kinel [1,*], Krzysztof Korbel [2], Piotr Janusz [3], Mateusz Kozinoga [3], Dariusz Czaprowski [2,4] and Tomasz Kotwicki [3]

1. Department of Rehabilitation, University of Medical Sciences in Poznan, 61-545 Poznan, Poland
2. Department of Physiotherapy, University of Medical Sciences in Poznan, 61-545 Poznan, Poland; kkorbel@ump.edu.pl (K.K.); dariusz.czaprowski@interia.pl (D.C.)
3. Department of Spine Disorders and Pediatric Orthopedics, University of Medical Sciences in Poznan, 61-545 Poznan, Poland; mdpjanusz@gmail.com (P.J.); mkozinoga@hotmail.com (M.K.); kotwicki@ump.edu.pl (T.K.)
4. Department of Health Sciences, Olsztyn University, Bydgoska 33, 10-243 Olsztyn, Poland
* Correspondence: ekinel@ump.edu.pl; Tel.: +48-61-831-0217

Abstract: The study aimed to carry on the process of the cultural adaptation of the Italian Spine Youth Quality of Life Questionnaire (ISYQOL) into Polish (ISYQOL-PL). The a priori hypothesis was: the ISYQOL-PL questionnaire is reliable and appropriate for adolescents with a spinal deformity. Fifty-six adolescents (mean age 13.8 ± 1.9) with idiopathic scoliosis (AIS) with a mean Cobb angle 29.1 (±9.7) and two with Scheuermann juvenile kyphosis (SJK) with a kyphosis angle 67.5 (±17.7) degrees were enrolled. All patients had been wearing a corrective TLSO brace for an average duration of 2.3 (±1.8) years. The Institutional Review Board approved the study. The cross-cultural adaptation of the ISYQOL-PL was performed following the guidelines set up by the International Quality of Life Assessment Project. The reliability was assessed using internal consistency (the Cronbach's alpha coefficient) and test–retest reliability (intraclass correlation coefficient $ICC_{2.1}$, CI = 95%); moreover, floor and ceiling effects were calculated. The internal consistency was satisfactory (Cronbach's alpha coefficient 0.8). The test–retest revealed high reliability with the value of $ICC_{2.1}$ for the entire group 0.90, CI (0.84 to 0.94). There was neither floor nor ceiling effect for the ISYQOL-PL overall score. The ISYQOL-PL is reliable and can be used in adolescents with spinal deformity.

Keywords: idiopathic scoliosis; health-related quality of life; cultural adaptation; Italian Spine Youth Quality of Life Questionnaire

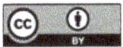

1. Introduction

The impact of the disease and the treatment applied on the quality of life of adolescents with spinal deformities, namely adolescent idiopathic scoliosis (AIS) or Scheuermann juvenile kyphosis (SJK), is considered to be multidimensional. This includes subjective perception, and changes in physical, psychological, and social well-being. Moreover, spinal deformities' progressive character can affect adolescents' health-related quality of life (HRQoL). Therefore, while evaluating AIS and SJK adolescents' treatment results, the changes in the HRQoL should be taken into account [1]. A variety of HRQoL questionnaires exist, dedicated to adolescents with spinal deformities having completed their treatment, e.g., Scoliosis Research Society—(SRS-22) or Scoliosis Quality of Life Index (SQLI) [2,3]. Vasiliadis et al. [4] developed the Brace Questionnaire (BrQ), an instrument for measuring the HRQoL specifically for scoliotic adolescents who are being treated conservatively by wearing a corrective brace, and the Polish version of BrQ has been validated [5]. There are questionnaires admitted to monitoring the level of stress induced by the deformity (Bad Sobernheim Stress Questionnaire, BSSQ—Deformity) and the stress induced by the treatment with a brace (Bad Sobernheim Stress Questionnaire, BSSQ—Brace) for patients with idiopathic scoliosis [6]. However, the BSSQ questionnaires do not evaluate the overall HRQoL. Recently, to address the limitations of existing HRQoL tools, the Italian Spine Youth Quality of Life (ISYQOL) questionnaire has been developed by the Italian Scientific Spine Institute. The ISYQOL questionnaire was built using Rasch analysis. The ISYQOL questionnaire measures HRQoL in all types of spinal deformities, including surgical curves [7,8]. The ISYQOL has been cross-culturally adapted and validated in English [9] and Spanish [10], but not yet in Polish. This paper aims to carry on the cultural adaptation of the ISYQOL questionnaire into Polish (ISYQOL-PL).

2. Materials and Methods

The a priori hypothesis was proposed as follows: the ISYQOL-PL questionnaire version is reliable and appropriate for adolescents with a spinal deformity.

2.1. Study Population

Fifty-eight patients with spinal deformities (56 AIS and 2 SJK) were enrolled to assess the ISYQOL-PL questionnaire version. The sample included 52 girls and six boys. The same specialist in orthopedics treated the patients. The following criteria for inclusion were applied: (1) patients at the age of 10–18 years; (2) AIS or SJK diagnosis; (3) who have been wearing the brace for at least three months for at least 12 h/24 h (4) AIS patients with a Cobb angle $\geq 20°$, SJK patients with a kyphosis angle $\geq 45°$. Exclusion criteria: (1) history of spine surgery; (2) combined spinal deformities (e.g., scoliosis plus spondylolysis), (3) a history of relevant diseases, surgery, or trauma, including a positive neurologic examination.

The mean age of the patients at the time of completing the questionnaire was 13.8 (± 1.9) years, the mean AIS patients' Cobb angle was 29.1 (± 9.7) degrees, and the SJK with kyphosis angle was 67.5 (± 17.7) degrees. All patients had been wearing a corrective TLSO brace with an average duration of 2.3 (± 1.8) years.

Twice within a one-week interval, patients were asked to fill in the questionnaire. The time needed to answer all questions during the first attempt to complete the questionnaire was measured. All the invited adolescents selected through the inclusion criteria participated in the study. The participants were left to fill in the questionnaire alone, being in a separate space, to minimize any influence from parents or medical staff. Data from the ISYQOL-PL were collected during November and December 2019.

The Institutional Review Board approved the study.

Before inclusion in the study, the parents and the patients awarded their informed consent.

2.2. Italian Spine Youth Quality of Life (ISYQOL) Questionnaire

The ISYQOL questionnaire is based on patients' concerns and has been shown to be particularly appropriate in AIS and SJK patients undergoing non-surgical management. The ISYQOL is a 20 items questionnaire. Each item is scored 0, 1, or 2. Items investigating the presence of spine-related problems (questions 1–4, 7–9, 11–12 and 14–20) are coded 0-1-2 (0: never; 1: sometimes; 2: often). Conversely, "items investigating the presence of positive thoughts" (question 5, 6, 10, 13) are coded 2-1-0 (2: never; 1: sometimes; 0: often). It provides a total score, with lower scores representing a higher quality of life. The ordinal ISYQOL total score is subsequently converted to an interval measure (i.e., ISYQOL measure), expressed on a 0–100% scale, where 100% indicates the highest quality of life.

The Rasch method used in the analysis allows for a comparison of the ISYQOL result of non-brace wearers (who answer only 13 of the 20 items) with brace wearers (who complete the entire questionnaire). The questionnaire is developmentally appropriate for ages 10–18 years and designed to be self-administered [7,8].

2.3. Adaptation Process

The process of the cross-cultural adaptation of the ISYQOL-PL was performed following the guidelines set up by the International Quality of Life Assessment (IQOLA) [11].

The implementation of this method includes the following steps: (1) forward translation, (2) back-translation and expert panel, (3) pre-testing and cognitive interviewing, (4) development of the final version. The total sample size was decided based on previous recommendations for validation studies [12].

2.4. Forward Translation

Two independent translators converted the original Italian version into Polish. Through the whole process of adaptation, one of the translators, who had a medical background, was involved. The second translator had a background outside of medicine.

2.5. Back-Translation and Expert Panel

A comparison of the original and two translated versions was achieved at this stage. The two translators, together with the authors, identified differences in translations and produced a combined version. Next, back-translation was carried out, where two independent translators, who were native in Italian, translated the Polish version into the original document's language (Italian). Both translators were not familiar with the original version. At the following step, a commission group combined of translators, a psychologist, a specialist in orthopedics, and a statistician, assessed the translations. The so-called pre-final version was drafted as a result of consensus.

2.6. Pre-Testing, and Cognitive Interviewing and Development of Final Version

Thirty-four adolescents with AIS and two with SJK patients (who met the study eligibility requirements described above) were checked for the pre-final questionnaire's comprehensiveness to ensure the adapted version was understandable. The participants were interviewed after completing the questionnaire in order to discuss their interpretation of each question and answer. The committee then reassessed this test's outcome, and the final form of the questionnaire was created (Supplemental Data File S1).

2.7. Statistical Analyses

All statistical analyses were carried out using the Real Statistics Resource Pack software (Release 4.7) with a significance level of $\alpha < 0.05$. The Shapiro–Wilk test for normality identified the data normally distributed; therefore, parametric tests were used.

Furthermore, statistical analysis included descriptive statistics in calculating means ± standard deviations (SD) for a given question and the second level of analysis, which was comparative, concerning reliability, floor, and ceiling effect.

2.8. Reliability

The reliability was assessed using the two most important properties: consistency and stability.

Internal consistency was assessed using Cronbach's alpha coefficient. Cronbach's alpha ranges from 0 (none of the items are correlated with one another) to 1 (reflects perfect internal consistency). Cronbach's alpha of at least 0.70 was chosen to indicate adequate internal consistency [13].

Test–retest reliability was evaluated using the intraclass correlation coefficient ($ICC_{2.1}$, CI = 95%), the most suitable and most commonly used reliability parameter for ordinal measures. $ICC_{2.1}$ concerns the variation in the population (interindividual variation) divided by total variation, which is the interindividual variation plus the intraindividual variation (measurement error), expressed as a ratio between 0 and 1. The sum of scores obtained per each question provided by all patients during the first time and second time and the sum of total scores obtained per each patient were used, respectively, for test–retest analysis. A positive rating for reliability is when the $ICC_{2.1}$ is at least 0.70 in a sample size of at least 50 patients [12]. To reduce the memory effect, there was a 7-day period between tests [12].

2.9. Measurement Error

The standard error of measurement (SEM) and minimal detectable change at the 90% level (MDC90) were employed. The sample included all patients ($n = 58$) who completed the ISYQOL-PL twice. The SEM was calculated as an element from the mean square error (MSE) from the analysis of variance, ANOVA. The MDC is the minimum change in a patient's score that ensures the change is not the result of measurement error. The MDC90 was calculated using the formula: MDC = SEM × 1.65 × $\sqrt{2}$, where 1.65 is the z-value that reflects the 90% CI of no change, [14] and $\sqrt{2}$ indicates two measurements assessing change [14].

2.10. Floor and Ceiling Effects

Floor and ceiling effects were calculated and considered to be high if >15% of patients reported the worst or best status, respectively [12]. The distribution of results indicates the number (percentage) of patients with a minimum score (floor effect) and the number (percentage) of patients with a maximum score (ceiling effect).

3. Results

The duration of completing the questionnaire was ≤10 min in all patients.
The lowest, highest, and mean scores (%) obtained using the ISYQOL-PL are presented in Table 1.

Table 1. Distribution of minimal, maximal, and mean total scores (%) of ISYQOL-PL.

Questionnaire	N	Min	Max	Mean	SD
ISYQOL-PL first trial	58	32.96%	62.83%	49.05%	3.15
ISYQOL-PL second trial	58	32.96%	66.29%	49.05%	3.15

Cronbach's alpha coefficient was 0.8, which indicates satisfactory internal consistency (Table 2).

Table 2. The Cronbach's alpha value coefficient of the ISYQOL-PL compared to the ISYQOL (original).

ISYQOL-PL	ISYQOL (Original)
Cronbach's alpha	Cronbach's alpha
0.8	0.83

The test–retest study revealed high reliability, and the value of $ICC_{2.1}$ for the entire group was high (0.90, CI ranged from 0.84 to 0.94) with SEM = 0.36 and MDC 90% CI = 0.84.

When completing the questionnaire for the first and the second time, there were no floor or ceiling effects for the ISYQOL-PL overall score. Cronbach's alpha, mean (%), and SD, floor and ceiling effects for each ISYQOL-PL domain are presented in Table 3.

Table 3. Cronbach's alpha, mean (%), and SD, floor and ceiling effects for each ISYQOL-PL domain.

ISYQOL-PL DOMAIN	Number of Items	Cronbach's Alpha	Mean	SD	Floor Effect	Ceiling Effect
SPINE HEALTH	13	0.79	56.88%	3.32	0 (0.0%)	0 (0.0%)
BRACE	7	0.77	68.21%	4	0 (0.0%)	1 (1.7%)

4. Discussion

This study presents a Polish adaptation of the ISYQOL, a new measure of HRQoL in adolescents with spinal deformities.

4.1. Statistical Relevance

Cronbach's alpha is considered a proper method for estimating multi-item scales' reliability, estimating internal consistency expressing the number of items and their average correlation [3]. Cronbach's alpha should be greater than 0.70 to prove good reliability [13]. The ISYQOL-PL had a good value of Cronbach's alpha coefficient (0.8), exceeding the minimum recommended value of 0.70 and indicating satisfactory internal consistency as a factor of satisfactory reliability of the ISYQOL-PL. The Cronbach's alpha score achieved by authors of the original version, Caronni et al. [7], was 0.83. The English version of the ISYQOL questionnaire had the value of Cronbach's alpha of 0.79 to 0.84 [9], indicating good internal consistency [1]. The Spanish version of the ISYQOL showed an acceptable internal consistency (0.77 Cronbach's alpha) [10] and is considered a reliable and valid tool to measure HRQoL admitted to Spanish-language-speaking adolescents with spinal deformity during conservative treatment (with or without a brace). There was neither floor nor ceiling effect for the ISYQOL-PL overall score. Sánchez-Raya et al. [10] reported similar results.

4.2. Clinical Relevance

The conservative treatment of adolescents with spinal deformities without or with a brace can significantly impact patients' subjective perception and social well-being and negatively affect their HRQoL [1]. Moreover, Wang et al. [15], in a recent review analyzing the impact of bracing on AIS patient's quality of life, indicated that self-image, mental health and vitality are the three most frequently reported affected domains.

The treatment's effectiveness has been demonstrated to depend on the patients' treatment compliance [16–18] and the quality of brace usage [18]. Additionally, the brace's impact on the self and body image is reported as a contributing factor for stress. The stress level determines compliance and can be assessed using the BSSQ questionnaire (BSSQ—Deformity, BSSQ—Brace). Kotwicki et al. [19] noticed that the BSSQ is a helpful method for determining the level of stress during conservative treatment for AIS patients. Lin et al. [20] found that female adolescents with idiopathic scoliosis who had undergone bracing were more vulnerable to depressive psychological status.

However, the international scientific Society on Scoliosis Orthopaedic and Rehabilitation Treatment (SOSORT) recommends the overall evaluation of adolescents with spinal deformities using HRQoL questionnaires [21]. The ISYQOL questionnaire, developed with Rasch analysis, fully complies with a fundamental measure (additivity, generalizability, and unidimensionality) [8]. The ISYQOL items were developed based on the concerns expressed by the patient and the clinician's input. Moreover, Caronni et al. showed high validity using HRQoL in adolescents with spinal deformities and better known-groups validity than the very often used SRS22 questionnaire [8]. Next of the ISYQOL questionnaire's strengths is the possibility to compare the measurement of the HRQoL in patients with AIS and SJK and patients wearing or not wearing a brace [7].

Our results indicate that an ISYQOL-PL questionnaire is a reliable tool for evaluating the HRQoL of adolescent patients with spinal deformities.

As a limitation, the ISYQOL-PL presented a lower sample than the Italian sample (402 Italian patients versus 58 Polish). Additionally, our group consisted of six boys and two patients with SJK, so it was impossible to analyze the per-gender and per-spinal deformities differences. Investigating this specific aspect at the larger sample size is under our ongoing study. Finally, in the future, the Polish version of the ISYQOL questionnaire could be tested in patients who had surgical treatment and adult patients, as recommended by Caronni et al. [8].

5. Conclusions

The ISYQOL-PL is a brief and practical tool for quantifying HRQoL in adolescents with a spine deformity. Filling in the questionnaire takes less than 10 minutes to be completed. The ISYQOL-PL questionnaire is reliable and can be used in adolescents with spinal deformities.

Supplementary Materials: The following are available online at https://www.mdpi.com/article/10.3390/jcm10102081/s1, (Supplemental Data File S1: ISYQOL-PL questionnaire).

Author Contributions: Conceptualization, E.K. and K.K.; methodology, E.K.; software, E.K.; validation, E.K., K.K.; formal analysis, E.K., K.K., P.J., M.K., D.C., T.K.; investigation, E.K., K.K., P.J., M.K., D.C.; resources, K.K., M.K., D.C.; data curation, K.K.; writing—original draft preparation, E.K.; writing—review and editing, E.K., T.K.; visualization, E.K.; supervision, T.K.; project administration, K.K.; funding acquisition, K.K. All authors have read and agreed to the published version of the manuscript.

Funding: This research received no external funding. The publication cost was partly covered by the Poznan University of Medical Sciences.

Institutional Review Board Statement: All subjects gave their informed consent for inclusion before they participated in the study. The study was conducted in accordance with the Declaration of Helsinki, and the Institutional Review Board of Poznan University of Medical Sciences approved the study (9 October 2018).

Informed Consent Statement: Informed consent was obtained from the parents and the patients involved in the study.

Data Availability Statement: The data presented in this study are available on request from the corresponding author.

Conflicts of Interest: The authors declare no conflict of interest.

References

1. Aulisa, A.G.; Guzzanti, V.; Perisano, C.; Marzetti, E.; Specchia, A.; Galli, M.; Giordano, M.; Aulisa, L. Determination of quality of life in adolescents with idiopathic scoliosis subjected to conservative treatment. *Scoliosis* **2010**, *5*, 21. [CrossRef] [PubMed]
2. Asher, M.; Lai, S.M.; Burton, D.; Manna, B. The influence of spine and trunk deformity on preoperative idiopathic scoliosis patients' health-related quality of life questionnaire responses. *Spine* **2004**, *29*, 861–868. [CrossRef] [PubMed]
3. Feise, R.J.; Donaldson, S.; Crowther, E.R.; Menke, J.M.; Wright, J.G. Construction and Validation of the Scoliosis Quality of Life Index in Adolescent Idiopathic Scoliosis. *Spine* **2005**, *30*, 1310–1315. [CrossRef] [PubMed]
4. Vasiliadis, E.; Grivas, T.B.; Gkoltsiou, K. Development and preliminary validation of Brace Questionnaire (BrQ): A new instrument for measuring quality of life of brace treated scoliotics. *Scoliosis* **2006**, *1*, 7. [CrossRef] [PubMed]
5. Kinel, E.; Kotwicki, T.; Podolska, A.; Białek, M.; Stryła, W. Polish validation of Brace Questionnaire. *Eur. Spine J.* **2012**, *21*, 1603–1608. [CrossRef] [PubMed]
6. Botens-Helmus, C.; Klein, R.; Stephan, C. The reliability of the Bad Sobernheim Stress Questionnaire (BSSQbrace) in adolescents with scoliosis during brace treatment. *Scoliosis* **2006**, *1*, 22. [CrossRef] [PubMed]
7. Caronni, A.; Sciumè, L.; Donzelli, S.; Zaina, F.; Negrini, S. ISYQOL: A Rasch-consistent questionnaire for measuring health-related quality of life in adolescents with spinal deformities. *Spine J.* **2017**, *17*, 1364–1372. [CrossRef] [PubMed]
8. Caronni, A.; Donzelli, S.; Zaina, F.; Negrini, S. The Italian Spine Youth Quality of Life questionnaire measures health-related quality of life of adolescents with spinal deformities better than the reference standard, the Scoliosis Research Society 22 questionnaire. *Clin. Rehabil.* **2019**, *33*, 1404–1415. [CrossRef] [PubMed]
9. ISYQOL. Available online: https://www.isyqol.org/ (accessed on 3 February 2021).
10. Sánchez-Raya, J.; D'Agata, E.; Donzelli, S.; Caronni, A.; Bagó, J.; Rigo, M.; Figueras, C.; Negrini, S. Spanish validation of Italian Spine Youth Quality of Life (ISYQOL) Questionnaire. *J. Phys. Med. Rehabil.* **2020**, *2*, 1–4. [CrossRef]
11. Beaton, D.E.; Bombardier, C.; Guillemin, F.; Ferraz, M.B. Guidelines for the Process of Cross-Cultural Adaptation of Self-Report Measures. *Spine* **2000**, *25*, 3186–3191. [CrossRef] [PubMed]
12. Terwee, C.B.; Bot, S.D.M.; de Boer, M.R.; van der Windt, D.A.W.M.; Knol, D.L.; Dekker, J.; Bouter, L.M.; de Vet, H.C.W. Quality criteria were proposed for measurement properties of health status questionnaires. *J. Clin. Epidemiol.* **2007**, *60*, 34–42. [CrossRef] [PubMed]
13. Tsang, S.; Royse, C.F.; Terkawi, A.S. Guidelines for developing, translating, and validating a questionnaire in perioperative and pain medicine. *Saudi J. Anaesth.* **2017**, *11*, S80–S89. [CrossRef] [PubMed]
14. de Vet, H.; Terwee, C.; Mokkink, L.; Knol, D. *Measurement in Medicine: A Practical Guide (Practical Guides to Biostatistics and Epidemiology)*; Cambridge: Cambridge University Press, 2011; ISBN 978-1-139-49781-7.
15. Wang, H.; Tetteroo, D.; Arts, J.J.C.; Markopoulos, P.; Ito, K. Quality of life of adolescent idiopathic scoliosis patients under brace treatment: A brief communication of literature review. *Qual. Life Res.* **2020**. [CrossRef] [PubMed]
16. Bunge, E.M.; Habbema, J.D.F.; de Koning, H.J. A randomised controlled trial on the effectiveness of bracing patients with idiopathic scoliosis: Failure to include patients and lessons to be learnt. *Eur. Spine J. Off. Publ. Eur. Spine Soc. Eur. Spinal Deform. Soc. Eur. Sect. Cerv. Spine Res. Soc.* **2010**, *19*, 747–753. [CrossRef] [PubMed]

17. Landauer, F.; Wimmer, C.; Behensky, H. Estimating the final outcome of brace treatment for idiopathic thoracic scoliosis at 6-month follow-up. *Pediatr. Rehabil.* **2003**, *6*, 201–207. [CrossRef] [PubMed]
18. Lou, E.H.M.; Hill, D.L.; Raso, J.V.; Moreau, M.; Hedden, D. How quantity and quality of brace wear affect the brace treatment outcomes for AIS. *Eur. Spine J.* **2016**, *25*, 495–499. [CrossRef] [PubMed]
19. Kotwicki, T.; Kinel, E.; Stryła, W.; Szulc, A. Estimation of the stress related to conservative scoliosis therapy: An analysis based on BSSQ questionnaires. *Scoliosis* **2007**, *2*, 1. [CrossRef] [PubMed]
20. Lin, T.; Meng, Y.; Ji, Z.; Jiang, H.; Shao, W.; Gao, R.; Zhou, X. Extent of Depression in Juvenile and Adolescent Patients with Idiopathic Scoliosis During Treatment with Braces. *World Neurosurg.* **2019**, *126*, e27–e32. [CrossRef] [PubMed]
21. Negrini, S.; Donzelli, S.; Aulisa, A.G.; Czaprowski, D.; Schreiber, S.; de Mauroy, J.C.; Diers, H.; Grivas, T.B.; Knott, P.; Kotwicki, T.; et al. 2016 SOSORT guidelines: Orthopaedic and rehabilitation treatment of idiopathic scoliosis during growth. *Scoliosis Spinal Disord.* **2018**, *13*, 3. [CrossRef] [PubMed]

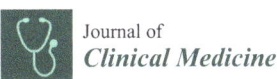

Review

The Effectiveness of Different Concepts of Bracing in Adolescent Idiopathic Scoliosis (AIS): A Systematic Review and Meta-Analysis

Lorenzo Costa, Tom P. C. Schlosser, Hanad Jimale, Jelle F. Homans, Moyo C. Kruyt and René M. Castelein *

Department of Orthopaedic Surgery, University Medical Center Utrecht, 3508 GA Utrecht, The Netherlands; L.Costa-2@umcutrecht.nl (L.C.); T.P.C.Schlosser@umcutrecht.nl (T.P.C.S.); h.jimale@students.uu.nl (H.J.); J.F.Homans-3@umcutrecht.nl (J.F.H.); M.C.Kruyt@umcutrecht.nl (M.C.K.)
* Correspondence: R.M.Castelein@umcutrecht.nl; Tel.: +31-(88)-755-4578; Fax: +31-(30)-251-06-38

Abstract: Brace treatment is the most common noninvasive treatment in adolescent idiopathic scoliosis (AIS); however it is currently not fully known whether there is a difference in effectiveness between brace types/concepts. All studies on brace treatment for AIS were searched for in PubMed and EMBASE up to January 2021. Articles that did not report on maturity of the study population were excluded. Critical appraisal was performed using the Methodological Index for Non-Randomized Studies tool (MINORS). Brace concepts were distinguished in prescribed wearing time and rigidity of the brace: full-time, part-time, and night-time, rigid braces and soft braces. In the meta-analysis, success was defined as $\leq 5°$ curve progression during follow-up. Of the 33 selected studies, 11 papers showed high risk of bias. The rigid full-time brace had on average a success rate of 73.2% (95% CI 61–86%), night-time of 78.7% (72–85%), soft braces of 62.4% (55–70%), observation only of 50% (44–56%). There was insufficient evidence on part-time wear for the meta-analysis. The majority of brace studies have significant risk of bias. No significant difference in outcome between the night-time or full-time concepts could be identified. Soft braces have a lower success rate compared to rigid braces. Bracing for scoliosis in Risser 0–2 and 0–3 stage of maturation appeared most effective.

Keywords: systematic review; meta-analysis; adolescent idiopathic scoliosis; brace therapy; brace concepts; rigid brace; night time brace

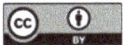

1. Introduction

Idiopathic scoliosis is a deviation from normal growth of the spine and trunk, with a prevalence of 2–4% in the general population [1]. Its management depends on the magnitude of the spinal curvature. Observation is indicated for mild curves and brace treatment is normally recommended in curves between 20° and 45° [2,3]. The application of many different brace concepts (distinguished in prescribed wearing time and rigidity of the brace: full-time, part-time, and night-time, rigid braces and soft braces) have been described in the literature. They all apply different degrees of external corrective forces to the trunk to correct the complex 3-D spinal deformity. Full time braces usually aim at in-brace correction of the curve to at least 50% of the original magnitude; nighttime braces are a bit more ambitious and aim to correct about 70% or an even higher percentage of the curve while the brace is worn [4,5].

The "Bracing in Adolescent Idiopathic Scoliosis Trial" (BRAIST) has provided high-quality evidence for the application of full-time rigid brace treatment in AIS patients with curves 20–40° before skeletal maturity [6]. For other concepts of bracing, most studies are retrospective and not controlled [7]. Despite the efforts of societies like SRS and SOSORT, high-quality evidence for the effectiveness of other concepts of bracing is still lacking. Furthermore, due to the development of multiple braces and non-standardized criteria, it is difficult to compare the results. Nevertheless, many studies provide insight in effectiveness [6,8,9].

The aim of this systematic review and meta-analysis is to evaluate the literature on the effectiveness of different concepts of brace treatment, in terms of effect on spinal curve magnitude. The questions are:

1. What is the most effective brace concept?
2. What is the most effective brace type (Boston brace, Providence brace, etc.)?
3. What is the effect of skeletal maturity on the effectiveness of different concepts of brace treatment?

Even though Randomized Control Trials (RCTs) are considered to be more reliable than observational studies when evaluating treatment effectiveness, RCTs are extremely demanding for these types of questions and often fail [10]. Meta-epidemiological research has shown that for non-pharmaceutical purposes, alternative study designs are not consistently more biased and should not be discarded. Therefore, we also included observational studies [11–14]. To allow assessment of this wide array of studies, tools are available to appraise study quality for non-comparative studies [15].

Lastly, many definitions of success rate such as $\leq 5°$, $\leq 10°$, or avoidance of surgery are used in scoliosis brace studies. As this heterogeneity would have affected the outcome of this review, the authors agreed to use, at least for the meta-analysis, the most used definition: $\leq 5°$ of curve progression as successful treatment.

2. Materials and Methods

2.1. Protocol

This systematic review was performed according to the PRISMA statement and is registered at PROSPERO with the ID CRD42020157636 [16].

2.2. Search Methods and Study Selections

A systematic search was undertaken to identify all studies reporting on bracing in AIS in PubMed and EMBASE till January 2021 (see Table 1). Inclusion criteria were shown in Table 2.

All studies that reported on spinal deformities other than AIS or with mixed-age population that did not report the outcomes for AIS separately were excluded. Since skeletal maturity is considered a significant parameter, if not stated, the studies were excluded from further analyses. Reviews, cross-sectional studies, and case series with less than 10 patients were also excluded (see Table 2). Title/abstract and full-text screening was done by two independent investigators. To ensure literature saturation, reference lists of included studies or relevant reviews identified through the search were reviewed.

Table 1. Strategy of the search in PubMed and Embase. There was no language restriction. Duplicates were removed in Rayyan [17].

PubMed	((((scoliosis [MeSH Terms] OR scolio * [Title/Abstract] OR spinal curvature [Title/Abstract] OR AIS [Title/Abstract]))) AND (((((brace [MeSH Terms] OR brace [Title/Abstract] OR bracing [Title/Abstract]))) AND ((time [Title/Abstract] OR parttime [Title/Abstract] OR nighttime [Title/Abstract] OR compliance [MeSH Terms] OR compliance [Title/Abstract] OR compliant [Title/Abstract] OR effect [Title/Abstract] OR treatment * [Title/Abstract] OR result [Title/Abstract] OR results [Title/Abstract] OR therap [Title/Abstract] OR mental disorder [Title/Abstract] OR hypersensitive [Title/Abstract] OR peer problem [Title/Abstract] OR depress [Title/Abstract]) OR psychologic [Title/Abstract] OR quality of life [Title/Abstract] OR quality of life [MeSH] OR life quality [Title/Abstract])))).
Medscape	('scoliosis': exp OR 'scolio *': ti, ab, kw OR 'spinal curvature *': ti, ab, kw OR 'AIS': ti, ab, kw) AND ('brace': exp OR 'brace *': ti, ab, kw OR 'braci *': ti, ab, kw) AND ('time': ti, ab, kw OR 'parttime': ti, ab, kw OR 'nighttime': ti, ab, kw OR 'compliance': exp OR 'compliance': ti, ab, kw OR 'compliant': ti, ab, kw OR 'effect *': ti, ab, kw OR 'treatment *': ti, ab, kw OR 'result': ti, ab, kw OR 'results': ti, ab, kw OR 'therap *': ti, ab, kw OR 'mental disorder *': ti, ab, kw OR 'hypersensitiv *': ti, ab, kw OR 'peer problem *': ti, ab, kw OR 'depress *': ti, ab, kw OR 'psychologic *': ti, ab, kw OR 'quality of life': ti, ab, kw OR 'quality of life': exp OR 'life quality': ti, ab, kw)

Table 2. Details regarding inclusion criteria.

1	Design	Longitudinal studies with at least one-year follow-up from brace initiation
2	Population	Patients with adolescent idiopathic scoliosis
3	Intervention	Specification of the concept(s) of brace (prescribed wearing time(s) and brace type(s)) used
4	Outcome	A definition of success rate (all definitions of success rate were accepted in the qualitative synthesis in this review)

2.3. Appraisal

Two authors independently assessed the quality and risk of bias of each included study using the validated Methodological Index for Non-Randomized Studies (MINORs) (see Table 3) [15]. For any disagreement, consensus was reached by discussion.

Table 3. The MINOR tool [15]. Items 1–8 are for both comparative and non-comparative studies. Items 9–12 are only for comparative studies. The items are scored 0 (not reported), 1 (reported but inadequate), or 2 (reported and adequate), the global ideal score being 16 for non-comparative studies and 24 for comparative studies. For comparative studies: <12 high risk of bias, 12–16 medium risk of bias, >16 low risk of bias. For non-comparative studies: <7 high risk of bias, 7–11 medium risk of bias, >11 low risk of bias.

1	A clearly stated aim	The question address should be precise and relevant.
2	Inclusions of consecutive patients	All patients potentially fit for inclusion had been included in the study.
3	Prospective collection data	Data were collected according to a protocol established before the beginning of the study.
4	Endpoints appropriate to the aim of the study	Unambiguous explanation of the criteria used to evaluate the main outcome.
5	Unbiased assessment of the study endpoint	Blind evaluation of objective end-points and double blind-evaluation of subjective endpoints. Other explanation of the reasons for not blinding.
6	Follow-up period appropriate to the aim of the study	The follow-up should be should be sufficiently long to allow the assessment of the main end-points.
7	Loss to follow-up less than 5%	All patients should be included in the follow-up. Otherwise, the proportion lost should not exceed the proportion experiencing the major end-points.
8	Prospective calculation of the study size	Information of the size of detectable difference of interest with a calculation of 95% confidence interval.
9	An adequate control group	Having a gold standard diagnostic test or therapeutic intervention recognized as the optimal intervention according to the available published data.
10	Contemporary groups	Control and studied group should be managed during the same time period.
11	Baseline equivalence of groups	The groups should be similar regarding criteria and studied end-point.
12	Adequate statistical analysis	Whether the statistics were in accordance with the type of study with calculation of confidence interval or relative risk.

2.4. Synthesis

Brace concepts and brace types, prescribed wearing time, actual wearing time (if reported), rigidity of the brace, maturity parameters, age, sex, curve magnitude, and outcomes (effect on curve magnitude and prevention of the need of surgery) were systematically collected and compared between the different brace concepts/types. Since heterogeneity in quality, methodology, and outcomes of the different studies was expected, a best-evidence-synthesis was performed in the form of a systematic qualitative synthesis [18]. The qualitative synthesis describes the outcomes of non-comparative and comparative studies on the different brace concepts/types. Because the majority of the studies report on success rates defined as ≤5° progression during study follow-up, success rates are reported according to this definition (otherwise indicated in the text). Follow-up is intended after at least 1 year of follow-up and/or after termination of brace treatment.

The meta-analysis was performed on the outcomes of studies with low risk-of-bias that reported on the effectiveness of different brace concepts or braces as defined as ≤5° coronal curve angle progression during study follow-up. In addition, the same was made with ≤50° of Cobb angle progression. OpenMeta Analyst was used to execute the analysis [19]. Mean success rate and 95% confidence intervals (95% CI) were calculated and compared between the concepts. Only the BRAIST study included data on untreated patients. Due to lack of other studies with control groups, two studies not included in this review on the natural history of AIS were used for calculation of the success rate of observation only (n = 267) [20,21].

The effect of skeletal maturity on the success of the brace treatment was analyzed using the same criteria as the meta-analysis. Outcomes were compared between studies with different skeletal maturity at inclusion: Risser sign 0–1, 0–2, 0–3, and 0–4.

3. Results
3.1. Search

The search yielded a total of 2609 papers. The PRISMA flowchart and reason for exclusion are shown in Figure 1. After title/abstract screening, 224 articles were selected for full-text reading. Reference tracking yielded no additional articles. After exclusions, a total of 33 articles were included in this study.

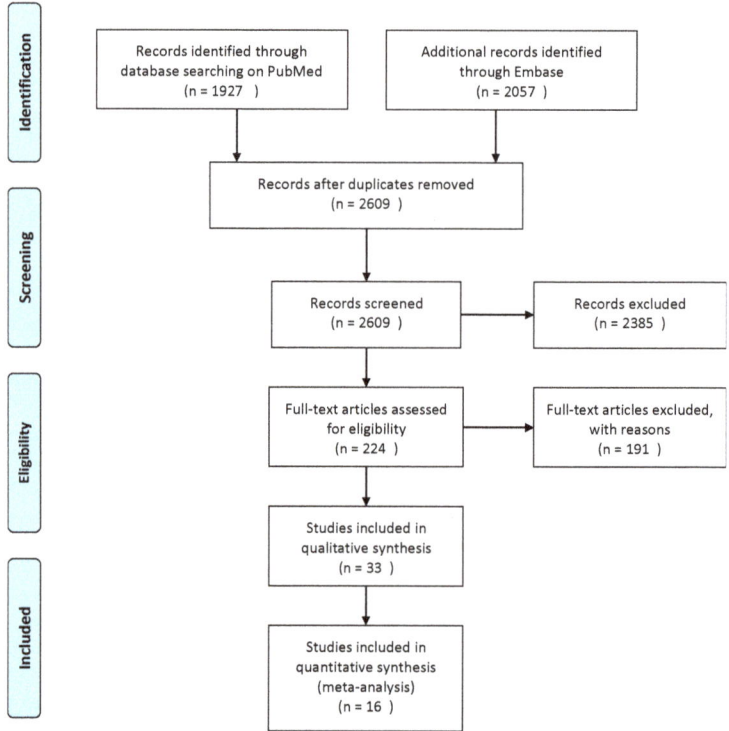

Figure 1. Flowchart of literature search.

3.2. Study Characteristic

In total, seven types of rigid, full-time braces; two types of rigid, part-time braces; two types of rigid, night-time braces; and one soft, full-time brace were described in the 33 studies (see Table 4).

Table 4. Overview of the different braces included in this systematic review.

Brace Type	Rigidity	Prescribed Wearing Time
Boston [22–24]	Rigid brace	Full-time/part-time
Cheneau brace [25–28]	Rigid brace	Full-time/part-time
PASB (Progressive Action Short Brace) [29]	Rigid brace	Full-time
Lyon brace [30]	Rigid brace	Full-time
Gensingen Brace [31]	Rigid brace	Full-time
OMC (Osaka Medical College) brace [32]	Rigid brace	Full-time
Pressure-adjustable orthosis [33]	Rigid brace	Full-time
Charleston brace [34,35]	Rigid brace	Night-time
Providence brace [5,36–39]	Rigid brace	Night-time
SpineCor [40,41]	Soft brace	Full-time

The study population varied between 23 and 843 patients per study. To one of the RCTs, patient preference cohorts were added during the inclusion period [6]. Seven studies (21%) recruited patients in Asia, seven (21%) in North-America and nineteen (58%) in Europe. All studies reported on prescribed wearing time and three studies reported on actual wearing time as assessed by a thermomonitor or by the orthoptist [6,42,43]. Concerning the Cobb angle, the inclusion criteria of the non-comparative studies were:

1. Rigid full-time braces (15 studies): 30% 20–40°, 30% 25–40°, 8% 25–45°, 8% $\geq$ 40°, 8% > 25°, 8% 0–45°.
2. Night-time braces (8 studies): 63% 25–40°, 13% 20–45°, 13% 25–49°, 13% < 25°.
3. Soft full-time braces (2 studies): 50% 25–40°, 50% 15–40°.

For the comparative studies (8 studies): 50% 25–40°, 26% > 25°, 13% 20–30°, 13% 15–30° for soft braces and >30° for rigid full-time braces.

At the inclusion, most of the studies reported a magnitude between 25–40° for the Cobb angle. Two papers presented a mean Cobb angle above 40° and one paper below 20°.

In total, 69% of the studies included thoracic, thoracolumbar, and lumbar curves; 25% included thoracolumbar curves; and 6% double major curves.

The radiographic skeletal maturity at initiation of the treatment was reported in all papers. Of the studies, 32 used the Risser sign and one study only used menarche as a proxy for maturity [39]. Of those, 3% used the Risser sign between 0–1 (as subgroup), 70% between 0–2, 18% between 0–3, 3% between 0–4, 3% used Risser 0–1 and Tanner between 2–3, and 3% used Risser 0–2 and menarche period as well (pre-menarche or 1 year post-menarche) (see Tables 5 and 6).

3.3. Study Quality

The critical appraisal results are shown in Tables 5 and 6. The mean quality score of the 3 RCTs was 14.5 (out of 24); of the 8 comparative cohort studies 10.7 (out of 24); and of the 24 non-comparative cohort studies, 8.1 (out of 16). Twelve studies had low quality and high risk-of-bias and six did not report on success defined as $\leq$5° progression. A total of sixteen papers were included in the meta-analysis. There was insufficient evidence available to include the part-time, rigid brace concept in the meta-analysis. Quality of the two studies added for the control group was 7/16 and 15/24 [20,21].

Table 5. Overview of the non-comparative studies. The studies lightened in bold are the ones included in the meta-analysis.

First Author	Year	Risk of Bias	Sample Size	Cobb Angle	Skeletal Maturity	Type of Brace	Brace	Timing	Follow-Up	Definition of Success Rate	Success Rate
Weinstein [6]	2014	14/24	146 96	20–40	Risser 0–2	Rigid Control group	TLSO	Full-time	7 years	>50°	72% 42%
Xu [22]	**2019**	**8/16**	**90**	**40–45**	**Risser 0–3 (divided in subgroups)**	**Rigid**	**Boston brace**	**Full-time**	**2 years**	**≤5°**	**51.1%**
Yrjonen [23]	2007	10/24	51 51	>25°	Risser 0–3	Rigid	Boston brace	Full-time	>1 year	≤5°	Girls 78.4% Boys 62.7%
Grivas [24]	**2003**	**7/16**	**28**	**20–40**	**Pre or <1 year post-menarche and Risser**	**Rigid**	**modified Boston brace**	**Full-time**	**mean of 2.3 years**	**≤5°**	**82%**
Pasquini [25]	2016	5/16	843	20–40	Risser 0–2	Rigid	modified Cheneau brace	Full-time	≥2 years	≤5°	81%
Fang [26]	2015	10/16	32	25–40	Risser 0–2	Rigid	Cheneau brace	Full-time	2 years	no curve progression ≥ 50°	81%
Pham [27]	2007	7/16	63	20–45	Risser 0–2	Rigid	Cheneau brace	Full-time	2 years after discontinuing brace therapy	<10°	85.7%
Zabrowska Sapeta [28]	2010	7/16	79	20–45	Risser 0–4	Rigid	Cheneau brace + exercises	Full-time	1–5 years	≤5°	48%
Maruyama [44]	**2015**	**9/16**	**33**	**25–40**	**Risser 0–2 and pre or 1 year post-menarche**	**Rigid**	**Rigo-Cheneau brace**	**Full-time**	**Mean 2.8 years**	**≤5°**	**76%**
Aulisa [29]	2009	6/16	50	25–40	Risser 0–2	Rigid	PASB	Full-time	>2 years	≤5°	100%
Aulisa [45]	**2020**	**12/16**	**163**	**20–60 mean 28**	**Risser 0–4**	**Rigid**	**PASB**		**10y after termination**	**≤5°**	**65.6%**
Aulisa [30]	2015	4/16	69	25–40	Risser 0–2	Rigid	Lyon brace	Full-time	2 years	≤5°	98.5%
Weiss [31]	**2017**	**9/16**	**25**	**≥40**	**Risser 0–2**	**Rigid**	**Gensingen Brace**	**Full-time**	**≥1.5 years**	**≤5°**	**92%**
Kuroki [32]	2015	10/16	31	20–40	Risser 0–2	Rigid	OMC brace	Full-time	2 years after discontinuing brace therapy	no curve progression ≥ 50°	67.8%
Yangmin Lin [33]	2020	6/16	24	20–40	Risser 0–2	Rigid	Pressure-adjustable orthosis		1 year	≤5°	100%
Lateur [46]	**2017**	**10/16**	**142**	**<25**	**Risser 0–3**	**Rigid**	**Night-time brace**	**Night-time**	**>1 year mean 3.75 y**	**≤5°**	**83%**

Table 5. Cont.

First Author	Year	Risk of Bias	Sample Size	Cobb Angle	Skeletal Maturity	Type of Brace	Brace	Timing	Follow-Up	Definition of Success Rate	Success Rate
Price [34]	1990	7/16	139	25–49	Risser 0–2	Rigid	Charleston brace	Night-time	>1 year	≤5°	83%
Lee [35]	2012	9/16	95	25–40	Risser 0–2	Rigid	Charleston brace	Night-time	>2 years after skeletal maturity	≤5°	84.2%
Davis [36]	2019	6/16	56	25–40	Risser 0–2	Rigid	Providence brace	Night-time	mean 2.21 years	≤5°	51.8%
Ohrt-Nissen [37]	2016	7/16	63	25–40	Risser 0–2	Rigid	Providence brace	Night-time	2 years	≤5°	57%
D' Amato [5]	2001	8/16	102	20–42	Risser 0–2	Rigid	Providence brace	Night-time	Min 2 y after stop bracing	≤5°	74%
Bohl [38]	2014	6/16	34	25–40	Risser 0–2	Rigid	Providence brace	Night-time	2 years after maturity	≤5° or >45 degrees	50% >5°, 59% >45°
Simony [39]	2019	10/16	80	20–45	Pre or <1 year post-menarche	Rigid	Providence brace	Night-time	Till 1 year after stop bracing	≤5°	89%
Coillard [40]	2007	8/16	170	25–40	Risser 0–2	Soft	SpineCor	Full-time	2 years after discontinuing brace therapy	≤5°	59.4%
Coillard [41]	2014	16/24	32	15–30	Risser 0–2	Soft	SpineCor brace	Full-time	5 years	≤5°	73%
			36				control group				57%

Table 6. Ovrview of the comparative studies between braces.e The studies lightened in bold are the ones included in the meta-analysis.

First Author	Year	Risk of Bias	Sample Size	Cobb Angle	Skeletal Maturity	Type of Brace	Brace	Timing	Follow-Up	Definition of Success Rate	Success Rate
Minsk [47]	2017	11/24	13	25–40	Risser 0–2	Rigid	Rigo-Cheneau	Full-time	>1 year	≤5°; no need of surgery	Spinal surgery: 0% >6°:31%
			93				Boston				Spinal surgery: 34%
Hanks [42]	1988	11/24	75	>25	Risser 0–4	Rigid	Wilmington Jacket	Full-time	1 year after discontinuing brace	<10°	Full-time 80%
			25					Part-time			84%
Katz [43]	2010	11/24	57	25–40	Risser 0–2	Rigid	Boston brace	Full-time	>1 year	≤5°	82% > 12 h
			43					Part-time			31% > 7 h
Yrjonen [4]	**2006**	**12/24**	**36**	**>25°**	**Risser sign 0–3**	**Rigid**	**Providence brace**	**Night-time**	**mean 1.8 years**	**≤5°**	**72%**
			36			**Rigid**	**Boston brace**	**Full-time**			**78%**
Janicki [48]	2007	10/24	35	25–40	Risser 0–2	Rigid	Providence brace	Night-time	>2 years	≤5°	31%
			48			Rigid	Custom TLSO	Full-time			15%
Ohrt-Nissen [49]	2019	13/24	40	25–40	Risser 0–2	Rigid	Providence brace	Night-time	2 years	≤5° (primary outcome); curve progression ≥45°	45%
			37			Rigid	Boston brace	Full-time			38%
Weiss [50]	2005	8/24	12	15–30 and >30 for rigid brace	Risser sign 0 (one exeption with 1) Tanner 2 or 3	Soft	SpineCor	Full-time	mean 3.5 years	≤5°	8%
			10			Rigid	Cheneau brace	Full-time			80%
Guo [51]	**2014**	**13/24**	**20**	**20–30**	**Risser 0–2 Pre or < 1 year post-menarche**	**Soft**	**SpineCor brace**	**Full-time**	**2 years after discontinuing brace therapy**	**≤5°**	**65%**
			18			**Rigid**	**TLSO**	**Full-time**			**94%**

3.4. Qualitative Analysis

- Full-time, rigid braces

Thirteen studies described the outcomes of six full-time, rigid braces. Six brace types were individually studied (see Table 4).

Weinstein et al. (n = 242) included rigid full-time TLSOs (thoraco-lumbo-sacral orthosis) in a study that was designed as RCT to which patient preference cohorts were added (68% was treated with Boston brace) [6]. This was one of the few studies that defined success as progression to no more than 50° Cobb angle and no surgical treatment. Brace treatment was successful in 72% of cases versus 42% in the observation only group [6].

The effectiveness of the Boston brace was investigated in three studies [22–24]. The success rate was 51–83% in a total of 169 patients [22,24]. Yrjönen et al. found that 63% of boys had a successful treatment compared to 78% of the girls [23]. The Chêneau brace was investigated in four studies: Pasquini et al. (low quality study) reported a success rate of 81%, Fang et al. of 81% (defined as no curve progression to >50°) and Pham et al. of 86% (defined as curve progression ≤10°) [25–27]. Pham et al. indicated that the Chêneau brace was most effective in the lumbar curves [27]. Zabrowska-Sapeta et al. (n = 79), studied the Cheneau brace in combination with physiotherapy. Treatment was successful in 48% of cases [28]. Maruyama et al. (n = 33) investigated the Rigo-Chêneau brace. Success was observed in 76% of the patients [44]. The progressive action short brace (PASB) was studied by Aulisa et al. in 69 and 163 patients. In this study with low quality (6/16), the reported success rate was between 65.6 and 100% [29,45]. Similarly, the Lyon brace was studied by Aulisa et al. in 69 patients and the reported success rate was 99% [30]. The Gensingen brace was studied by Weiss et al. (n = 25). The percentage of successful treatment was 92% [31].

The Osaka Medical College Brace was studied by Kuroki et al. (n = 31). Treatment was successful in 68% of the patients [32].

Pressure-adjustable orthosis was developed by Yangmin Lin et al. in 2020 (n = 24). The reported treatment success was 100% after 1 year of treatment [33].

- Part-time, rigid braces

There were no non-comparative studies.

- Night-time, rigid braces

Eight studies focused on rigid, night-time braces with a total of 762 patients treated with the Charleston or Providence brace. Lauteur et al. (n = 142) studied the night-time brace concept. The treatment was successful in 83% of cases [46].

The Charleston brace was studied by Lee et al. (n = 95) and Price et al. (n = 139) with a success rate of 83% and 84% [34,35]. Price et al. noticed that patients with double curves treated with Charleston brace should be observed closely for the risk of increase in compensatory curves [34].

The Providence brace was studied in four non-comparative studies with low to moderate quality (total n = 56 + 63 + 102 + 34 + 80) [5,36–39]. Success rates were between 52% and 89% [36,39].

- Full-time soft braces

Two studies by Coillard et al. reported on one type of full-time soft braces (SpineCor), one RCT (n = 68) compared to controls (study quality = 16/24) and one non-comparative cohort (n = 101).

With 5 years follow-up or follow-up to more than 2 years after discontinuation, the brace treatment was successful in 59–73% of the patients [40,41].

- Comparative studies

Minsk et al. (n = 108) compared the Rigo-Chêneau brace and a thoraco-lumbo-sacral orthosis (TLSO). Success rate was defined as curve ≤5° and failure defined as need of surgery [47]. No patients with the Rigo-Chêneau needed surgery compared to 34% of patients with the TLSO brace that needed surgical intervention [47].

Two studies compared full-time with part-time braces (part-time was considered: ≤16 h—Hanks et al., as prescribed wearing time—or 7–12 h—Katz et al., as actual wearing time) [42,43]. Wilmington Jacket (Hanks et al. n = 100, success rate defined as curve progression ≤10°) and Boston brace (Katz et al. n = 100) were identified. The Wilmington Jacket full-time group had a success of 80%, while the part-time group had a successful treatment in 84% of the cases [42]. Boston full-time bracing wear had a success of 82% and the part-time worn brace of 31% [43].

Three studies, Yrjönen et al. (n = 72), Janicki et al. (n = 83), and Ohrt-Nissen et al. (n = 77), prospectively compared the Providence brace and the full-time TLSO [4,48,49]. Success rate was defined as curve progression ≤5° or residual curve < 45° [49]. Providence brace was successful in 31%, when the full-time TLSO was in 15% [4,48].

Two studies, Weiss et al. (n = 22) and Guo et al. (RCT n = 38), focused on the SpineCor brace vs TLSO [50,51]. Success was between 8 and 65% for the SpineCor and between 80% and the 94.4% for the TLSO [50,51].

3.5. Meta-Analysis

Sixteen studies had medium or low risk-of-bias, with defined success as progression ≤ 5° and were included in the meta-analysis. The rigid full-time brace had a success of 73.2% (95% CI 60.9–85.5%), the night-time of 78.7% (95% CI 72.4–85%), and soft braces of 62.4% (95% CI 55.1–69.6%) (see Figure 2). The success rate of observation was only 50% (95%, CI 44–56%) [20,21,41]. In addition, three studies over rigid full-time bracing with medium or low risk-of-bias, when success is defined as progression ≤ 50°, were separately included in the analysis. The success was of 73.2% (95% CI, 67.2–79.2%). The bubble plot shows no relation between the study quality and reported success rates (Figure 3).

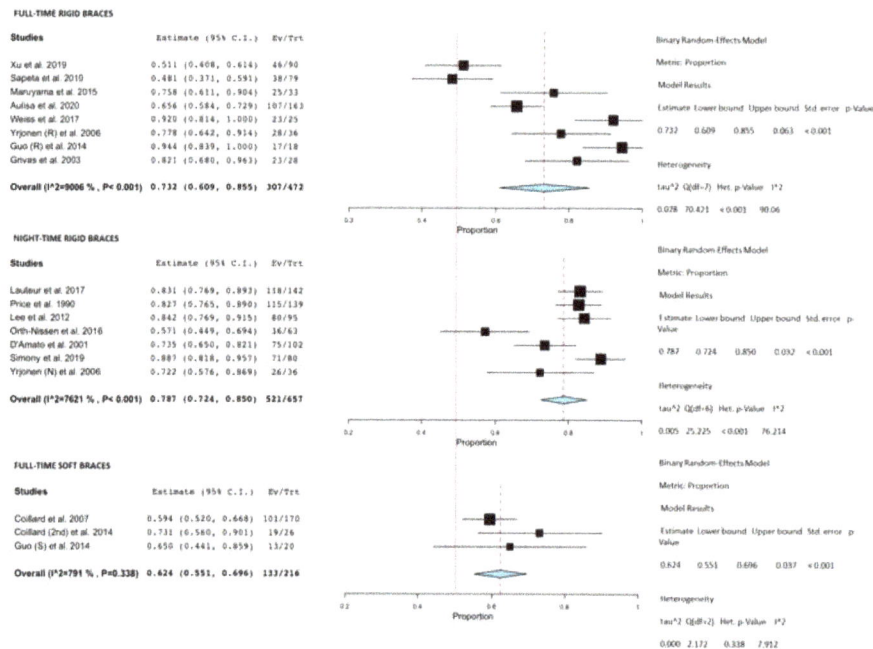

Figure 2. Forest plot of the studies divided per type of concept. Control groups were selected based on type of scoliosis (AIS). A success rate (≤5°) and reviews or case reports (<10 pt.) were excluded. The red line represents successes in the case control group (50%) [4,5,22,24,28,31,34,35,37,39–41,44–46,51].

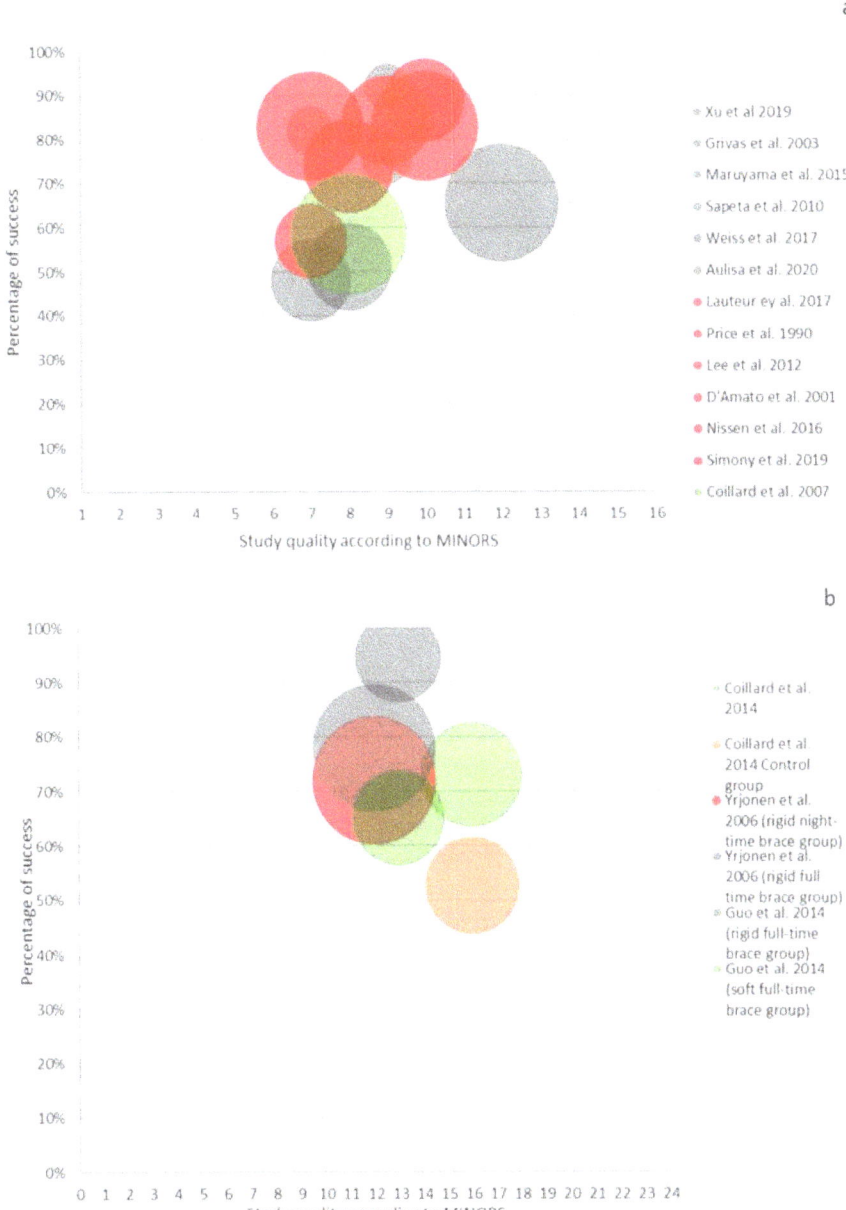

Figure 3. The bubble graph represents the proportion of the population with less than 5° Cobb angle progression (Y axis) relative to the MINORS score (X axis) and sample size (diameter of the circle). Thirteen non-comparative studies are represented in (**a**) and three comparative studies in (**b**). The grey color represents the rigid full-time concept, the red color the night-time concept, the green one the soft concept, and the orange color represents the control group [4,5,22,24,28,31,34,35,37,39–41,44–46,51].

3.6. The Role of Skeletal Maturity

Fourteen studies were included for the assessment of efficacy in relation to the Risser sign at initiation of brace therapy. Xu et al. divided their study group already based on Risser stage at initiation, so these subgroups were used separately for each category. For the category Risser 0–1, one paper could be used and the success rate was low, 42% (95%CI not applicable because there was only one study). For patients included with Risser 0–2, 10 papers reported a success rate of 71% (68–74%). The 0–3 category yielded 3 papers with a success rate of 75% (70–80%). The category that included all Risser stages at initiation of therapy showed a little lower success rate of 60% (54–66%) (see Figure 4).

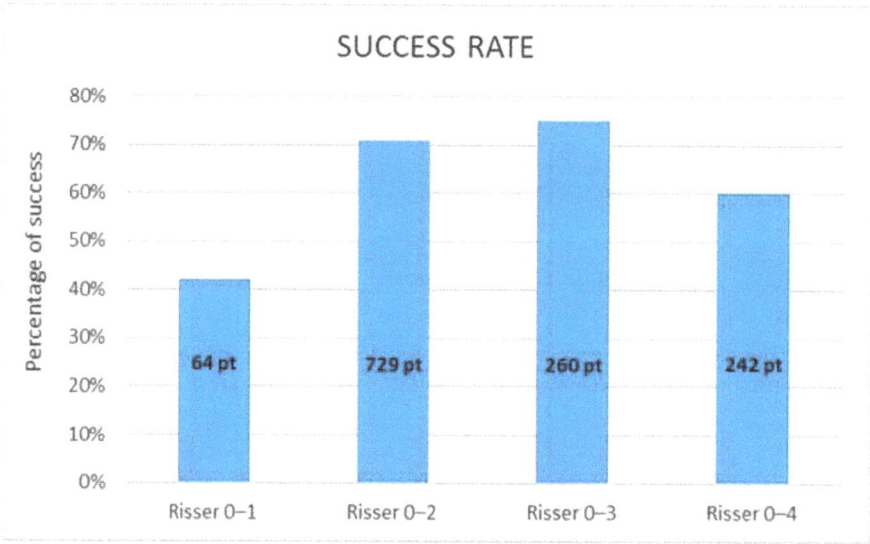

Figure 4. Mean success rate related to maturity. All studies used the Risser sign for assessment of skeletal maturity for initiation of brace treatment and used ≤5° as definition of successful treatment.

4. Discussion

This systematic review and meta-analysis aimed to compare the effectiveness of different concepts of bracing for treatment of AIS. Comparison of the effectiveness between the different brace concepts revealed that rigid braces have better outcomes than soft braces and that night-time braces have comparable effectiveness compared to full-time braces. Rigid part-time bracing data were too limited to be included in the meta-analysis [4,42,48–51]. Most of the studies used as curve type thoracic, thoraco-lumbar, and lumbar curves with no subgroups organization. Therefore, it was not possible to detect differences in brace efficacy between different curve types. Nevertheless, most of the papers reported curves between 25–40° Cobb angle (no subgroups) as well as the Risser sign between 0–2 at initiation of the study and differences between brace types could be analyzed as seen in the results section.

A clear distinction can be made between rigid braces with a constant shape that force the body in a certain position and soft or dynamic orthoses that exert a constant force [52,53]. Another distinction is the prescribed wearing time. Full-time is the most used concept, where the patient should wear the brace 18 to 23 h per day. Part-time bracing is normally prescribed for less than 16 h per day. Night-time bracing is a different concept that aims to provide better correction because of the reduction of axial loading on the supine spine. [4,39].

Thirty-four studies could be selected for the purpose of this systematic review. Important reasons to exclude studies were: unclear or not stated range of coronal Cobb angle, etiology, assessment of maturity at inclusion, type of brace, follow-up time, time in brace, and the success/failure rate. The vast majority of the studies had a moderate to high risk of bias, as also shown by Negrini et al. in their review and SOSORT guidelines [8,18]. First, due to the nature of the treatment it is not possible to conduct trials in which patients are blinded. Second, it is difficult to perform RCTs in this kind of treatment because the risk of selection bias [54–56]. In 2008, Bunge et al. tried to perform an RCT study, however with no success since "it is harder to perform a RCT that abolishes or postpones a treatment than a RCT that adds a new treatment" [57]. In 2013, the BRAIST study was published (started as an RCT and ended as an RCT combined with patient preference cohorts). The patient's/parent's preference had led to a substantial proportion of patients refusing randomization and therefore decreasing the external validity. Nevertheless, the efficacy of bracing is generally accepted now because of this trial [6]. In the present study, we included 31 cohort studies and 3 RCTs. In general, estimates of treatment effectiveness are predominantly affected by the quality measures of the study design. In RCTs, for example, if randomization is not adequate, the effects of the treatment are overestimated [58,59]. Interestingly, methodological research has indicated that especially for non-pharmaceutical treatments the validity of observational studies is not necessarily inferior [60,61].

In line with the aim of bracing, success means the avoidance of surgery, as was used in the BRAIST study. However, since criteria for surgery vary between institutes and countries that definition of success is difficult for comparison. The most often used proxy for effectiveness in the available literature is the prevention of progression ($\leq 5°$). Despite its shortcomings, this outcome can be used for comparisons of different brace concepts and brace types. Ideally, future brace studies should report on (1) the percentage of patients who have $\leq 5°$ curve progression per year, at skeletal maturity and two years after ending brace, and the percentage of patients who have $>5°$ progression up to skeletal maturity, (2) the percentage of patients with coronal curve angle exceeding $45°$ at skeletal maturity, (3) the percentage who have had surgery recommended/undertaken and (4) skeletal maturity parameters [62,63].

Skeletal maturity analysis show that the Risser grade, particularly stages 0–2, is still the most used classification for skeletal maturity assessment. This should be considered as the parameter for more homogeneous inclusion criteria in future studies. Moreover, our results highlight the correlation between maturity and chance of curve progression.

Furthermore, it is interesting to notice that if rigid full-time braces with success defined as no more than $5°$ progression is compared with the data of the same brace concept with definition of success as no more than $50°$ of ultimate Cobb angle, the results are comparable. This should need further analyses to understand its relevance since it is hard to objectively compare them.

In our opinion, this systematic review and meta-analysis provides a valuable addition to the existing literature.

To avoid heterogeneity of the data, future studies should also perform stratifications of the subjects related to initial Cobb angle, type of curve, sex, and skeletal maturity.

5. Conclusions

Bracing is effective in AIS treatment. Rigid full-time braces, rigid night-time braces, and full-time soft braces are more effective than observation only in terms of halting curve progression. The reported effectiveness of night-time braces is comparable to full-time rigid braces; soft braces perform less well. The Risser sign is still the most used parameter for bone maturity.

Supplementary Materials: The following are available online at https://www.mdpi.com/article/10.3390/jcm10102145/s1, The data presented in this study are available in "Supplementary materials The Effectiveness of Different Concepts of Bracing in Adolescent Idiopathic Scoliosis (AIS) A Systematic Review and Meta-Analysis".

Author Contributions: Conceptualization, R.M.C., M.C.K., L.C., T.P.C.S.; methodology, L.C., T.P.C.S., J.F.H.; validation, R.M.C., M.C.K., L.C., T.P.C.S.; formal analysis, L.C., H.J.; investigation, L.C., H.J.; resources, L.C., H.J.; data curation, L.C., T.P.C.S.; writing—original draft preparation, L.C.; writing—review and editing, R.M.C., M.C.K., T.P.C.S.; visualization, L.C.; supervision, R.M.C., M.C.K., T.P.C.S. All authors have read and agreed to the published version of the manuscript.

Funding: This research received funding from the EU's H2020 research and innovation program under Marie S. Curie cofound RESCUE grant agreement No 801540.

Institutional Review Board Statement: Not applicable.

Informed Consent Statement: Not applicable.

Data Availability Statement: Data is contained within the article or Supplementary Material. The data presented in this study are available in "Supplementary Materials The Effectiveness of Different Concepts of Bracing in Adolescent Idiopathic Scoliosis (AIS) A Systematic Review and Meta-Analysis".

Conflicts of Interest: The authors declare no conflict of interest. The funders had no role in the design of the study; in the collection, analyses, or interpretation of data; in the writing of the manuscript, or in the decision to publish the results.

References

1. Konieczny, M.R.; Senyurt, H.; Krauspe, R. Epidemiology of adolescent idiopathic scoliosis. *J. Child. Orthop.* **2013**, *7*, 3–9. [CrossRef] [PubMed]
2. Lonstein, J.E. Scoliosis: Surgical versus nonsurgical treatment. *Clin. Orthop. Relat. Res.* **2006**, *87*, 248–259. [CrossRef] [PubMed]
3. Weinstein, S.L.; Dolan, L.A.; Cheng, J.C.; Danielsson, A.; Morcuende, J.A. Adolescent idiopathic scoliosis. *Lancet* **2008**, *371*, 1527–1537. [CrossRef]
4. Yrjönen, T.; Ylikoski, M.; Schlenzka, D.; Kinnunen, R.; Poussa, M. Effectiveness of the Providence nighttime bracing in adolescent idiopathic scoliosis: A comparative study of 36 female patients. *Eur. Spine J.* **2006**, *15*, 1139–1143. [CrossRef] [PubMed]
5. D'Amato, C.R.; Griggs, S.; McCoy, B. Nighttime bracing with the Providence brace in adolescent girls with idiopathic scoliosis. *Spine* **2001**, *26*, 2006–2012. [CrossRef]
6. Weinstein, S.L.; Dolan, L.; Wright, J.G.; Dobbs, M.B. Effect of bracing adolescent idiopathic scoliosis. *New Engl. J. Med.* **2014**, *369*, 1512–1521. [CrossRef]
7. Lenssinck, M.L.B.; Frijlink, A.C.; Berger, M.Y.; Bierma-Zeinstra, S.M.; Verkerk, K.; Verhagen, A.P. Effect of bracing and other conservative Interventions in the Treatment of Idiopathic Scoliosis in Adolescents: A Systematic Review of clinical trials. *Phys. Ther.* **2005**, *85*, 1329–1339. [CrossRef] [PubMed]
8. Negrini, S.; Donzelli, S.; Aulisa, A.G.; Czaprowski, D.; Schreiber, S.; De Mauroy, J.C.; Diers, H.; Grivas, T.B.; Knott, P.; Kotwicki, T.; et al. 2016 SOSORT guidelines: Orthopaedic and rehabilitation treatment of idiopathic scoliosis during growth. *Scoliosis Spinal Disord.* **2018**, *13*, 1–48. [CrossRef] [PubMed]
9. Guyatt, G.; Oxman, A.D.; Akl, E.A.; Kunz, R.; Vist, G.; Brozek, J.; Norris, S.; Falck-Ytter, Y.; Glasziou, P.; Debeer, H.; et al. GRADE guidelines: 1. Introduction – GRADE evidence profiles and summary of findings tables. Washington (DC): National Academies P. *BMJ* **2011**, *16*, 1–13. [CrossRef]
10. McKee, M.; Britton, A.; Black, N.; McPherson, K.; Sanderson, C.; Bain, C. Methods in health services research: Interpreting the evidence: Choosing between randomised and non-randomised studies. *Br. Med. J.* **1999**, *319*, 312–315. [CrossRef] [PubMed]
11. Houwert, R.; Verhofstad, M.; Hietbrink, F.; Kruyt, M. De conventionele RCT voor trauma- en orthopedisch chirurgen: Geen heilige graal. *Ned. Tijdschr. Voor Traumachirurgie* **2016**, *24*, 2–5. [CrossRef]
12. Abraham, N.S.; Byrne, C.J.; Young, J.M.; Solomon, M.J. Meta-analysis of well-designed nonrandomized comparative studies of surgical procedures is as good as randomized controlled trials. *J. Clin. Epidemiol.* **2010**, *63*, 238–245. [CrossRef] [PubMed]
13. Jacobs, W.C.; Kruyt, M.C.; Verbout, A.J.; Oner, F.C. Spine surgery research: On and beyond current strategies. *Spine J.* **2012**, *12*, 706–713. [CrossRef] [PubMed]
14. Jacobs, W.C.; Kruyt, M.C.; Moojen, W.A.; Verbout, A.J.; Öner, F. C No evidence for intervention-dependent influence of methodological features on treatment effect. *J. Clin. Epidemiol.* **2013**, *66*, 1347–1355.e3. [CrossRef] [PubMed]
15. Slim, K.; Nini, E.; Forestier, D.; Kwiatkowski, F.; Panis, Y.; Chipponi, J. Methodological index for non-randomized studies (Minors): Development and validation of a new instrument. *ANZ J. Surg.* **2003**, *73*, 712–716. [CrossRef]
16. Liberati, A.; Altman, D.; Jennifer, T. The PRISMA Statement for Reporting Systematic Reviews and Meta-Analyses of Studies That Evaluate Health Care Interventions: Explanation and Elaboration. *PLoS Med.* **2009**, *6*, 50931. [CrossRef] [PubMed]
17. Ouzzani, M.; Hammady, H.; Fedorowicz, Z.; Elmagarmid, A. Rayyan-a web and mobile app for systematic reviews. *Syst. Rev.* **2016**, *5*, 1–10. [CrossRef] [PubMed]

18. Negrini, S.; Minozzi, S.; Bettany-Saltikov, J.; Chockalingam, N.; Grivas, T.B.; Kotwicki, T.; Maruyama, T.; Romano, M.; Zaina, F. Braces for idiopathic scoliosis in adolescents (Review) summary of findings for the main comparison. *Cochrane Database Syst. Rev.* **2015**. [CrossRef]
19. Wallace, B.C.; Trikalinos, T.A.; Lau, J.; Trow, P.; Schmid, C.H. Closing the Gap between Methodologists and End-Users: R as a Computational Back-End. *J. Stat. Softw.* **2012**, *49*, 1–15. [CrossRef]
20. Picault, C.; Demauroy, J.C.; Mouilleseaux, B.; Diana, G. Natural history of idiopathic scoliosis in girls and boys. *Spine* **1986**, *11*, 777–778. [CrossRef]
21. Nachemson, A.L.; Peterson, L. E Effectiveness of tretment with a brace in girls who have adolescent idiopathic scoliosis. *J. Bone Joint Surg. Am.* **1995**, *77*, 815–822. [CrossRef] [PubMed]
22. Xu, L.; Yang, X.; Wang, Y.; Wu, Z.; Xia, C.; Qiu, Y.; Zhu, Z. Brace Treatment in Adolescent Idiopathic Scoliosis Patients with Curve Between 40° and 45°: Effectiveness and Related Factors. *World Neurosurg.* **2019**, *126*, e901–e906. [CrossRef]
23. Yrjönen, T.; Ylikoski, M.; Schlenzka, D.; Poussa, M. Results of brace treatment of adolescent idiopathic scoliosis in boys compared with girls: A retrospective study of 102 patients treated with the Boston brace. *Eur. Spine J.* **2007**, *16*, 393–397. [CrossRef] [PubMed]
24. Grivas, T.B.; Vasiliadis, E.; Chatziargiropoulos, T.; Polyzois, V.D.; Gatos, K. The effect of a modified Boston brace with anti-rotatory blades on the progression of curves in idiopathic scoliosis: Aetiologic implications. *Pediatr. Rehabil.* **2003**, *6*, 237–242. [CrossRef] [PubMed]
25. Pasquini, G.; Cecchi, F.; Bini, C.; Molino-Lova, R.; Vannetti, F.; Castagnoli, C.; Paperini, A.; Boni, R.; Macchi, C.; Crusco, B.; et al. The outcome of a modified version of the Cheneau brace in adolescent idiopathic scoliosis (AIS) based on SRS and SOSORT criteria: A retrospective study. *Eur J Phys Rehabil Med* **2016**, *52*, 618–629. [PubMed]
26. Fang, M.-Q.; Wang, C.; Xiang, G.-H.; Lou, C.; Tian, N.-F.; Xu, H.-Z. Long-term effects of the Chêneau brace on coronal and sagittal alignment in adolescent idiopathic scoliosis. *J. Neurosurg. Spine* **2015**, *23*, 505–509. [CrossRef]
27. Pham, V.-M.; Herbaux, B.; Schill, A.; Thevenon, A. Evaluation of the Chêneau brace in adolescent idiopathic scoliosis. *Évaluation du résultat du corset Chêneau dans la scoliose idiopathique l'adolescent* **2007**, *50*, 125–133.
28. Zabrowska-Sapeta, K.; Kowalski, I.M.; Protasiewicz-Fałdowska, H.; Wolska, O. Evaluation of the effectiveness of Chêneau brace treatment for idiopathic scoliosis—Own observations. *Pol. Ann. Med.* **2010**, *17*, 44–53. [CrossRef]
29. Aulisa, A.G.; Guzzanti, V.; Galli, M.; Perisano, C.; Falciglia, F.; Maggi, G.; Aulisa, L. Treatment of lumbar curves in adolescent females affected by idiopathic scoliosis with a progressive action short brace (PASB): Assessment of results according to the SRS committee on bracing and nonoperative management standardization criteria. *J. Orthop. Traumatol.* **2009**, *12*, S38. [CrossRef]
30. Aulisa, A.G.; Guzzanti, V.; Falciglia, F.; Giordano, M.; Marzetti, E.; Aulisa, L. Lyon bracing in adolescent females with thoracic idiopathic scoliosis: A prospective study based on SRS and SOSORT criteria Orthopedics and biomechanics. *BMC Musculoskelet. Disord.* **2015**, *16*. [CrossRef] [PubMed]
31. Weiss, H.-R.; Tournavitis, N.; Seibel, S.; Kleban, A. A Prospective Cohort Study of AIS Patients with 40° and More Treated with a Gensingen Brace (GBW): Preliminary Results. *Open Orthop. J.* **2017**, *11*, 1558–1567. [CrossRef] [PubMed]
32. Kuroki, H.; Inomata, N.; Hamanaka, H.; Higa, K.; Chosa, E.; Tajima, N. Predictive factors of Osaka Medical College (OMC) brace treatment in patients with adolescent idiopathic scoliosis. *Scoliosis* **2015**, *10*, 11. [CrossRef] [PubMed]
33. Lin, Y.; Lou, E.; Lam, T.P.; Cheng, J.C.-Y.; Sin, S.W.; Kwok, W.K.; Wong, M.S. The Intelligent Automated Pressure-Adjustable Orthosis for Patients With Adolescent Idiopathic Scoliosis: A Bi-Center Randomized Controlled Trial. *Spine* **2020**, *45*, 1395–1402. [CrossRef] [PubMed]
34. Price, C.T.; Scott, D.S.; Reed, F.E.; Riddick, M.F. Nighttime bracing for adolescent idiopathic scoliosis with the Charleston bending brace. Preliminary report. *Spine* **1990**, *15*, 1294–1299. [CrossRef]
35. Lee, C.S.; Hwang, C.J.; Kim, D.-J.; Kim, J.H.; Kim, Y.-T.; Lee, M.Y.; Yoon, S.J.; Lee, D.-H. Effectiveness of the Charleston night-time bending brace in the treatment of adolescent idiopathic scoliosis. *J. Pediatr. Orthop.* **2012**, *32*, 368–372. [CrossRef] [PubMed]
36. Davis, L.; Murphy, J.S.; Shaw, K.A.; Cash, K.; Devito, D.P.; Schmitz, M.L. Nighttime bracing with the Providence thoracolumbosacral orthosis for treatment of adolescent idiopathic scoliosis: A retrospective consecutive clinical series. *Prosthet. Orthot. Int.* **2019**, *43*, 158–162. [CrossRef] [PubMed]
37. Ohrt-Nissen, S.; Hallager, D.W.; Gehrchen, M.; Dahl, B. Flexibility Predicts Curve Progression in Providence Nighttime Bracing of Patients With Adolescent Idiopathic Scoliosis. *Spine* **2016**, *41*, 1724–1730. [CrossRef]
38. Bohl, D.D.; Telles, C.J.; Golinvaux, N.S.; Basques, B.A.; DeLuca, P.A.; Grauer, J.N. Effectiveness of Providence nighttime bracing in patients with adolescent idiopathic scoliosis. *Orthopedics* **2014**, *37*, e1085-90. [CrossRef]
39. Simony, A.; Beuschau, I.; Quisth, L.; Jespersen, S.M.; Carreon, L.Y.; Andersen, M.O. Providence nighttime bracing is effective in treatment for adolescent idiopathic scoliosis even in curves larger than 35°. *Eur. Spine J.* **2019**, *28*, 2020–2024. [CrossRef]
40. Coillard, C.; Vachon, V.; Circo, A.B.; Beauséjour, M.; Rivard, C.H. Effectiveness of the SpineCor brace based on the new standardized criteria proposed by the scoliosis research society for adolescent idiopathic scoliosis. *J. Pediatr. Orthop.* **2007**, *27*, 375–379. [CrossRef]
41. Coillard, C.; Circo, A.B.; Rivard, C.H. A prospective randomized controlled trial of the natural history of idiopathic scoliosis versus treatment with the SpineCor brace. Sosort Award 2011 winner. *Eur. J. Phys. Rehabil. Med.* **2014**, *50*, 479–487.
42. Hanks, G.A.; Zimmer, B.; Nogi, J. TLSO treatment of idiopathic scoliosis. An analysis of the Wilmington jacket. *Spine* **1988**, *13*, 626–629. [CrossRef]

43. Katz, D.E.; Herring, J.A.; Browne, R.H.; Kelly, D.M.; Birch, J.G. Brace wear control of curve progression in adolescent idiopathic scoliosis. *J. Bone Joint Surg. Am.* **2010**, *92*, 1343–1352. [CrossRef] [PubMed]
44. Maruyama, T.; Kobayashi, Y.; Miura, M.; Nakao, Y. Effectiveness of brace treatment for adolescent idiopathic scoliosis. *Scoliosis* **2015**, *10*, S12. [CrossRef] [PubMed]
45. Aulisa, A.G.; Giordano, M.; Toniolo, R.M.; Aulisa, L. Long term results after brace treatment with PASB in adolescent idipathic scoliosis. *Minerva Anestesiol.* **2020**. [CrossRef]
46. Lateur, G.; Grobost, P.; Gerbelot, J.; Eid, A.; Griffet, J.; Courvoisier, A. Efficacy of nighttime brace in preventing progression of idiopathic scoliosis of less than 25°. *Orthop. Traumatol. Surg. Res.* **2017**, *103*, 275–278. [CrossRef]
47. Minsk, M.K.; Venuti, K.D.; Daumit, G.L.; Sponseller, P.D. Effectiveness of the Rigo Chêneau versus Boston-style orthoses for adolescent idiopathic scoliosis: A retrospective study. *Scoliosis Spin. Disord.* **2017**, *12*, 1–6. [CrossRef] [PubMed]
48. Janicki, J.A.; Poe-Kochert, C.; Armstrong, D.G.; Thompson, G.H. A comparison of the thoracolumbosacral orthoses and providence orthosis in the treatment of adolescent idiopathic scoliosis: Results using the new SRS inclusion and assessment criteria for bracing studies. *J. Pediatr. Orthop.* **2007**, *27*, 369–374. [CrossRef]
49. Ohrt-Nissen, S.; Lastikka, M.; Andersen, T.B.; Helenius, I.; Gehrchen, M. Conservative treatment of main thoracic adolescent idiopathic scoliosis: Full-time or nighttime bracing? *J. Orthop. Surg.* **2019**, *27*, 1–8. [CrossRef]
50. Weiss, H.-R.; Weiss, G.M. Brace treatment during pubertal growth spurt in girls with idiopathic scoliosis (IS): A prospective trial comparing two different concepts. *Pediatr. Rehabil.* **2005**, *8*, 199–206. [CrossRef]
51. Guo, J.; Lam, T.P.; Wong, M.S.; Ng, B.K.W.; Lee, K.M.; Liu, K.L.; Hung, L.H.; Lau, A.H.Y.; Sin, S.W.; Kwok, W.K.; et al. A prospective randomized controlled study on the treatment outcome of SpineCor brace versus rigid brace for adolescent idiopathic scoliosis with follow-up according to the SRS standardized criteria. *Eur. Spine J.* **2014**, *23*, 2650–2657. [CrossRef]
52. Emans, M.J.B.; Hresko, M.D.M.T.; Hall, M.D.J.E.; Hedequist, C.D.; Karlin, M.D.L.; Miller, M.D.J.; Miller, R.R.; Magin, C.P.O.M.; McCarthy, R.N.C.; Cassella, R.M.; et al. *Reference Manual for the Boston Scoliosis Brace*; 2003; Available online: https://www.bostonoandp.com/Customer-Content/www/CMS/files/BostonBraceManual.pdf (accessed on 12 January 2021).
53. Fayssoux, R.S.; Cho, R.H.; Herman, M.J. A history of bracing for idiopathic scoliosis in north America. *Clin. Orthop. Relat. Res.* **2010**, *468*, 654–664. [CrossRef]
54. Donzelli, S.; Zaina, F.; Minnella, S.; Lusini, M.; Negrini, S. Consistent and regular daily wearing improve bracing results: A case-control study. *Scoliosis spinal Disord.* **2018**, *13*, 16. [CrossRef]
55. Misteroska, E.; Glowacki, J.; Głowacki, M.; Okręt, A. Long-term effects of conservative treatment of Milwaukee brace on body image and mental health of patients with idiopathic scoliosis. *PLoS ONE* **2018**, *13*. [CrossRef]
56. Aulisa, A.G.; Guzzanti, V.; Falciglia, F.; Galli, M.; Pizzeti, P.; Aulisa, L. Curve progression after long-term brace treatment in adolescent idiopathic scoliosis: Comparative results between over and under 30 Cobb degrees—SOSORT 2017 award winner. *Scoliosis Spin. Disord.* **2017**, *12*. [CrossRef]
57. Bunge, E.M.; De Koning, H.J. Bracing patients with idiopathic scoliosis: Design of the Dutch randomized controlled treatment trial. *BMC Musculoskelet. Disord.* **2008**, *9*, 1–7. [CrossRef] [PubMed]
58. Kunz, R.; Oxman, A.D. The unpredictability paradox: Review of empirical comparisons of randomised and non-randomised clinical trials. *BMJ* **1998**, *317*, 1185–1190. [CrossRef] [PubMed]
59. Vandenbroucke, J.P. Why do the results of randomised and observational studies differ? Statistical theory conflicts with empirical findings in several areas of research. *BMJ* **2011**, *343*, 1128. [CrossRef]
60. Ioannidis, J.P.; Lau, J. Completeness of Safety Reporting in Randomized Trials. *JAMA* **2001**, *285*, 437. [CrossRef] [PubMed]
61. Concato, J. Randomized controlled trial, observational studies and the hierarchy of research designs. *Int. J. Biol. Markers* **2000**, *15*, 79–83. [CrossRef] [PubMed]
62. Richards, B.S.; Bernstein, R.M.; D'Amato, C.R.; Thompson, G.H. Standardization of criteria for adolescent idiopathic scoliosis brace studies: SRS Committee on Bracing and Nonoperative Management. *Spine* **2005**, *30*, 2068–2075. [CrossRef] [PubMed]
63. Upadhyay, S.S.; Nelson, I.W.; Ho, E.K.; Hsu, L.C.; Leong, J.C. New Prognostic Factors to Predict the Final Outcome of Brace Treatment in Adolescent Idiopathic Scoliosis. *Spine* **1995**. [CrossRef] [PubMed]

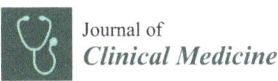

Comment

Comment on Costa et al. The Effectiveness of Different Concepts of Bracing in Adolescent Idiopathic Scoliosis (AIS): A Systematic Review and Meta-Analysis. *J. Clin. Med.* 2021, 10, 2145

Hans-Rudolf Weiss

Schroth Best Practice Academy, 55546 Neu-Bamberg, Germany; hr.weiss@koob-skoliose.com

I read the above-mentioned work with great interest, and I would like to thank the authors for considering two papers from our working group. However, I wonder why our paper containing the preliminary results of the treatment with the Gensingen Brace [1] was taken into account within this systematic review but not the final results that were first published online in 2020 [2]. The latter paper with the final results would have had a lower risk of bias than the paper containing the preliminary results.

The authors seem committed to finding the most effective concept of bracing or even the most effective brace model. In my opinion, however, they have chosen the wrong study design for this because one cannot find this through averaging and can only find it through an individual case analysis.

Surprisingly, in their systematic review regarding night-time brace treatment, the authors came to completely different conclusions than the authors of another current systematic review on the subject [3]. Ruffilli et al. [3] concluded that *"the current available literature does not permit us to draw conclusions about night-time braces. The low methodological quality of the studies examined makes it impossible to compare the effectiveness of the night-time braces with that of traditional TLSOs"*.

In fact, the results of night-time bracing are very diverse. As early as 1997, there was a meta-analysis that showed that part-time or night bracing was clearly inferior to full-time brace treatment [4]. Further studies on this topic clearly show that wearing time and the correction effect are the two main criteria for success [5,6]. The greater the corrective effect of a brace and the longer the wearing time, the greater the success rate [5,6]. However, the authors do not discuss these important parameters in their study.

The question is how the authors of this systematic review, compared to Ruffilli et al. [3], came to such different conclusions:

One study on the Providence Brace included by the authors has an exceptionally high success rate [7], while other studies on the Providence Brace tend to conclude with success rates of between 50% and 60% [8]. One study cited by the authors has a success rate of over 70%, but this is a more mature and therefore prognostically more favorable cohort (Risser 0–3) [9].

A success rate of 89% in a night-time brace is very exceptional [7]. However, if one reads the study carefully, one will find the following passage on the subject of inclusion criteria: *"We included all patients, diagnosed with AIS who fulfilled the following criteria, age >10 years at time of diagnosis, less than 12 months post-menarche, Cobb 20°–42°, no prior scoliosis treatment, initial in-brace curve correction >60% and follow-up including radiographs at least 12 months after brace termination. The patients were braced according to the SRS criteria"*.

Accordingly, this study [7] is a selective study with favorable inclusion criteria. No statement can be found in the paper on the outcome of the patients with a correction effect of <60°. Interestingly, this particular patient selection is addressed neither in the abstract nor further elaborated in the discussion. In addition, the collective of Simony et al. [7] also failed to meet the SRS inclusion criteria for brace studies. The Risser sign, as an essential

Citation: Weiss, H.-R. Comment on Costa et al. The Effectiveness of Different Concepts of Bracing in Adolescent Idiopathic Scoliosis (AIS): A Systematic Review and Meta-Analysis. *J. Clin. Med.* 2021, 10, 2145. *J. Clin. Med.* 2022, 11, 752. https://doi.org/10.3390/jcm11030752

Academic Editor: Theodoros B. Grivas

Received: 28 October 2021
Accepted: 27 January 2022
Published: 30 January 2022

Publisher's Note: MDPI stays neutral with regard to jurisdictional claims in published maps and institutional affiliations.

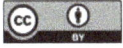

Copyright: © 2022 by the author. Licensee MDPI, Basel, Switzerland. This article is an open access article distributed under the terms and conditions of the Creative Commons Attribution (CC BY) license (https://creativecommons.org/licenses/by/4.0/).

part of the SRS inclusion criteria, was not recorded, and the cohort was also significantly older than in comparable studies on the topic [1,2]. This was—among other things—already discussed in a letter to the editor by Dr. Potts [10].

The problem was thus known, and yet, this work with a considerable selection bias [7] was included by the authors in their systematic review with meta-analysis and was related to other studies without correspondingly favorable patient selection. This systematic review with meta-analysis by Costa et al., therefore, has a systematic selection bias and should not have been published in the present form. This all too positive outlier with a success rate of 89% [7] has a significant influence on the results of this review. Without the inclusion of the Simony paper [7], one would not come to the conclusion that the results of night-time bracing are on a par with full-time bracing.

Finally, the authors did not indicate a conflict of interest (René M. Castelein, Stryker Spine (a, d), found in the programs of the SRS Conferences 2020 and 2021, [11,12]).

The fact that publications contaminated by errors coexist with their healthy counterparts in different databases, and in the worst-case scenario, multiply in systematic reviews and meta-analyses, is well recognized [13]. And this is just what has happened in the paper addressed within this comment.

Conclusions

1. The goal of finding the most effective bracing concept or even the most effective brace model was not achieved and was not further discussed in this work.
2. The unveiled findings cannot be reconciled with the study design of a systematic review with meta-analysis. The study shows features of a narrative review with a pronounced selection bias, which significantly influences the conclusions.
3. The fact that the described original work with a considerable selection bias [7] was included by the authors in their so-called systematic review with meta-analysis despite extensive discussion in the literature [9] raises doubts about a simple oversight as the cause.

Funding: This research received no external funding.

Institutional Review Board Statement: Not applicable.

Informed Consent Statement: Not applicable.

Data Availability Statement: Not applicable.

Conflicts of Interest: The author currently serves as the senior consultant for Koob Scolitech GmbH, Neu-Bamberg, Germany. The company is held by the spouse of the author. He has held a patent on a sagittal realignment brace (EP 1 604 624 A1).

References

1. Weiss, H.R.; Tournavitis, N.; Seibel, S.; Kleban, A. A Prospective Cohort Study of AIS Patients with 40° and More Treated with a Gensingen Brace (GBW): Preliminary Results. *Open Orthop. J.* **2017**, *11*, 1558–1567. [CrossRef] [PubMed]
2. Weiss, H.R.; Lay, M.; Seibel, S.; Kleban, A. Is it possible to improve treatment safety in the brace treatment of scoliosis patients by using standardized CAD algorithms? *Orthopäde* **2021**, *50*, 435–445. (In German) [CrossRef] [PubMed]
3. Ruffilli, A.; Fiore, M.; Barile, F.; Pasini, S.; Faldini, C. Evaluation of night-time bracing efficacy in the treatment of adolescent idiopathic scoliosis: A systematic review. *Spine Deform.* **2021**, *9*, 671–678. [CrossRef] [PubMed]
4. Rowe, D.E.; Bernstein, S.M.; Riddick, M.F.; Adler, F.; Emans, J.B.; Gardner-Bonneau, D. A meta-analysis of the efficacy of non-operative treatments for idiopathic scoliosis. *J. Bone Joint Surg. Am.* **1997**, *79*, 664–674. [CrossRef] [PubMed]
5. Landauer, F.; Wimmer, C.; Behensky, H. Estimating the final outcome of brace treatment for idiopathic thoracic scoliosis at 6-month follow-up. *Pediatr. Rehabil.* **2003**, *6*, 201–207. [CrossRef] [PubMed]
6. van den Bogaart, M.; van Royen, B.J.; Haanstra, T.M.; de Kleuver, M.; Faraj, S.S.A. Predictive factors for brace treatment outcome in adolescent idiopathic scoliosis: A best-evidence synthesis. *Eur. Spine J.* **2019**, *28*, 511–525. [CrossRef] [PubMed]
7. Simony, A.; Beuschau, I.; Quisth, L.; Jespersen, S.M.; Carreon, L.Y.; Andersen, M.O. Providence nighttime bracing is effective in treatment for adolescent idiopathic scoliosis even in curves larger than 35°. *Eur. Spine J.* **2019**, *28*, 2020–2024. [CrossRef] [PubMed]

8. Davis, L.; Murphy, J.S.; Shaw, K.A.; Cash, K.; Devito, D.P.; Schmitz, M.L. Nighttime bracing with the Providence thoracolumbosacral orthosis for treatment of adolescent idiopathic scoliosis: A retrospective consecutive clinical series. *Prosthet. Orthot. Int.* **2019**, *43*, 158–162. [CrossRef] [PubMed]
9. Yrjönen, T.; Ylikoski, M.; Schlenzka, D.; Kinnunen, R.; Poussa, M. Effectiveness of the Providence nighttime bracing in adolescent idiopathic scoliosis: A comparative study of 36 female patients. *Eur. Spine J.* **2006**, *15*, 1139–1143. [CrossRef] [PubMed]
10. Potts, M.A. Letter to the editor concerning "Providence nighttime bracing is effective in treatment for adolescent idiopathic scoliosis even in curves larger than 35°" by Simony A, Beuschau I, Quisth L, et al. (Eur Spine J; [2019]:. https://doi.org/10.1007/s00586-019-06077-z). *Eur. Spine J.* **2020**, *29*, 641–642. [CrossRef] [PubMed]
11. Scoliosis Research Society Virtual 55th Annual Meeting. p. 17. Available online: https://www.srs.org/UserFiles/file/AM20-FinalProgram.pdf (accessed on 3 December 2021).
12. Scoliosis Research Society 56th Annual Meeting 22–25 September 2021, St. Louis, MI, USA. p. 29. Available online: https://www.srs.org/UserFiles/file/AM21_FinalProgram.pdf (accessed on 3 December 2021).
13. Stamm, T. From honest mistakes to fake news—Approaches to correcting the scientific literature. *Head Face Med.* **2020**, *16*, 6. [CrossRef] [PubMed]

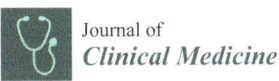

Reply

Reply to Weiss, H.-R. Comment on "Costa et al. The Effectiveness of Different Concepts of Bracing in Adolescent Idiopathic Scoliosis (AIS): A Systematic Review and Meta-Analysis. *J. Clin. Med.* 2021, *10*, 2145"

Lorenzo Costa, Tom P. C. Schlösser, Moyo C. Kruyt and René M. Castelein *

Department of Orthopaedic Surgery, University Medical Center Utrecht, 3508 GA Utrecht, The Netherlands; l.costa-2@umcutrecht.nl (L.C.); t.p.c.schlosser@umcutrecht.nl (T.P.C.S.); m.c.kruyt@umcutrecht.nl (M.C.K.)
* Correspondence: r.m.castelein@umcutrecht.nl; Tel.: +31-(88)-755-45-78; Fax: +31-(30)-251-06-38

We would like to thank you for the opportunity to reply to the comments in regard of the letter by Dr. Weiss [1]. We acknowledge the author's valuable contribution in this field as reflected by the presence of some of his papers in both our systematic review and meta-analysis.

Most of the criticism seems to stem from a disagreement with our conclusion that the night-time brace concept may be comparable to full-time bracing. Several methodological aspects of our search and selection are mentioned as potential bias in favor of night-time braces. We strongly object to this suggestion. This study was done strictly according to the PRISMA statement with a predetermined objective and quality assessment. A threshold for all papers that were included in the meta-analysis was applied.

We do not agree with the argument that individual case analysis is the correct design to compare brace models. The strength of a systematic review and meta-analysis on this topic is that it can answer a question that cannot be posed by individual studies and can improve the precision of the estimation of effect.

During title and abstract screening, both the title and conclusion suggested that this study, "*Is it possible to improve treatment safety in the corset care of scoliosis patients by applying standardized CAD algorithms?*" should not be included [2]. Nevertheless, reading the full paper, it appears that the aim of the manuscript was to study the *effectiveness* (and not the *safety*) of the Gensingen brace, so in that sense we regret that this paper was not selected. Unfortunately, this kind of error is inherent to the methodology of title and abstract screening, which was performed by two independent researchers [3]. Including a paper post hoc would introduce a potential bias and, therefore, should not be done. Besides the methodological inaccuracy, including the paper would lead to an overlap with the population of another study by the same author, from 2017, that we included in both the systematic review and meta-analysis [4].

Our study was compared with a systematic review by Ruffilli et al. which had a similar aim and Rowe et al. that yielded different results [5,6]. However, Ruffilli et al. only selected comparative studies which resulted in a different and much smaller patient sample. The paper by Rowe et al. (1997), was performed more than 20 years ago in a period where much less studies were present in the literature and the methodology had serious limitations including no strict guidelines for inclusion criteria [6].

One of the aims of this work was to study the effect of skeletal maturity on the effectiveness of brace treatment. Therefore, papers with a Risser grade higher than 2 were also included. Indeed, for this analysis, we only included papers that documented the Risser grade. In the other analyses of effectiveness of braces, all maturation parameters such as menarche (but not only) were included. Furthermore, menarche is considered a valuable tool that is often used as mentioned by Richards et al. in 2005 [7]. Moreover, it

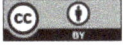

is important to notice that also studies on full-time braces with Risser 0–3 or 0–4 were included in the systematic review and meta-analysis [8,9].

We are aware of the letter by Potts et al. in 2020 and their concern regarding the Simony et al. paper [10,11]. They were concerned that the Risser stage was not assessed. Nevertheless, Tanner scale, time of menarche in girls and continued height gain in boys were used [12]. We took both letters into consideration [11,12].

We disagree with the claim that because timing is a key point for brace treatment, it is not possible that the Simony paper has such a positive result [10]. Other studies on night time bracing (which did include Risser sign as a parameter of maturity) showed similar good results [13–15]. Therefore, Simony paper is not the first nor the only one. We agree that this result is in the higher range [10]. However, with sufficient quality, the reported outcome cannot be a reason to discard a paper.

The author expresses concern about the variability of the Providence results. We agree that high variability generally weakens the reliability. However, this high variability is not a prerogative of night-time brace concept, but more a general problem of brace studies as was reported in the discussion sections by Ruffilli et al., our article and mentioned by the author himself (specifically focusing on the Cheneau brace) [2,5].

According to the *JCM* Guidelines for authors, "*authors must disclose all relationships or interests that could inappropriately influence or bias their work*". The analysis was performed according to the above-described and pre-established criteria. One of the authors has received a research grant for studies into scoliosis etiology, but this is unrelated to the current project. Furthermore, the senior author recently founded the Dutch Scoliosis Center. In retrospect, it would have been better to mention this new disclosure, although it had no influence on this particular study. As highlighted in the funding section, this study was supported by funding from the EU's H2020 research and innovation program under Marie S. Curie cofound RESCUE grant agreement No 801540.

To conclude, we would like to thank the author for highlighting the findings of his previous work and showing his concerns in matter of our systematic review. Nevertheless, we believe that the study was conducted according to widely accepted pre-determined criteria and shows a valid result. This conclusion should not be interpreted as an absolute statement, but is meant to bring awareness in the limitations of the current literature and possibilities of these devices. As we wrote in our discussion, further studies with higher criteria and standards should be done in order to better understand the best treatment and management for AIS patients.

Author Contributions: Conceptualization, L.C., T.P.C.S., M.C.K. and R.M.C.; methodology, L.C., T.P.C.S., M.C.K. and R.M.C.; investigation, L.C.; writing—original draft preparation, L.C.; writing—review and editing, L.C., T.P.C.S., M.C.K. and R.M.C.; visualization, L.C., T.P.C.S., M.C.K. and R.M.C.; supervision, T.P.C.S., M.C.K. and R.M.C. All authors have read and agreed to the published version of the manuscript.

Funding: This research received funding from Marie S. Curie cofound RESCUE grant agreement No 801540.

Conflicts of Interest: The senior author R.M. Castelein is founder of the Dutch Scoliosis Center. He received grants, unrelated to the topic of this study, from Stryker Spine, Fundation Yves Cotrel. He is in collaboration with Telefield Medical Imaging Ltd. (Hong Kong) and MRI guidance. R.M. Castelein and M.C. Kruyt are co-founders of Cresco Spine. There are no other conflict of interest.

References

1. Weiss, H.-R. Comment on Costa et al. The Effectiveness of Different Concepts of Bracing in Adolescent Idiopathic Scoliosis (AIS): A Systematic Review and Meta-Analysis. *J. Clin. Med.* 2021, *10*, 2145. *J. Clin. Med.* **2022**, *11*, 752. [CrossRef]
2. Weiss, H.-R.; Lay, M.; Seibel, S.; Kleban, A. Is it possible to improve treatment safety in the brace treatment of scoliosis patients by using standardized CAD algorithms? *Orthopade* **2021**, *50*, 435–445. [CrossRef] [PubMed]
3. Wang, Z.; Nayfeh, T.; Tetzlaff, J.; O'Blenis, P.; Murad, M.H. Error rates of human reviewers during abstract screening in systematic reviews. *PLoS ONE* **2020**, *15*, e0227742. [CrossRef] [PubMed]

4. Weiss, H.-R.; Tournavitis, N.; Seibel, S.; Kleban, A. A Prospective Cohort Study of AIS Patients with 40° and More Treated with a Gensingen Brace (GBW): Preliminary Results. *Open Orthop. J.* **2017**, *11*, 1558–1567. Available online: https://www.ncbi.nlm.nih.gov/pubmed/29399229 (accessed on 25 December 2021). [CrossRef] [PubMed]
5. Ruffilli, A.; Fiore, M.; Barile, F.; Pasini, S.; Faldini, C. Evaluation of night-time bracing efficacy in the treatment of adolescent idiopathic scoliosis: A systematic review. *Spine Deform.* **2021**, *9*, 671–678. [CrossRef] [PubMed]
6. Rowe, D.E.; Bernstein, S.M.; Riddick, M.F.; Adler, F.; Emans, J.B.; Gardner-Bonneau, D. A Meta-Analysis of the Efficacy of Non-Operative Treatments for Idiopathic Scoliosis. *J. Bone Jt. Surg.* **1997**, *79*, 664–674. [CrossRef] [PubMed]
7. Richards, B.S.; Bernstein, R.M.; D'Amato, C.R.; Thompson, G.H. Standardization of Criteria for Adolescent Idiopathic Scoliosis Brace Studies: SRS Committee on Bracing and Nonoperative Management. *Spine* **2005**, *30*, 2068–2075. [CrossRef] [PubMed]
8. Xu, L.; Yang, X.; Wang, Y.; Wu, Z.; Xia, C.; Qiu, Y.; Zhu, Z. Brace Treatment in Adolescent Idiopathic Scoliosis Patients with Curve Between 40° and 45°: Effectiveness and Related Factors. *World Neurosurg.* **2019**, *126*, e901–e906. Available online: https://www.ncbi.nlm.nih.gov/pubmed/30872192 (accessed on 25 December 2021). [CrossRef] [PubMed]
9. Aulisa, A.G.; Giordano, M.; Toniolo, R.M.; Aulisa, L. Long term results after brace treatment with PASB in adolescent idipathic scoliosis. *Eur. J. Phys. Rehabil. Med.* **2020**, *57*, 406–413. [CrossRef] [PubMed]
10. Simony, A.; Beuschau, I.; Quisth, L.; Jespersen, S.M.; Carreon, L.Y.; Andersen, M. Providence nighttime bracing is effective in treatment for adolescent idiopathic scoliosis even in curves larger than 35°. *Eur. Spine J.* **2019**, *28*, 2020–2024. [CrossRef] [PubMed]
11. Potts, M.A. Letter to the editor concerning 'Providence nighttime bracing is effective in treatment for adolescent idiopathic scoliosis even in curves larger than 35°' by Simony A, Beuschau I, Quisth L; et al. (Eur Spine J; [2019]. https://doi.org/10.1007/s00586-019-06077-z). *Eur. Spine J.* **2020**, *29*, 641–642. [CrossRef] [PubMed]
12. Simony, A. Answer to the Letter to the Editor of M. A. Potts concerning "Providence nighttime bracing is effective in treatment for adolescent idiopathic scoliosis even in curves larger than 35°" by Simony A, Beuschau I, Quisth L; et al. [Eur Spine J; (2019): https://doi.org/10.1007/s00586-019-06077-z]. *Eur. Spine J.* **2020**, *29*, 643–645. [CrossRef] [PubMed]
13. D'Amato, C.R.; Griggs, S.; McCoy, B. Nighttime Bracing with the Providence Brace in Adolescent Girls with Idiopathic Scoliosis. *Spine* **2001**, *26*, 2006–2012. [CrossRef] [PubMed]
14. Price, C.T.; Scott, D.S.; Reed, F.E.; Riddick, M.F. Nighttime Bracing for Adolescent Idiopathic Scoliosis with the Charleston Bending Brace. *Spine* **1990**, *15*, 1294–1299. Available online: https://www.ncbi.nlm.nih.gov/pubmed/2281373 (accessed on 25 December 2021). [CrossRef] [PubMed]
15. Lee, C.S.; Hwang, C.J.; Kim, D.-J.; Kim, J.H.; Kim, Y.-T.; Lee, M.Y.; Yoon, S.J.; Lee, D.-H. Effectiveness of the Charleston Night-time Bending Brace in the Treatment of Adolescent Idiopathic Scoliosis. *J. Pediatr. Orthop.* **2012**, *32*, 368–372. Available online: http://www.embase.com/search/results?subaction=viewrecord&from=export&id=L364863882 (accessed on 25 December 2021). [CrossRef] [PubMed]

Article

Ossification and Fusion of the Vertebral Ring Apophysis as an Important Part of Spinal Maturation

Lorenzo Costa, Steven de Reuver, Luc Kan, Peter Seevinck, Moyo C. Kruyt, Tom P. C. Schlosser and René M. Castelein *

Department of Orthopaedic Surgery, University Medical Center Utrecht, 3584CX Utrecht, The Netherlands; l.costa-2@umcutrecht.nl (L.C.); S.deReuver-4@umcutrecht.nl (S.d.R.); l.p.m.vankan@students.uu.nl (L.K.); p.seevinck@umcutrecht.nl (P.S.); M.C.Kruyt@umcutrecht.nl (M.C.K.); T.P.C.Schlosser@umcutrecht.nl (T.P.C.S.)
* Correspondence: R.M.Castelein-3@umcutrecht.nl; Tel.: +31-88-755-4578; Fax: +31-30-251-0638

Abstract: In scoliosis, most of the deformity is in the disc and occurs during the period of rapid growth. The ring apophyses form the insertion of the disc into the vertebral body, they then ossify and fuse to the vertebrae during that same crucial period. Although this must have important implications for the mechanical properties of the spine, relatively little is known of how this process takes place. This study describes the maturation pattern of the ring apophyses in the thoracic and lumbar spine during normal growth. High-resolution CT scans of the spine for indications not related to this study were included. Ossification and fusion of each ring apophysis from T1 to the sacrum was classified on midsagittal and midcoronal images (4 points per ring) by two observers. The ring apophysis maturation (RAM) was compared between different ages, sexes, and spinal levels. The RAM strongly correlated with age (R = 0.892, $p < 0.001$). Maturation differed in different regions of the spine and between sexes. High thoracic and low lumbar levels fused earlier in both groups, but, around the peak of the growth spurt, in girls the mid-thoracic levels were less mature than in boys, which may have implications for the development of scoliosis.

Keywords: ring apophysis; maturation; ossification; fusion; scoliosis

1. Introduction

The majority of pediatric spinal deformities develop during puberty when the body weight and dimensions increase rapidly, as the skeleton matures into its adult form.

Recent studies have demonstrated the significant contribution of the intervertebral discs to the deformation of the spine in scoliosis [1–3]. For undisturbed and harmonious spinal development, rapidly increasing loads during the growth spurt require adequate maturation of the spine's stabilizers, of which the disc is an essential component [4]. Skeletal maturity is traditionally assessed on X-rays of the iliac crest, the hand, and wrists, or other growth cartilages remote from the spine. The most used classifications are the Risser grade based on ossification and fusion of the iliac apophysis and the Sanders simplified skeletal maturity scoring system, based on the maturation of the hand epiphyses [5,6]. Another classification is the Proximal Humerus Ossification System (PHOS) [7]. This classification is a five-stage system that uses the proximal humeral physis in assessing skeletal maturity. These skeletal maturation scoring systems correlate with the Peak Height Velocity (PHV) during pubertal growth and the curve acceleration phase in scoliosis, however, they do not necessarily assess the maturation of different regions of the spine itself [6,8–10].

After the formation of the three primary ossification centers for each vertebra (one for the body and two for the vertebral arch), the maturation of the spine continues with the closure of the neurocentral synchondroses from age 4–8 [11]. The secondary ossification centers are the ring apophyses and the tips of the transverse and spinous processes [12]. The ring apophyses are not inside the epiphyseal plate and are not involved in the longitudinal growth of the spine [13]. During growth, they encircle the inferior and superior surfaces of the vertebral bodies. The outermost fibers of the annulus fibrosus, the Sharpey's fibers, insert into the ring apophysis and thus anchor the intervertebral disc to the two adjacent vertebrae (Figure 1) [14–18]. During skeletal maturation, these initially cartilaginous insertions of the disc ossify and ultimately fuse to the vertebral bodies [19]. This process has important implications for the mechanical stability of the disc-vertebral body complex at a time when spinal loading increases rapidly, but very little is known about its different phases during growth [20,21].

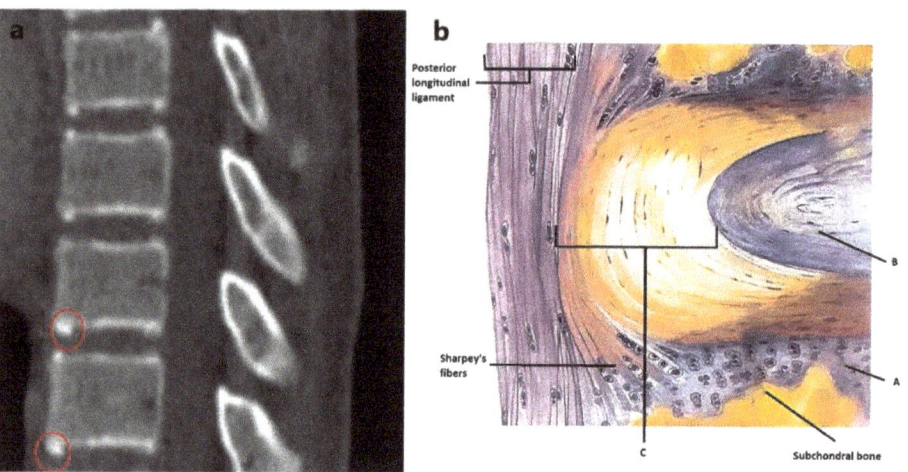

Figure 1. (a) A view of the ossified rings and the start of the fusion (red circles) to the vertebral body; (b) schematic anatomical view of the IVD and the attachment of the Sharpey's fibers to cartilage tissue. A: cartilaginous endplate. B: Nucleus pulposus. C: Anulus fibrosus.

2. Materials and Methods

2.1. Study Population

After a waiver from the ethical review board (ERB) for formal review of this retrospective study, pre-existing high-resolution Computed Tomography (CT) scans of the thorax and/or abdomen acquired from a tertiary pediatric hospital for indications not related to this study (e.g., trauma screening, pulmonary disease, and gastro-enteric disorders) were included from our local patient archiving and communications system (PACS). Inclusion criteria were patients between 6 and 21 years of age and available high-resolution images of the spine (slice thickness ≤ 1 mm and slice interval ≤ 1.5 mm). The ages of 6 and 21 were chosen based on previous studies by Woo et al. and Uys et al. [13,19]. Exclusion criteria were the presence of spinal pathology, bone disorders (e.g., Scheuermann's disease), syndromes associated with growth disorders, growth hormone treatment, and insufficient CT-scan quality including movement artifacts. According to all available information, subjects represented healthy adolescents. A minimum of 10 subjects per age cohort was included. Age, sex, Risser grade, and proximal humeral ossification system (PHOS) were collected on the coronal survey scans.

2.2. CT-Scan Analysis

The included CT scans were analyzed independently by two trained observers, who scored each vertebra separately blinded from each other. Multiplanar images of the exact mid-sagittal and mid-coronal plane of each individual vertebra were reconstructed, using the RadiAnt DICOM viewer© (RadiAnt, Poznan, Poland) (Figure 2).

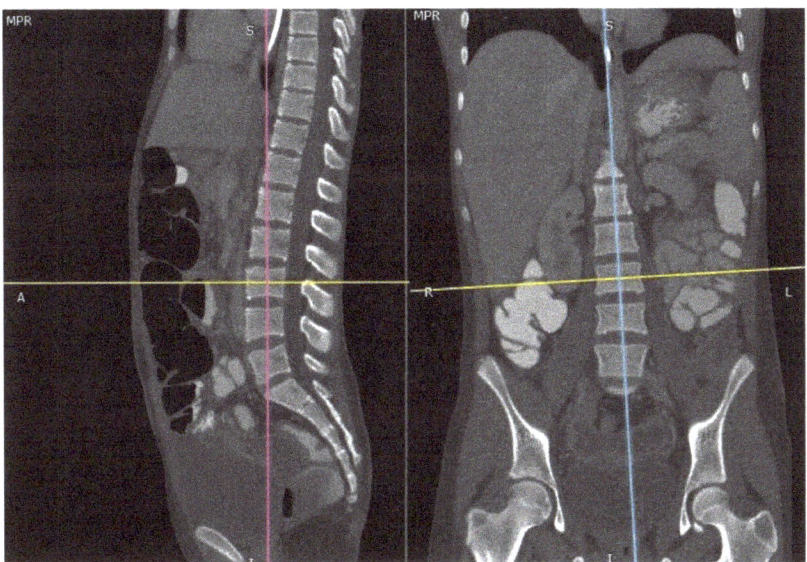

Figure 2. Mid-sagittal and mid-coronal reconstructions were used for each spinal level to describe the presence of ossification and fusion in four areas of each ring.

The window level was set to the bone. Ossification and/or fusion of the anterior, posterior, and lateral parts of each superior and inferior apophyseal ring was classified. If needed, the two observers viewed adjacent slices to confirm that suspected ossified structures were part of the ring apophysis, and discrepancies were resolved by consensus.

According to previous observations by Uys et al., and confirmed following a pilot study performed, the ossification and fusion of each region of interest (ROI) of the ring apophyses were scored as shown in Figure 3 [19]:

- Phase 0: Ring not detectable.
- Phase 1: Ring detectable.
- Phase 2: Fusion not completed.
- Phase 3: Fusion completed.

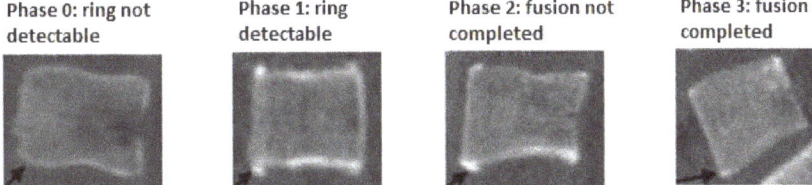

Figure 3. The four phases of maturation of the ring apophysis on mid-sagittal images. In phase 0 the rings are still in a cartilaginous stage and are not detectable on CT scans. In phase 1 the rings are ossified and can be seen on CT scans but have not yet started to fuse. In phase 2 the rings are starting to fuse with the bodies. In phase 3 the rings are completely fused with the vertebral bodies.

Next, the overall ring apophysis maturation (RAM) of each ring was classified as:

- Stage 0: no ossification (phase 0) in all 4 ROI.
- Stage 1: Beginning of ossification (phase 1 in 1–3 ROI).
- Stage 2: Complete ossification (phase 1 in all 4 ROI).
- Stage 3: Incomplete fusion (phase 3 in 1–3 ROI).
- Stage 4: Complete fusion at all 4 points (phase 3 in all 4 ROI).

Intraclass correlation coefficients (kappa value) were calculated for the assessment of intra- and inter-observer reliability.

2.3. Statistical Analysis

Statistical analyses were performed using SPSS 25.0 for Windows (IBM, Armonk, NY, USA). The median, range, and IQR of the RAM were calculated for each age and spinal level for both sexes. The normality of distribution of the RAM within the study population was analyzed via Q-Q plots. The correlation between the RAM and age was tested with a non-parametric Spearman's rank test as well as for different areas of the rings. In the ring ossification stage (phase 1), the authors compared the sagittal plane (both anterior and posterior) with the coronal plane, with a standard t-test. The same procedure was done for fusion (phase 3). Different growth patterns between the lower thoracic and thoracolumbar spine and the other spinal sections were calculated through a generalized linear model. The correlation between the median RAM of the whole spine and the conventional skeletal maturity scores (Risser and PHOS) was analyzed with a Spearman's rank test. The p-value was set at 0.05.

3. Results

3.1. Study Population

Out of 4775 available CT scans, 456 could be included in this study. Most exclusions were due to insufficient image quality. Of the included subjects, 50% were females. The CT scan images analyzed were 289 (63%) full-body, 82 (18%) thoracic, and 85 (19%) abdominal. Descriptive statistics of patients and CT scans are shown in Table 1.

Table 1. Patient demographics.

	Population	
Age	Males	Females
6	15	17
7	18	16
8	13	13
9	13	11
10	11	12
11	16	16
12	17	20
13	17	15
14	14	19
15	14	17
16	16	12
17	14	13
18	12	14
19	14	13
20	12	11
21	11	10
Total (percentage)	227 (49.7%)	229 (50.3%)
Mean age	13.22	13.15
SD	4.52	4.44
Range	6–21	6–21
	CT scans	
Selected CT scans	456	
Total-body n (%)	289 (63%)	
Thoracic n (%)	82 (18%)	
Abdominal n (%)	85 (19%)	

3.2. Ring Apophysis Maturation

Maturation of the ring apophysis is a process that varies for each age at different levels of the spine and differs between sexes. Furthermore, it does not strictly follow the same patterns and timing of the most common physes used for skeletal maturity assessment such as iliac apophysis (Risser), hand epiphysis (Sanders), and proximal humeral physis (PHOS).

Ossification occurred from age 9–15 in males and 7–15 in females, fusion from 14–19 and 13–19, respectively.

RAM correlated significantly with age (R = 0.892, Figure 4) and both ossification and fusion occurred earlier in females (p = 0.002, Figure 4).

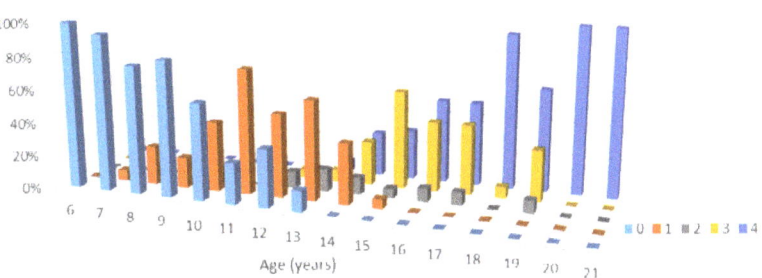

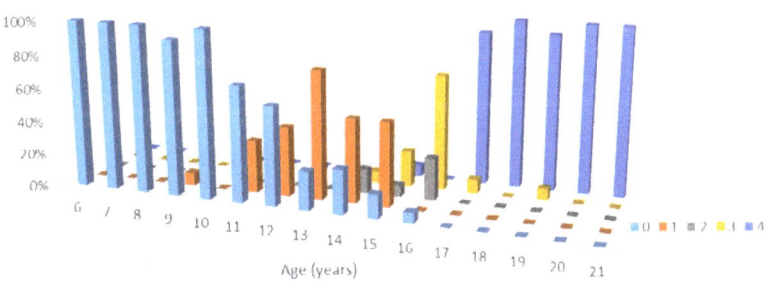

Figure 4. A 3-D histogram showing the percentiles of the different maturation stages of the apophyseal ring in females and males at different ages.

At age 21, 98% of the rings were completely fused (stage 4). Whereas ossification and fusion occurred on average between 9 and 19 in males and 7 and 19 in females, important differences were observed per spinal level, especially when related to the average age of the PHV (13 years of age in females and 15 in males) as can be seen in Table 2 and Figure 5. Most differences between the sexes could be detected in the thoracic levels. In females at the age of 13, the median of RAM was stage 0 between T1 and T6 and stage 1 between T7 and T12. In 15-year old males, the median of maturation in spinal sections was stage 3 for T1 and T2 and stage 1 between T3 and T12.

For both males and females, the ossification of the inferior ring was earlier than the superior ring. In contrast, fusion occurred earlier in the superior ring. Furthermore, maturation of one ring does not appear to occur in all areas at the same time: ossification (phase 1) and fusion (phase 3) occurred half a year later (between 11 and 12 years, median 12) in the coronal than the sagittal plane (p = 0.031). Finally, the high thoracic and low lumbar levels ossified later but fused earlier (while the growth spurt was ceasing in females and was mid-way in males) than the thoracolumbar levels (after the growth spurt has ceased in females and was ceasing in males).

Table 2. The differences in mean maturation of the apophyseal ring in males (in blue) and females (in red) for each spinal level.

							M 0	1	2	3	4								
							F 0	1	2	3	4								
AGE	10	11	12	13	14	15	16	17	18	AGE	10	11	12	13	14	15	16	17	18
T1										T1									
T2										T2									
T3										T3									
T4										T4									
T5										T5									
T6										T6									
T7										T7									
T8										T8									
T9										T9									
T10										T10									
T11										T11									
T12										T12									
L1										L1									
L2										L2									
L3										L3									
L4										L4									
L5										L5									
S1										S1									

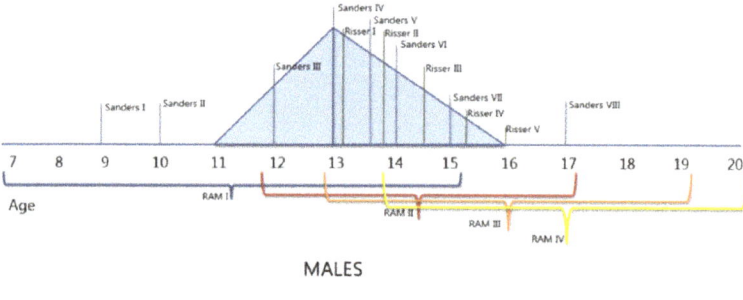

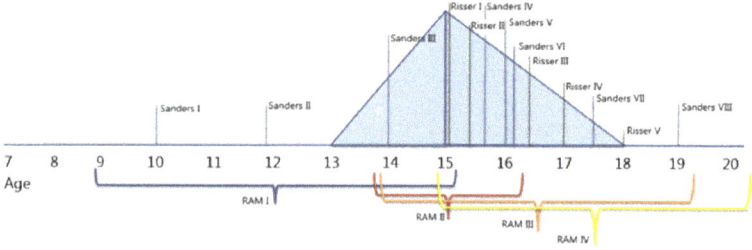

Figure 5. Figure based on Di Meglio et al. (2011) in which Sanders, Risser, and RAM classifications are correlated to growth velocity (and peak height velocity) in females and males [22].

3.3. Correlation with Other Skeletal Maturity Parameters

Although ring maturation varies per level studied, the overall RAM presented a clear correlation with the other two classifications. The Spearman's test between the RAM and Risser grade was 0.900 and between RAM and PHOS was 0.908.

4. Discussion

This study provides a CT-based analysis of the maturation of the disc's fixation to the vertebral body, the ring apophysis, related to age, sex, and spinal levels. Knowledge of the maturation pattern of the ring apophysis is important in the management and etiologic understanding of developmental spine problems since the disc is considered the primary passive stabilizer of the spine [4,23,24]. Whether it is anchored to bone or cartilage during a period in life when body weight and dimensions increase rapidly is supposed to make a major difference for the mechanical properties of the system.

Unlike what all traditional maturation parameters that Risser, PHOS, and Sanders suggest, spinal maturation differs per spinal level. Overall, ossification occurred from age 9–15 years in males and 7–15 in females, fusion from 14–19 and 13–19. Between 12–15 in females and 13–16 years old in males, the ring apophysis undergoes a massive change [25,26]. In girls, around their growth spurt, fewer vertebrae have started the maturation process than in boys, who, in general, have a growth spurt around two years later (Table 2) [22].

The anterior and posterior parts, compared to the lateral parts, ossified and fused half a year earlier and the high thoracic and low lumbar levels fused earlier than the mid-thoracic and thoracolumbar.

We observed an earlier fusion of the superior ring compared to the inferior ring as was also observed in earlier radiography studies [16,19]. Moreover, the observations that the inferior ring ossifies earlier than the superior one, that they have the same level of maturation at the age of 15–16, and finally that the superior ring overcomes the inferior one during the fusion stage is in line with the findings by Woo et al. [13].

Not all of the spinal areas mature at the same time. This study showed a later fusion in the mid thoracic and thoracolumbar spine in both sexes, which is similar to the closure pattern of the Neuro Central Junction [11]. Interestingly, the most common curve type in Adolescent Idiopathic Scoliosis (AIS) patients is in the same region where the maturation of the ring apophysis is slower [27].

As mentioned previously, understanding the maturation of the spine is of key importance for the management of disturbances of its harmonious development. Nowadays, the most used technique to determine bone maturation is the Risser grade even though its accuracy is debated since the Risser stages do not reflect the exact growth activity in the vertebral endplates [6,9,10,28,29]. Even though other classifications such as Sanders are shown to be more reliable, a specific, spine-based classification of spine maturation is lacking. Furthermore, the spine continues to mature after Risser 4 and 5. Similar discrepancies have already been demonstrated by James et al. in 1958 in which in most cases of the studied x-rays, Risser 5 was not synchronous with the end of the ring maturation [18]. This delayed maturation, as compared to most of the long bones, may be relevant to better understand the response of the spine to the increased loads of the adolescent body during the growth spurt. This topic is nicely displayed in the paper by Sanders et al. (2020) [30]. The authors explained that the spine continues to grow longer than the lower extremities [30]. Di Meglio et al. provided similar results in two of their studies, showing differences in yearly height gain velocity between the trunk and the lower limbs [22,31]. Furthermore, as the pelvis reflects the lower extremities more, it is clear that the Risser grade is not deeply connected to the growth of the spine which continues after the lower limb's growth has ceased [30]. Moreover, it is clear that Risser 1 occurs after the peak height velocity as shown previously by Di Meglio et al. and in Figure 5 while ring apophysis maturation varies, depending on spinal level, for each Risser stage [22].

Finally, inter- and intra-observer reliability of RAM was highly positive, resulting in a substantial agreement. Nevertheless, many differences between the RAM and other classifications could be detected. This might be due to the necessity to form age groups of the subjects.

This study gives an important insight into the maturation of the spine itself, showing interesting differences between the sexes and different anatomical areas. The area of the spine in which most common types of idiopathic scoliosis develop appears to mature later than the rest of the spine. Sharpey's fibers insert into the ring apophysis and thus anchor the intervertebral disc to the two adjacent vertebrae [19]. As it is a weak point, this ossification and fusion process might have important implications for the mechanical stability of the disc–vertebral body complex of the mid-thoracic and thoraco-lumbar sections at a time when spinal loading increases rapidly due to the growth spurt [20,21]. This may be important for understanding the patho-mechanism of idiopathic scoliosis. Furthermore, around the PHV females appear to have less matured rings if compared to males at the PHV. As most adolescent spine deformities occur mainly in this period and females have a less-matured spine, this could partly explain why the onset of these deformities is more common in females.

This study used an existing CT database to analyze ossification and fusion of the ring apophysis, obviously, this cannot be used in clinical practice because of radiation hygiene [32]. We are presently working on the further development of bone-MRIs, a new radiation-free technique, which uses MRI to create synthetic CT images based on deep-learning processes [33,34]. Possibly, in the near future, it can also be applied to the scoliotic spine, providing a true spine-based assessment of spinal maturation per level of the spine in a patient group that often undergoes MRI scanning as a regular procedure.

5. Conclusions

This study describes the maturation of the ring apophysis as the attachment of the disc to the vertebral body on CT images and shows that they ossify and fuse later in the mid-thoracic and thoraco-lumbar spine. Furthermore, related to the timing of their growth spurt, the female spine appears to be less mature than the male spine.

Author Contributions: Conceptualization, R.M.C., L.C. and S.d.R.; methodology, R.M.C., T.P.C.S. and M.C.K.; software, P.S., L.C., L.K. and S.d.R.; validation, L.C., M.C.K., L.K., and P.S.; formal analysis, S.d.R., T.P.C.S. and L.C.; investigation, L.C., L.K. and T.P.C.S.; resources, L.C.; data curation, S.d.R. and L.C.; writing—original draft preparation, L.C.; writing—review and editing, L.C., M.C.K. and R.M.C.; visualization, L.C.; supervision, R.M.C., M.C.K. and T.P.C.S.; project administration, R.M.C., M.C.K. and T.P.C.S. All authors have read and agreed to the published version of the manuscript.

Funding: This research received funding from the EU's H2020 research and innovation program under the Marie S. Curie cofound RESCUE grant agreement No 801540.

Institutional Review Board Statement: For the current study, an existing CT scan research database from one tertiary children's hospital was used. The Institutional Review Board (IRB) approved an exemption for patient-informed consent for this retrospective cross-sectional comparative study (PROTOCOL CODE 19/642 AND DATE OF APPROVAL 8 October 2019).

Informed Consent Statement: As the authors used existing data, informed consent was not necessary.

Data Availability Statement: The data presented in this study are available on request from the corresponding author. The data are not publicly available due to ethical and privacy reasons.

Conflicts of Interest: The authors declare no conflict of interest. The funders had no role in the design of the study; in the collection, analyses, or interpretation of data; in the writing of the manuscript, or in the decision to publish the results.

References

1. Schlösser, T.P.; Shah, S.A.; Reichard, S.J.; Rogers, K.; Vincken, K.L.; Castelein, R.M. Differences in early sagittal plane alignment between thoracic and lumbar adolescent idiopathic scoliosis. *Spine J.* **2014**, *14*, 282–290. [CrossRef]

2. Will, R.E.; Stokes, I.; Qiu, X.; Walker, M.R.; Sanders, J.O. Cobb Angle Progression in Adolescent Scoliosis Begins at the Intervertebral Disc. *Spine* **2009**, *34*, 2782–2786. [CrossRef]
3. Grivas, T.B.; Vasiliadis, E.; Malakasis, M.; Mouzakis, V.; Segos, D. Intervertebral disc biomechanics in the pathogenesis of idiopathic scoliosis. *Stud. Health Technol. Inform.* **2006**, *123*, 80–83. [PubMed]
4. Castelein, R.M.; Pasha, S.; Cheng, J.C.; Dubousset, J. Idiopathic Scoliosis as a Rotatory Decompensation of the Spine. *J. Bone Miner. Res.* **2020**, *35*, 1850–1857. [CrossRef]
5. Risser, J.C. The Iliac Apophysis:An Invaluable Sign in the Management of Scoliosis. *Clin. Orthop. Relat. Res.* **1958**, *11*, 111–119.
6. Vira, S.; Husain, Q.; Jalai, C.; Paul, J.; Poorman, G.W.; Poorman, C.; Yoon, R.S.; Looze, C.; Lonner, B.; Passias, P.G. The Interobserver and Intraobserver Reliability of the Sanders Classification Versus the Risser Stage. *J. Pediatr. Orthop.* **2017**, *37*, e246–e249. [CrossRef] [PubMed]
7. Li, D.; Cui, J.J.; DeVries, S.; Nicholson, A.D.; Li, E.; Petit, L.; Kahan, J.B.; Sanders, J.O.; Liu, R.W.; Cooperman, D.R.; et al. Humeral Head Ossification Predicts Peak Height Velocity Timing and Percentage of Growth Remaining in Children. *J. Pediatr. Orthop.* **2018**, *38*, e546–e550. [CrossRef] [PubMed]
8. Sanders, J.O.; Khoury, J.G.; Kishan, S.; Browne, R.H.; Mooney, J.F.; Arnold, K.D.; McConnell, S.J.; Bauman, J.A.; Finegold, D. Predicting Scoliosis Progression from Skeletal Maturity: A Simplified Classification during Adolescence. *J. Bone Jt. Surg. Am. Vol.* **2008**, *90*, 540–553. [CrossRef]
9. Modi, H.N.; Modi, C.H.; Suh, S.W.; Yang, J.-H.; Hong, J.-Y. Correlation and comparison of Risser sign versus bone age determination (TW3) between children with and without scoliosis in Korean population. *J. Orthop. Surg. Res.* **2009**, *4*, 36. [CrossRef] [PubMed]
10. Noordeen, M.H.H.; Haddad, F.S.; Edgar, M.A.; Pringle, J. Spinal Growth and a Histologic Evaluation of the Risser Grade in Idiopathic Scoliosis. *Spine* **1999**, *24*, 535–538. [CrossRef]
11. Schlösser, T.P.; Vincken, K.L.; Attrach, H.; Kuijf, H.J.; Viergever, M.A.; Janssen, M.M.; Castelein, R.M. Quantitative analysis of the closure pattern of the neurocentral junction as related to preexistent rotation in the normal immature spine. *Spine J.* **2013**, *13*, 756–763. [CrossRef]
12. Skórzewska, A.; Grzymisławska, M.; Bruska, M.; Łupicka, J.; Woźniak, W. Ossification of the vertebral column in human foetuses: Histological and computed tomography studies. *Folia Morphol.* **2013**, *72*, 230–238. [CrossRef] [PubMed]
13. Woo, T.D.; Tony, G.; Charran, A.; Lalam, R.; Singh, J.; Tyrrell, P.N.M.; Cassar-Pullicino, V.N. Radiographic morphology of normal ring apophyses in the immature cervical spine. *Skelet. Radiol.* **2018**, *47*, 1221–1228. [CrossRef]
14. Taylor, J.R. Growth of human intervertebral discs and vertebral bodies. *J. Anat.* **1975**, *120*, 49–68. [PubMed]
15. Bernick, S.; Cailliet, R.; Levy, B. The Maturation and Aging of the Vertebrae of Marmosets. *Spine* **1980**, *5*, 519–524. [CrossRef] [PubMed]
16. Edelson, J.G.; Nathan, H. Stages in the Natural History of the Vertebral End-Plates. *Spine* **1988**, *13*, 21–26. [CrossRef] [PubMed]
17. Melrose, J.; Smith, S.M.; Little, C.; Moore, R.J.; Vernon-Roberts, B.; Fraser, R.D. Recent advances in annular pathobiology provide insights into rim-lesion mediated intervertebral disc degeneration and potential new approaches to annular repair strategies. *Eur. Spine J.* **2008**, *17*, 1131–1148. [CrossRef]
18. Zaoussis, A.L.; James, J.I.P. The iliac apophysis and the evolution of curves in scoliosis. *J. Bone Jt. Surg. Br. Vol.* **1958**, *40-B*, 442–453. [CrossRef] [PubMed]
19. Uys, A.; Bernitz, H.; Pretorius, S.; Steyn, M. Age estimation from anterior cervical vertebral ring apophysis ossification in South Africans. *Int. J. Leg. Med.* **2019**, *133*, 1935–1948. [CrossRef]
20. Makino, T.; Kaito, T.; Sakai, Y.; Kashii, M.; Yoshikawa, H. Asymmetrical ossification in the epiphyseal ring of patients with adolescent idiopathic scoliosis. *Bone Jt. J.* **2016**, *98*, 666–671. [CrossRef]
21. Cheng, J.; Castelein, R.M.; Chu, W.; Danielsson, A.J.; Dobbs, M.B.; Grivas, T.; Gurnett, C.; Luk, K.D.; Moreau, A.; Newton, P.O.; et al. Adolescent idiopathic scoliosis. *Nat. Rev. Dis. Prim.* **2015**, *1*, 15030. [CrossRef]
22. Dimeglio, A.; Bonnel, F.; Canavese, F. Normal Growth of the Spine and Thorax. *Eur. Spine J.* **2011**, 13–42. [CrossRef]
23. Takeuchi, T.; Abumi, K.; Shono, Y.; Oda, I.; Kaneda, K. Biomechanical Role of the Intervertebral Disc and Costovertebral Joint in Stability of the Thoracic Spine. *Spine* **1999**, *24*, 1414–1420. [CrossRef]
24. Waxenbaum, J.A.; Reddy, V.; Futterman, B.; Williams, C. Anatomy, Back, Intervertebral Discs. In *StatPearls [Internet]*; StatPearls Publishing: Treasure Island, FL, USA, 2021.
25. Gerver, W.; De Bruin, R. Growth velocity: A presentation of reference values in Dutch children. *Horm. Res.* **2003**, *60*, 181–184. [CrossRef] [PubMed]
26. Tanner, J.; Davies, P.S. Clinical longitudinal standards for height and height velocity for North American children. *J. Pediatr.* **1985**, *107*, 317–329. [CrossRef]
27. Choudhry, M.N.; Ahmad, Z.; Verma, R. Adolescent Idiopathic Scoliosis. *Open Orthop. J.* **2016**, *10*, 143–154. [CrossRef] [PubMed]
28. Sanders, J.O.; McConnell, S.J.; Margraf, S.A.; Browne, R.H.; Cooney, T.E.; Finegold, D.N. Maturity Assessment and Curve Progression in Girls with Idiopathic Scoliosis. *J. Bone Jt. Surg. Am. Vol.* **2007**, *89*, 64–73. [CrossRef]
29. Little, D.G.; Sussman, M.D. The Risser Sign. *J. Pediatr. Orthop.* **1994**, *14*, 569–575. [CrossRef] [PubMed]
30. Sanders, J.O.; Karbach, L.E.; Cai, X.; Gao, S.; Liu, R.W.; Cooperman, D.R. Height and Extremity-Length Prediction for Healthy Children Using Age-Based Versus Peak Height Velocity Timing-Based Multipliers. *J. Bone Jt. Surg. Am. Vol.* **2021**, *103*, 335–342. [CrossRef]

31. DiMeglio, A. Growth in Pediatric Orthopaedics. *J. Pediatr. Orthop.* **2001**, *21*, 549–555. [CrossRef]
32. Ron, E. Cancer risks from medical radiation. *Health Phys.* **2003**, *85*, 47–59. [CrossRef] [PubMed]
33. Florkow, M.C.; Zijlstra, F.; Willemsen, K.; Maspero, M.; Berg, C.A.T.V.D.; Kerkmeijer, L.G.W.; Castelein, R.M.; Weinans, H.; Viergever, M.A.; Van Stralen, M.; et al. Deep learning–based MR-to-CT synthesis: The influence of varying gradient echo–based MR images as input channels. *Magn. Reson. Med.* **2020**, *83*, 1429–1441. [CrossRef] [PubMed]
34. Edmondston, S.; Song, S.; Bricknell, R.; Davies, P.; Fersum, K.; Humphries, P.; Wickenden, D.; Singer, K. MRI evaluation of lumbar spine flexion and extension in asymptomatic individuals. *Man. Ther.* **2000**, *5*, 158–164. [CrossRef] [PubMed]

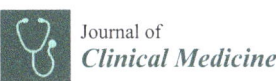

Article

The ISJ 3D Brace, a Providence Brace Evolution, as a Surgery Prevention Method in Idiopathic Scoliosis

Luis González Vicente [1], María Jiménez Barrios [2,*], Josefa González-Santos [2,*], Mirian Santamaría-Peláez [2], Raúl Soto-Cámara [2], Juan Mielgo-Ayuso [2], Diego Fernández-Lázaro [3,4] and Jerónimo J. González-Bernal [2]

1. Orthopedic Department, Institut Sant Joan SL, 08009 Barcelona, Spain; luisgonzalez555@hotmail.com
2. Department of Health Sciences, University of Burgos, 09001 Burgos, Spain; mspelaez@ubu.es (M.S.-P.); rscamara@ubu.es (R.S.-C.); jfmielgo@ubu.es (J.M.-A.); jejavier@ubu.es (J.J.G.-B.)
3. Department of Cellular Biology, Histology and Pharmacology, Faculty of Health Sciences, Campus of Soria, University of Valladolid, 42003 Soria, Spain; diego.fernandez_lazaro@uva.es
4. Neurobiology Research Group, Faculty of Medicine, University of Valladolid, 47002 Valladolid, Spain
* Correspondence: mariajb@ubu.es (M.J.B.); mjgonzalez@ubu.es (J.G.-S.)

Abstract: Background: The high incidence of idiopathic scoliosis worldwide as well as the serious health problems it can cause in adulthood, make it necessary to seek effective treatments to prevent the progression of the disease to more aggressive treatments such as surgery and improve patients' quality of life. The use of night braces, besides a less severe influence on the patient's quality of life, is effective in stopping the progression of the curve in idiopathic scoliosis. Methods: A longitudinal study was performed with an experimental population of 108 participants who attended orthotic treatment at the University Hospital of Barcelona, with ages between 4 and 15 years old, with a main curvature greater than 25 degrees and a Risser between 0 and 3. The participants received treatment with Providence ISJ-3D night braces until their pubertal change (mean duration of 2.78 years for males and 1.97 years for females). Results: The implementation of night-time orthotic treatment in children with idiopathic scoliosis is effective in slowing the progression of the curve and in the prevention of more aggressive treatments such as surgery, maintaining the patient's quality of life. Conclusions: The use of night braces is efficacious in the treatment of idiopathic scoliosis, although new studies including more sociodemographic data as well as curves from 20 degrees of progression are necessary.

Keywords: idiopathic scoliosis; nighttime orthotic treatment; surgery; quality of life

1. Introduction

Idiopathic scoliosis, with a worldwide incidence ranging from 0.47% to 5.2% [1], is the most common type of scoliosis in children and adolescents during their growth phase, without an apparent cause. It is defined as any deformity of the spine characterized by a lateral deviation greater than 10 degrees (Cobb angle) [2] combined with a spinal rotation and generally associated with a hypociphosis. Depending on the age of onset, it can be classified as infantile up to two years old, juvenile, between three and nine years old, and adolescent, from ten years old or higher [3–5].

Factors such as the patient's chronological and bone age, Risser's sign, and menarche have been linked to the patient's growth, and thus to the progression of scoliosis [6]. The Risser sign determines the skeletal maturity of the child, providing an estimate of how much skeletal growth remains, due to it classifies the progress of bone fusion of the iliac process. Risser degrees range from 0 to 5 where: 0 means no ossification, degree 1 up to 25% ossification, degree 2 between 26% and 50% ossification, degree 3 between 51% and 75% ossification, degree 4 between 76% and 100% ossification and degree 5 is related to the complete bone fusion of the process [6–9]. The severity of scoliosis is assessed by the Cobb angle or degrees of spinal curvature [7], so that if this angle exceeds the "critical threshold" (30°–50° at the end of the growth stage), there is a greater risk of health problems, decreased quality of life, aesthetic deformity, disability, pain and functional limitations in adulthood [6].

One of the most effective conservative techniques in the treatment of scoliosis is the use of a brace, which improves the patient's balance and stabilizes the curvature, preventing its progression, especially in the higher risk phases: Risser's sign of 0–1 or pre-menarchal phase in the female, and Risser's sign 3 in the male [10–13].

On the other hand, surgery is indicated in those cases in which the child or adolescent presents a structured primary curve with a Cobb angle greater than 45°, that is to say, unacceptable curves in an adult due to the effect they could have of different physiological functions [7,14].

With regard to orthopedic treatment, there are different types of braces depending on aspects such as the material they are made of, the time of use or the body region they cover. Regarding the time of use, a distinction is made between daytime braces (20–23 h) and nighttime braces (8–10 h), which are similarly effective in the treatment of scoliosis, the only difference being that nighttime braces have less impact on the quality of life and less psychosocial impact, which in practice translates into greater adherence to and better compliance with treatment [15–23].

The Providence brace is a night-time scoliosis correction system, designed and manufactured through a computer-assisted CAD-CAM system, which makes it easy to use and increases patient comfort [16,24]. The ISJ 3D brace, designed through the Rodin computer system, is an evolution of the Providence brace, which like that one, is based on the correction of deformities through compression forces at three or four points, improving the result of the treatment by avoiding the appearance of secondary curves. The brace is made through the CAD-CAM system starting from the lumbar point or 0 point, located between the iliac crest and the twelfth rib, applying a lateral-rotational pressure on the patient's spine. This system allows obtaining a personalized module for each patient, with a precise virtual correction for its subsequent manufacture [25].

The operation of this brace is based on the premise that scoliosis has a biomechanical mode of deformity progression based on the Hueterr Volkamann principle, whereby greater axial compression slows growth of the deformity and less axial compression accelerates growth [26].

The double curve design of the night brace produces a controlled application of opposite, direct, lateral and rotational forces on the trunk that leads to a push of the apexes of the curves towards the midline or more. In addition to these pressure points, it also has empty or hollow areas that allow to mantained the shell in continuity. The carbon fiber reinforced braces included in this type of corset offer greater patient comfort because the empty areas space is reduced. On the other hand, this three-point system also helps to control double curves allowing the treatment of curves with apex at the height of T6 without the need for a neck extension [27].

Depending on the location of the curve, derotation occurs differently. The lumbar pad that the corset presents between the iliac crest and the twelfth rib performs the segmental derotation of the curve at the lumbar level [27]. Derotation of the thoracic part is facilitated by the position that the patient adopts in the supine or prone position on the bed, since his own weight is transferred in the form of pressure to the costovertebral joints producing a change in the curvature of the spine [28]. Derotation of this section of the device is achieved thanks to the CAD/CAM model whereby at first the thoracic section is separated from the lumbar section and then the thoracic portion is rotated a certain amount to realign with the lumbar section [27].

Given that there is no effective method for the detection of scoliosis progression and that the use of full time braces has been shown to have variable adherence as a consequence of the psychosocial wear and tear they produce, the present study has been designed with the objective of verifying the effectiveness of the ISJ 3D Night Brace, a Providence evolution, in the treatment of idiopathic scoliosis as a method of preventing surgery.

2. Materials and Methods

2.1. Design and Study Sample

A non-controlled clinical trial was designed with a single intervention group ($n = 108$), whose study population was made up of all patients of both sexes, aged between 4 and 15 years, who during the development of the study attended the Orthopedic Surgery and Traumatology Outpatient Service of the University Hospital (Barcelona, Spain), and who met the following inclusion criteria: they had been diagnosed with idiopathic scoliosis, had a main curvature greater than 25° (the upper limit of curvature included in the study is 47 degrees ($n = 1$), and three other users had 44 degrees), with a Risser's sign of 0 to 3, and had not previously received any surgical treatment. Cases of neuromuscular or congenital scoliosis (they usually do not tolerate the use of the corset and require other types of orthopedic measures), those presenting a Risser's sign of 4–5 or those who had already completed the bone growth stage were excluded.

2.2. Procedure

All of volunteers were invited to participate in the study, having to sign the informed consent if they accepted, thus respecting the confidentiality and anonymity of each participant, in accordance with the Organic Law 15/1999 on the protection of personal data, being assigned to each of them an ethical identification code of the San Joan de Deu Foundation.

After the general physical analysis, the spine was examined and the characteristics of the deformity were recorded, using a plummet to measure the imbalance of the trunk in relation to the pelvis [29].

A radiographic evaluation (one at the beginning, one with the corset in place, and then every 6 months, up to one year after the removal of the corset) was carried out using the Cobb method [30]. According to the International Scientific Society for Orthopedic and Rehabilitation Treatment of Scoliosis (SOSORT) a curve progression of less than 5° is considered a successful treatment [31]. Based on the topography elaborated by means of the structured light technique, the Posterior Trunk Symmetry Index (POTSI) and the Deformity in the Horizontal Plane Index (DHOPI) were determined [32].

After the initial assessment, CAD-CAM measurements were taken using the latest generation of digital scanners.

The evaluation was carried out at three timepoints: a first evaluation before starting the treatment, a second evaluation at the end of the treatment and a final evaluation one year after its completion. This evaluation consisted of the measurement according to the Cobb method of the different types of curves (PT, MT, TL/L), identification of the apex of each main curve, classification of the different curves according to Lenke, as well as the measurement of the Risser degree. In addition, at the end of the treatment, the CAVIDRA quality of life scale was administered to people with spinal deformity, in order to check how the use of the corset has influenced the patients' quality of life.

2.3. Outcome Measures

Through the results obtained from primary curvature as the main variable of the study, the participants who would require surgery were determined. The magnitude of this curve was established by Cobb angle measurements carried out by a group of specialists who followed a previously established protocol.

The magnitude of the curve was determined by measuring the Cobb angle, derived from an X-ray of the standing spine. The Cobb angle is the angle formed by a line drawn perpendicular to the top of the upper vertebrae of the scoliotic curve and a similar perpendicular line drawn along the bottom of the lower vertebrae [33]. The result obtained is a numerical value that allows both the comparison of the magnitude of each curve, and the comparison between each of them. A curve progression of 6 or more degrees would be considered treatment failure [31,34].

To carry out the evaluation, on the one hand, Lenke's classification was determined considering the pattern of the curve, specifying the limits and name of the scoliosis according to the segment involved, six curve types are distinguished in this system based on whether the Proximal Thoracic (PT), Main Thoracic (MT), and Thoracolumbar/Lumbar (TL/L) regions are major, minor structural, or nonstructural including: Type 1, MT; Type 2, Double Thoracic (DT); Type 3, Double Major (DM); Type 4, Triple Major (TM); Type 5, TL/L; Type 6, TL/L-MT.; On the other hand, taking into account the convexity of the main curve, it was possible to distinguish whether the curve was right or left, and finally, the degree of bone growth (Risser) was established [35].

2.4. Statistical Analysis

The total sample consisted of 108 patients (94 females and 14 males). The mean age of the participants at the beginning of the treatment was 10.14 for the boys (DS ± 2.77), and 11.17 for the girls (DS ± 2.28), 72.22% of the total were between 10 and 13 years old. To verify the relationship between the different variables analyzed, the data was analyzed using the Pearson Correlation. The means obtained at the different time points were compared through the Wilcoxon and Manova test. Statistical analysis was carried out with the IBM SPSS Statistics, Version 25.0 (IBM Corp, Armonk, NY, USA) using a value of 0.05 as the limit of statistical significance.

3. Results

First, data were obtained from a total of 326 cases, but after a purging process, those whose questionnaires were incomplete, that is, they lacked data in some of the evaluations, were discarded in order to obtain as faithful and clean a sample as possible.

A total of 108 participants received treatment with the ISJ-3D Night Brace, which they had to wear between 8 and 10 h a night (M = 9.25 h; SD ± 2.18) every day until reaching Risser 4 in the girls and Risser 5 in the boys, which would establish the end of the treatment. The average age at treatment completion was 13.73 years for boys (SD ± 1.19) and 13.74 years for girls (SD ± 1.21) except for one patient who completed treatment at 11 years because she underwent the change prematurely at age 9. The data at the beginning of the treatment were: mean height 144.96 (SD ±12.99), mean weight 41.69 (SD ±7.83), mean BMI 19.62 (SD ±1.45). The Cobb angle of the main curve was M = 2932 SD ± 539 at pretest, and M = 3200, SD = 1307 at the end of treatment. The duration of treatment with the brace has been 2.78 years for boys (SD ± 1.85) and 1.97 years for girls (SD ± 1.19). The follow-up time was one year after the end of the treatment. The adherence of the brace was mesured by an Orthotimer, an electronic wearing time system that thoroughly documents the wearing time of the device. Each brace has a built-in a small sensor with a unique individual ID number and can be automatically connected to the patients registered in the database. This sensor is controlled with a wireless reading device which is connected with the computer via a USB plug and the saved wearing time dates are transferred to the software. The wear time is presented in various charts. A total wear time overview or an individually selected range extracted from the entire monitoring period of time can be observed [18,24,36].

The descriptive statistics for topographic and radiographic variables of initial assessment 1 and final assessment 2 are summarized in Table 1.

The values obtained in the different types of curves (PT, MT, TL/L) before and after treatment with the night brace are summarized in Table 2.

When the pre-test values were compared with the post-test values of the degrees of the different types of curves at the beginning and end of the treatment, statistically significant differences were observed in the PT (Z = 3.42; $p = 0.001$), MT (Z = 3.47; $p = 0.001$) and TL/L (Z = 2.26; $p = 0.024$) curves, in such a way that the degrees of all the curves have increased, although in no case reaching 6 degrees. When checking the percentage of users who improved, meaning that the degrees at the end of the treatment are lower than at the beginning of the treatment, the proximal dorsal curves are the ones that improved the most with this orthopedic treatment, obtaining an improvement in 40% of the cases (43 of 108 patients). The MT curves were the ones that improved the least after the treatment, with a greater improvement observed in 29% of the cases (31 of 108 patients). With respect to the lumbar curves after finishing the treatment, 33% (38 of 108 patients) of the participants improved.

Table 1. Descriptive statistics (initial assessment 1-final assessment 2) for topographic and radiographic variables.

	Evaluation	M	SD
ATR thoracic hump	1	5.22	3.51
	2	5.67	4.22
ATR lumbar hump	1	4.65	2.57
	2	5.01	3.55
Main cobb	1	29.32	5.39
	2	32.00	13.07
Vertebral rotation	1	8.53	5.22
	2	8.90	5.36
Thoracic kyphosis angle	1	27.48	7.31
	2	27.66	7.66
Lumbar lordosis angle	1	45.21	7.75
	2	46.89	8.61
DIHP	1	6.22	1.33
	2	6.86	1.61
PTSI	1	20.01	8.63
	2	20.91	8.88
CP	1	40.33	8.05
	2	41.05	8.17

ART = angle of rotation of the trunk; Cobb princ. = Cobb angle of the main curve of scoliosis; Rot. apex = angle of rotation of the apical vertebra of the main curve of scoliosis. DIHP = deformity index in the horizontal plane; CP = columnar profile; PTSI = posterior trunk symmetry index.

Table 2. Values and comparison of the degrees of each type of curve, before and after performing brace intervention (Mean = 2.07 years, SD = 1.3).

	Pre-Intervention		Post-Intervention		Student's T	p-Value
	M	SD	M	SD		
(PT)	12.12	8.13	15.44	10.60	3.58	0.001
(MT)	27.26	7.19	32.48	15.56	3.84	0.000
(TL/L)	21.85	8.26	25.36	12.66	2.73	0.008

PT = Proximal Thoracic; MT = Main Thoracic; TL = Thoracolumbar; L = Lumbar; M: mean; SD: standard deviation; p-value < 0.05.

All the curves (PT, MT, TL/L) evolved less than 6 degrees ($1.59 < \bar{x} < 5.53$), with no significant differences according to the type of curve ($p = 0.95$), that is, the orthotic treatment is equally effective on the PT, MT and TL/L curves. In the same way, the results indicated statistically significant changes ($p = 0.000$) in the evaluation carried out one year after finishing the treatment in relation to the evaluation made at the beginning of the treatment, in such a way that the main curve increased until reaching 36.11 degrees of average (SD ± 14.33) against 29.72 (SD ± 5.45) obtained at the end of the treatment. With respect to the overall curve, 28% showed an improvement of 5°. On the other hand, the ANCOVA according to the type of Lenke indicated that there were no significant differences, between the post-test and the pre-test ($F_{(5, 101)} = 0.34$, $p = 0.883$). It is observed that Lenke type 5 that reduces the degrees, and Lenke type 1, are the types that best respond to treatment (Table 3).

Table 3. Ancova test, differential score between the post-test and the pre-test (2-1), Lenke clasification.

LENKE Type	Mean	Std. Deviation	N
1	1.34	6.99	29
2	2.90	326	11
3	6.28	15.65	21
4	5.69	8.66	23
5	−0.25	6.48	12
6	5.58	14.39	12
Total	3.68	10.32	108

$p = 0.883$.

The descriptive results showed that the MT curves increased in Risser 0 and 1 and decreased in Risser 2 and 3, in the same way as occurred with the TL/L curves (Table 4).

Table 4. Differential score between the post-test and the pre-test (2-1), on the main curve.

Risser	Mean	Std. Deviation	N
0	4.40	11.25	82
1	2.86	6.25	15
2	0.00	6.52	8
3	−2.00	4.35	3
Total	3.68	10.32	108

13% of the participants who received the night brace treatment required surgery. Of all of them, 50% correspond to juvenile scoliosis and the other 50% to adolescent scoliosis, with the average age of treatment initiation being 10–50 years. Of the 14 patients who needed surgery, 11 were women and three were men. It is important to highlight the similarity between the 14 surgical curves, since 13 of them were double curves, right dorsal, left lumbar and one of them right dorsal-lumbar. In all of them, the predominant surgical curve was the right dorsal thoracic curve (Figure 1).

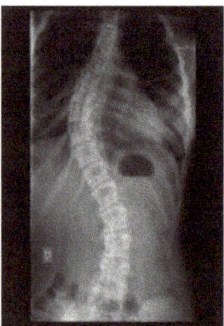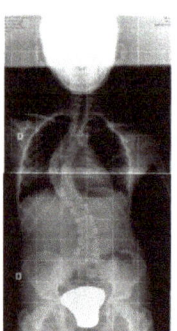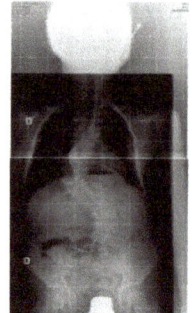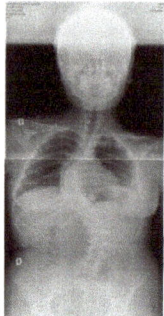

Figure 1. *Cont.*

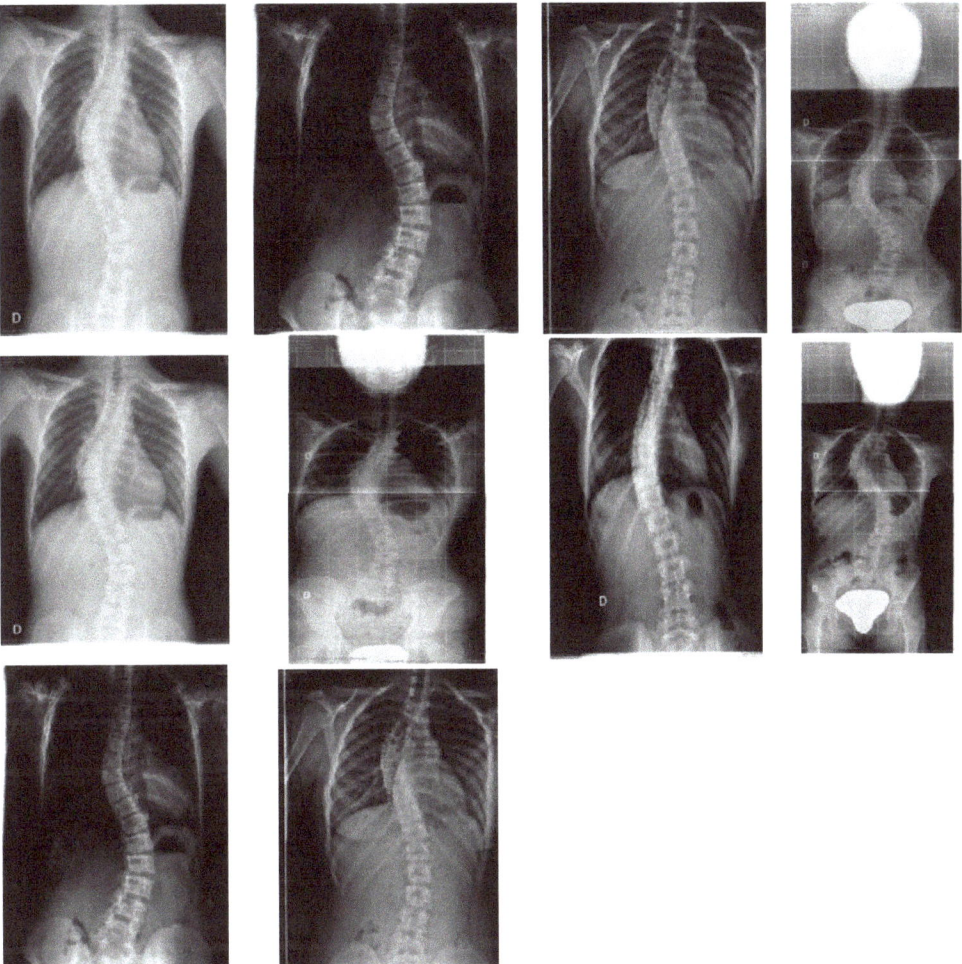

Figure 1. X-ray of the 14 participants who required surgery.

With respect to the secondary measures, the Quality of life in Spinal Deformities (CAVIDRA) or Quality of Life Profile for Spinal Deformities (QLPSD), developed in Spain by Climent in 1995, was used to measure the quality of life in patients with spinal deformities at growth age. It is a self-administered questionnaire consisting of a total of 21 items distributed in five dimensions: psychosocial functioning, sleep disorders, back pain, body image and spinal mobility. The patient shows his or her agreement or disagreement degree on a five-grade on a Likert type scale, being able to obtain a total score between 21 and 105, where a higher score means a greater impact on the quality of life. The reliability obtained from the scale for this study was 0.910 [37,38].

The results of the evaluation of the quality of life according to the Cavidra scale showed that the incidence of the ISJ-3D corset evolution of the Providence brace on the patients' quality of life is very low, since a mean score of 1.42 over 5 has been obtained (SD ± 0.42). In the same way, the domains of the scale in an unidividualized way presented little repercussion on the quality of life, being the highest incidence in the domain of body image with a mean of 1.81 (SD ± 0.84) and the lowest in the psychosocial functioning with a mean of 1.23 (SD ± 0.27). On the other hand, no statistically significant differences ($p = 0.00$)

were observed in the results of the Cavidra in relation to the degrees of the main curve measured in the three temporalis moments (beginning, end and at the year of treatment). In the results obtained, a significant correlation was observed between the degrees of the main curve and the scores of the different dimensions and the totals of the Cavidra scale ($p = 0.001$), in such a way that higher grades are related to higher scores in the scale, which means a worse quality of life (Table 5).

Table 5. Values of Pearson's correlation between degrees of main curve and Cavidra scale values.

	Main Curve		
	Pearson's Correlation	p-Value	N
Cavidra total	0.95	0.001	108
Psychosocial functioning	0.78	0.001	108
Sleep disorder	0.87	0.001	108
Back pain	0.74	0.001	108
Body image	0.88	0.001	108
Mobility	0.83	0.001	108

p-value < 0.05.

Table 6 presents the quality of life scores according to the Lenke classification, it is observed that the lowest scores correspond to type 1 (1.20, SD = 0.20) and type 5 (M = 1.24, SD = 0.45), which they are the groups that improve the most. The differences are significant, $F_{(5, 102)} = 5.28, p = 0.001$.

Table 6. Anova, Outcome measures related to the CAVIDRA score (QLPSD) according to the type of curve in the Lenke classification.

Lenke	N	Mean	SD
1	29	1.20	0.20
2	11	1.36	0.34
3	21	1.47	0.44
4	23	1.61	0.45
5	12	1.24	0.45
6	12	1.73	0.44
Total	108	1.42	0.42

$p = 0.001$.

4. Discussion

The choice of treatment for idiopathic soliosis is mainly based on the size and location of the deformity. Different studies have shown the effectiveness of orthopaedic appliances in stopping curve progression and correcting it [39,40]. The prescription of the brace treatment is directed to patients with a curve between 24° and 40° still growing, curves less than 25° and progression from 5° to 10° in six months or patients with scoliosis between 20° and 25° with skeletal immaturity (Risser 0) [41].

In the study carried out in the United States and Canada, the effectiveness of the Boston-type thoracolumbosacral orthosis in the progression of idiopathic scoliosis was verified. A total of 242 patients participated in the trial, of which 60% received braces and 40% were only observed. The brace was prescribed for 18 h per day. The treatment failure rate was 25% with an average time of brace use of 12.1 ± 6.5 h per day. The study concluded that this type of device reduces the progression of the curves and a greater number of hours of corset use is associated with greater benefits [42].

According to these results, in other studies carried out to verify the effectiveness of Wilmington and Boston braces with a sample of 36 patients with a mean age of 12 years and a sample of 395 with a mean age of 13.2, respectively, concluded that the progression of the curve was reduced only in those participants who use the brace for more than 20 h per day [43,44].

In the same way, in the study conducted by Sanders et al., where the use of the brace was prescribed between 17 and 23 h per day in 126 patients with adolescent idiopathic scoliosis, the results obtained showed that this treatment can avoid surgery in patients provided that the treatment regimen is followed. However, only 31% of the participants wore the brace for 10 h or more and 17% for more than 14 h. Among the factors that can influence compliance with treatment, the discomfort of wearing it, the social problems it causes, and poor self-image stand out, with patients choosing to assume the risk of progression to surgery rather than wear an orthopedic appliance for that number of hours. Thus the weak evidence of the effectiveness of bracing can be explained in part by poor compliance with the brace use [44,45].

With respect to the efficacy of nighttime orthotic treatments, the study by Lee et al., verified the efficacy of the Charleston night brace for the treatment of idiopathic scoliosis in 95 patients aged 10–16 years with curves between 25 and 40 degrees and concluded that 84.2% of patients had 5 degrees or less progression of the curve, 15.8% had a progression of 6 or more degrees and only 7.8% progressed to surgery [46]. According to these results in the study carried out by Simony et al., which verified the effectiveness of treatment with the Providence night brace in curves between 20 and 42 degrees, concluded that it was effective in preventing the progression of the curve in 71 of 80 patients and only five participants were referred to surgery, making these results comparable to the full-time treatment with the Boston corset [24].

In a study by Yrjönen et al., the effectiveness of the full-time Boston-style corset and the Providence night-time corset was compared in a total of 72 patients. The average correction of prone positioning braces was 92% for the Providence night brace and 50% for the foot X-ray group and only one of the patients treated with the Providence device progressed to surgery, which is in agreement with the results obtained in the present study [16].

With respect to the psychosocial study of the present study, the results showed that the use of the night brace was effective in the treatment of the progression of the curve without influencing the patient's quality of life, unlike other full time orthopedic devices with which the same results are achieved in the progression of the curve only if the time of use prescribed is complied with, having a great influence on the patient's quality of life [11,16,36,47].

The results obtained in this research with the use of the ISJ-3D evolution of Providence night brace coincide with those obtained by other authors in which they demonstrate the same results as full-time Boston-type orthoses, but unlike these, night braces do not influence the patient's quality of life, which makes treatment adherence greater. In addition, due to the rotational component of the ISJ-3D night brace, it is able to achieve better scoliosis corrections than other night braces such as the Charleston that do not have this component [18,24,39,43,48,49].

The results obtained in the study by Bonilla et al., showed that the different evaluation instruments designed to evaluate the quality of life of patients with idiopathic scoliosis, such as the SRS-22r and CAVIDRA, present adequate psychometric properties with regard to the domain of perceived self-image [50]. However, according to the studies carried out by Rezaei et al. or Liu et al. other assessment instruments such as the Bad Sobernheim stress questionnaire (BSSQ) or the Braces Questionnaire (BrQ), are more specific for measuring the quality of life of patients with brace treatment in adolescent idiopathic scoliosis, present adequate reliability and validation psychometric properties and are excellent tools to measure this aspect [51,52].

The study's findings should be considered within the context of its strengths and limitations. Among its strengths is the collection of data from a homogeneous sample in terms of age, Risser degree and degrees of progression of the curve or its longitudinal design following up one year after the completion of treatment. With regard to the limitations of the study, the absence of a control group for observation or treatment with orthopedic apparatus on a full-time basis that would allow the results to be compared stands out, as well as the lack of data collection such as the body mass index, the socio-demographic state or the vertebral rotation. In addition, the CAVIDRA assessment was used to evaluate the quality of life because of its high reliability and its validation into Spanish however, it has not been specifically evaluated, validated or analyzed for this pathology. Nevertheless, this tool is not specific for patients who receiving conservative orthopedic treatment such as BRQ or BSSQ, which will be taken into account for future studies.

5. Conclusions

The fundamental idea of night braces is to reduce the negative effects of full brace use on the quality of life without worsening the end results of treatment. The results obtained with the ISJ-3D night brace, an evolution of the Providence night brace, showed the great effectiveness of this type of orthosis since only 13% of the participants required surgery and the average increase in the curves in no case exceeded 6 degrees, without affecting the patient's quality of life. The results also showed the same efficacy of the treatment regardless of which curve was predominant.

Taking into account these results and the scarce number of studies evaluating the efficacy of this type of orthosis, the development of new research on this subject is justified, with representative samples, with a Risser 0 and in curves between 20 and 40 degrees.

Author Contributions: Conceptualization, L.G.V. and D.F.-L.; methodology, R.S.-C. and J.J.G.-B.; sowtware D.F.-L., J.J.G.-B., and M.J.B.; validation J.M.-A., J.G.-S., J.J.G.-B. and L.G.V.; fomarl analysis, M.S.-P., D.F.-L., J.J.G.-B. and R.S.-C.; investigation, L.G.V., J.M.-A., and D.F.-L.; resources J.J.G.-B., J.G.-S. and L.G.V.; data curation, M.J.B., J.J.G.-B., R.S.-C. and M.S.-P.; writing—original draft preparation, M.J.B., D.F.-L., M.S.-P. and L.G.V.; writing—review and editing, J.J.G.-B.; R.S.-C. and J.G.-S.; visualization, L.G.V., D.F.-L. and J.M.-A.; supervision, J.J.G.-B.; J.G.-S., L.G.V. and M.J.B.; proyect administration, J.J.G.-B.; J.M.-A., D.F.-L. and L.G.V.; funding acquisition, J.J.G.-B. All authors have read and agreed to the published version of the manuscript.

Funding: This research received no external funding.

Institutional Review Board Statement: All subjects gave their informed consent for inclusion before they participated in the ISJ brace study. The study was conducted in accordance with the Declaration of Helsinki, and the protocol was approved by the San Joan de Deu Foundation (approval code: PIC-33-17).

Informed Consent Statement: Informed consent was obtained from all subjects involved in the study.

Data Availability Statement: The data that support the findings of this study are available from the corresponding author upon reasonable request.

Conflicts of Interest: The authors declare no conflict relevant to the content of this manuscript.

References

1. Lo, Y.F.; Huang, Y.C. Bracing in adolescent idiopathic scoliosis. *J. Nurs.* **2017**, *64*, 117–123. [CrossRef]
2. Cobb, J.R. Outline for the study os scoliosis. *Instr. Course Lect.* **1948**, *5*, 261–275.
3. Horne, J.P.; Flannery, R.; Usman, S. Adolescent Idiopathic Scoliosis: Diagnosis and Management. *Am. Fam. Physician* **2014**, *89*, 193–198.
4. Choudhry, M.N.; Ahmad, Z.; Verma, R. Adolescent Idiopathic Scoliosis. *Open Orthop. J.* **2016**, *10*, 143–154. [CrossRef]
5. Kuznia, A.L.; Hernandez, A.K.; Lee, L.U. Adolescent Idiopathic Scoliosis: Common Questions and Answers. *Am. Fam. Physician* **2020**, *101*, 19–23.
6. Ylikoski, M. Growth and progression of adolescent idiopathic scoliosis in girls. *J. Pediatr. Orthop.* **2005**, *14*, 320–324. [CrossRef]
7. Zhu, Z.; Xu, L.; Jiang, L.; Sun, X.; Qiao, J.; Qian, B.-P.; Mao, S.; Qiu, Y. Is Brace Treatment Appropriate for Adolescent Idiopathic Scoliosis Patients Refusing Surgery with Cobb Angle Between 40 and 50 Degrees. *Clin. Spine Surg.* **2017**, *30*, 85–89. [CrossRef]
8. Roach, J.W. Adolescent idiopathic scoliosis. *Orthop. Clin. North Am.* **1999**, *30*, 353–365. [CrossRef]
9. Hacquebord, J.H.; Leopold, S.S. In brief: The Risser Classification: A classic tool for the clinician trating Adolescent Idiopathic Scoliosis. *Clin. Orthop. Relat. Res.* **2012**, *470*, 2335–2338. [CrossRef]
10. Kotwicki, T.; Chowanska, J.; Kinel, E.; Czaprowski, D.; Janusz, P.; Tomaszewski, M. Optimal management of idiopathic scoliosis in adolescence. *Adolesc. Health Med. Ther.* **2013**, *4*, 59–73. [CrossRef]

11. Pham, V.M.; Herbaux, B.; Schill, A.; Thevenon, A. Evaluation of the Chêneau brace in adolescent idiopathic scoliosis. *Ann. Readapt. Med. Phys.* **2007**, *50*, 125–133. [CrossRef]
12. Negrini, S.; Aulisa, A.G.; Aulisa, L.; Circo, A.B.; De Mauroy, J.C.; Durmala, J.; Grivas, T.B.; Knott, P.; Kotwicki, T.; Maruyama, T.; et al. 2011 SOSORT guidelines: Orthopaedic and Rehabilitation treatment of idiopathic scoliosis during growth. *Scoliosis* **2012**, *7*, 3. [CrossRef]
13. Kwiatkowski, M.; Mnich, K.; Karpiński, M.; Domański, K.; Milewski, R.; Popko, J. Assessment of Idiopathic Scoliosis Patients' Satisfaction with Thoracolumbar Brace Treatment. *Ortop. Traumatol. Rehabil.* **2015**, *17*, 111–119. [CrossRef]
14. Dickson, J.; Mirkovic, S.; Noble, P.; Nalty, T.; Erwin, W. Results of operative treatment of Idiopathic Scoliosis in Adults. *J. Bone Jt. Surg.* **1998**, *77*, 513–523. [CrossRef]
15. Rożek, K.; Potaczek, T.; Zarzycka, M.; Lipik, E.; Jasiewicz, B. Effectiveness of Treatment of Idiopathic Scoliosis by SpineCor Dynamic Bracing with Special Physiotherapy Programme in SpineCor System. *Ortop. Traumatol. Rehabil.* **2016**, *18*, 425–434. [CrossRef]
16. Yrjönen, T.; Ylikoski, M.; Schlenzka, D.; Kinnunen, R.; Poussa, M. Effectiveness of the Providence nighttime bracing in adolescent idiopathic scoliosis: A comparative study of 36 female patients. *Eur. Spine J.* **2006**, *15*, 1139–1143. [CrossRef]
17. Miller, D.J.; Franzone, J.M.; Matsumoto, H.; Gomez, J.A.; Avendaño, J.; Hyman, J.E.; Roye, D.P., Jr.; Vitale, M.G. Electronic Monitoring Improves Brace-Wearing Compliance in Patients with Adolescent Idiopathic Scoliosis: A randomized clinical trial. *Spine* **2012**, *37*, 717–721. [CrossRef]
18. Rahman, T.; Sample, W.; Yorgova, P.; Neiss, G.; Rogers, K.; Shah, S.; Gabos, P.; Kritzer, D.; Bowen, J.R. Electronic monitoring of orthopedic brace compliance. *J. Child. Orthop.* **2015**, *9*, 365–369. [CrossRef]
19. Chalmers, E.; Lou, E.; Hill, D.; Zhao, H.V. An advanced compliance monitor for patients undergoing brace treatment for idiopathic scoliosis. *Med. Eng. Phys.* **2015**, *37*, 203–209. [CrossRef]
20. Lou, E.; Hill, D.; Hedden, D.; Mahood, J.; Moreau, M.; Raso, J. An objective measurement of brace usage for the treatment of adolescent idiopathic scoliosis. *Med. Eng. Phys.* **2011**, *33*, 290–294. [CrossRef]
21. Morton, A.; Riddle, R.; Buchanan, R.; Katz, D.; Birch, J. Accuracy in the prediction and estimation of adherence to bracewear before and during treatment of adolescent idiopathic scoliosis. *J. Pediatr. Orthop.* **2008**, *28*, 336–341. [CrossRef] [PubMed]
22. Helfenstein, A.; Lankes, M.; Öhlert, K.; Varoga, D.; Hahne, H.-J.; Ulrich, H.W.; Hassenpflug, J. The Objective Determination of Compliance in Treatment of Adolescent Idiopathic Scoliosis with Spinal Orthoses. *Spine* **2006**, *31*, 339–344. [CrossRef] [PubMed]
23. Nicholson, G.P.; Ferguson-Pell, M.W.; Smith, K.; Edgar, M.; Morley, T. The Objective Measurement of Spinal Orthosis Use for the Treatment of Adolescent Idiopathic Scoliosis. *Spine* **2003**, *28*, 2243–2250. [CrossRef] [PubMed]
24. Simony, A.; Beuschau, I.; Quisth, L.; Jespersen, S.M.; Carreon, L.Y.; Andersen, M.O. Providence nighttime bracing is effective in treatment for adolescent idiopathic scoliosis even in curves larger than 35°. *Eur. Spine J.* **2019**, *28*, 2020–2024. [CrossRef] [PubMed]
25. González Vicente, L. *El Corsé Nocturno ISJ 3D en el Tratamiento de las Escoliosis*; Tesis Ciencias de la Salud: Burgos, Spain, 2017. [CrossRef]
26. Stokes, I.A. Analysis and simulation of progressive adolescent scoliosis by biomechanical growth modulation. *Eur. Spine J.* **2007**, *16*, 1621–1628. [CrossRef]
27. Grivas, T.B.; Rodopoulos, G.I.; Bardakos, N.V. Night-time braces for treatment of Adolescent Idiopathic Scoliosis. *Disabil. Rehabil. Assist. Technol.* **2009**, *3*, 120–129. [CrossRef]
28. Grivas, T.B.; Rodopoulos, G.I.; Bardakos, N.V. Biomechanical and clinical perspectives on nighttime bracing for adolescent idiopathic scoliosis. *Stud. Health Technol. Inform.* **2008**, *135*, 279–290.
29. Zambudio Periago, R. *Prótesis, Ortesis y Ayudas Técnicas*, 1st ed.; Elsevier Masson: Issy-les-Moulineaux, France, 2009.
30. Langensiepen, S.; Semler, O.; Sobottke, R.; Fricke, O.; Franklin, J.; Schönau, E.; Eysel, P. Measuring procedures to determine the Cobb angle in idiopathic scoliosis: A systematic review. *Eur. Spine J.* **2013**, *22*, 2360–2371. [CrossRef]
31. Negrini, S.; Donzelli, S.; Aulisa, A.G.; Czaprowski, D.; Schreiber, S.; De Mauroy, J.C.; Diers, H.; Grivas, T.B.; Knott, P.; Kotwicki, T.; et al. 2016 SOSORT guidelines: Orthopaedic and rehabilitation treatment of idiopathic scoliosis during growth. *Scoliosis* **2018**, *13*, 3. [CrossRef]
32. Buendía, M.; Salvador, R.; Cibrián, R.; Laguia, M.; Sotoca, J.M. Determination of the object surface function by structured light: Application to the study of spinal deformities. *Phys. Med. Biol.* **1999**, *44*, 75–86. [CrossRef]
33. Reamy, B.V.; Slakey, J.B. Adolescent Idiopathic Scoliosis: Review and Current Concepts. *Am. Fam. Physician* **2001**, *64*, 111–117. [PubMed]
34. Negrini, S.; Negrini, F.; Fusco, C.; Zaina, F. Idiopathic scoliosis patients with curves more than 45 Cobb degrees refusing surgery can be effectively treated through bracing with curve improvements. *Spine J.* **2011**, *11*, 369–380. [CrossRef] [PubMed]
35. Lenke, L.G.; Edwards, C.C.; Bridwell, K.H. The Lenke classification of adolescent idiopathic scoliosis: How it organizes curve patterns as a template to perform selective fusions of the spine. *Spine* **2003**, *28*, 199–207. [CrossRef] [PubMed]
36. Takemitsu, M.; Bowen, J.R.; Rahman, T.; Glutting, J.J.; Scott, C.B. Compliance monitoring of brace treatment for patients with idiopathic scoliosis. *Spine* **2004**, *29*, 2070–2074. [CrossRef]
37. Schulte, T.L.; Thielsch, M.T.; Gosheger, G.; Boertz, P.; Terheyden, J.H.; Wetterkamp, M. German validation of the quality of life profile for spinal disorders (QLPSD). *Eur. Spine J.* **2018**, *27*, 83–92. [CrossRef] [PubMed]
38. Pham, V.M.; Houlliez, A.; Carpentier, A.; Herbaux, B.; Schill, A.; Thevenon, A. Determination of the influence of the Chêneau brace on the quality of life of adolescents with idiopathic scoliosis. *Ann. Readapt. Med. Phys.* **2008**, *51*, 3–15. [CrossRef]

39. Asher, M.A.; Burton, D.C. Adolescent idiopathic scoliosis: Natural history and long term treatment effects. *Scoliosis* **2006**, *1*, 2. [CrossRef]
40. Rowe, D.E.; Bernstein, S.M.; Riddick, M.F.; Adler, F.; Emans, J.B.; Gardner-Bonneau, D. A meta-analysis of the efficacy of non-operative treatments for idiopathic scoliosis. *J. Bone Jt. Surg. Am.* **1997**, *79*, 664–674. [CrossRef]
41. Landauer, F.; Wimmer, C.; Behensky, H. Estimating the final outcome of brace treatment for idiopathic thoracic scoliosis at 6-month follow-up. *Pediatr. Rehabil.* **2003**, *6*, 201–207. [CrossRef]
42. Weinstein, S.L.; Dolan, L.A.; Wright, J.G.; Dobbs, M.B. Effects of Bracing in Adolescents with Idiopathic Scoliosis. *N. Engl. J. Med.* **2013**, *369*, 1512–1521. [CrossRef]
43. Brox, J.I.; Lange, J.E.; Gunderson, R.B.; Steen, H. Good brace compliance reduced curve progression and surgical rates in patients with idiopathic scoliosis. *Eur. Spine J.* **2012**, *21*, 1957–1963. [CrossRef] [PubMed]
44. Rahman, T.; Bowen, J.R.; Takemitsu, M.; Scott, C. The Association Between Brace Compliance and Outcome for Patients With Idiopathic Scoliosis. *J. Pediatr. Orthop.* **2005**, *25*, 420–422. [CrossRef]
45. Sanders, J.O.; Newton, P.O.; Browne, R.H.; Katz, D.E.; Birch, J.G.; Herring, J.A. Bracing for idiopathic scoliosis: How many patients require treatment to prevent one surgery? *J. Bone Jt. Surg.* **2014**, *96*, 649–653. [CrossRef] [PubMed]
46. Lee, C.S.; Hwang, C.J.; Kim, D.-J.; Kim, J.H.; Kim, Y.-T.; Lee, M.Y.; Yoon, S.J.; Lee, D.-H. Effectiveness of the Charleston Night-time Bending Brace in the Treatment of Adolescent Idiopathic Scoliosis. *J. Pediatr. Orthop.* **2012**, *32*, 368–372. [CrossRef]
47. Sapountzi-Krepia, D.S.; Valavanis, J.; Panteleakis, G.P.; Zangana, D.T.; Vlachojiannis, P.C.; Sapkas, G.S. Perceptions of body image, happiness and satisfaction in adolescents wearing a Boston brace for scoliosis treatment. *J. Adv. Nurs.* **2001**, *35*, 683–690. [CrossRef]
48. De Giorgi, S.; Piazzolla, A.; Tafuri, S.; Borracci, C.; Martucci, A.; De Giorgi, G. Chêneau brace for adolescent idiopathic scoliosis: Long-term results. Can it prevent surgery? *Eur. Spine J.* **2013**, *22*, 815–822. [CrossRef]
49. Kaelin, A.J. Adolescent idiopathic scoliosis: Indications for bracing and conservative treatments. *Ann. Transl. Med.* **2020**, *8*. [CrossRef]
50. Bonilla Carrasco, M.I.; Solano Ruiz, M.C. Perceived self-image in adolescent idiopathic scoliosis: An integrative review of the literature. *Rev. Esc. Enferm. USP* **2014**, *48*, 748–757. [CrossRef]
51. Rezaei Montlagh, F.; Pezham, H.; Babaee, T.; Saeedi, H.; Hedayatu, Z.; Kamali, M. Persian adaptation of the Bad Sobernheim stress questionnaire for adolescent with idiopathic scoliosis. *Disabil. Rehabil.* **2020**, *42*, 562–566. [CrossRef]
52. Liu, S.; Zhou, G.; Xu, N.; Mai, S.; Wang, Q.; Zeng, L.; Du, C.; Du, Y.; Zeng, Y.; Yu, M.; et al. Translation and validation of the Chinese version of Brace Questionnaire (BrQ). *Transl. Pediatr.* **2021**, *1*, 598–603. [CrossRef]

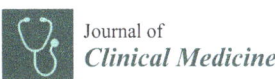

Article

Long-Term Influence of Paraspinal Muscle Quantity in Adolescent Idiopathic Scoliosis Following Deformity Correction by Posterior Approach

Hong Jin Kim [1,†], Jae Hyuk Yang [2,†], Dong-Gune Chang [1,*], Se-Il Suk [1], Seung Woo Suh [2], Yunjin Nam [2], Sang-Il Kim [3] and Kwang-Sup Song [4]

[1] Department of Orthopedic Surgery, Inje University Sanggye Paik Hospital, College of Medicine, Inje University, Seoul 01757, Korea; hongjin0925@naver.com (H.J.K.); seilsuk@unitel.co.kr (S.-I.S.)
[2] Department of Orthopedic Surgery, Korea University Guro Hospital, College of Medicine, Korea University, Seoul 08308, Korea; kuspine@naver.com (J.H.Y.); spine@korea.ac.kr (S.W.S.); nam.yunjin@gmail.com (Y.N.)
[3] Department of Orthopedic Surgery, College of Medicine, The Catholic University of Korea, Seoul 06591, Korea; sang1kim81@gmail.com
[4] Department of Orthopedic Surgery, Chung-Ang University Hospital, College of Medicine, Chung-Ang University, Seoul 06973, Korea; ksong70@cau.ac.kr
* Correspondence: dgchangmd@gmail.com; Tel.: +82-2-950-1284
† Hong Jin Kim and Jae Hyuk Yang equally contributed to this work, and should be considered as co-first author.

Abstract: Pedicle screw instrumentation (PSI) through posterior approach has been the mainstay of deformity correction for adolescent idiopathic scoliosis (AIS). However, changes in the quantity of paraspinal muscles after AIS surgery has remained largely unknown. The aim of this study was to investigate long-term follow-up changes in paraspinal muscle volume in AIS surgery via a posterior approach. Forty-two AIS patients who underwent deformity correction by posterior approach were analyzed through a longitudinal assessment of a cross-sectional area (CSA) in paraspinal muscles with a minimum five-year follow-up. The CSA were measured using axial computed tomography images at the level of the upper endplate L4 by manual tracing. The last follow-up CSA ratio of the psoas major muscle (124.5%) was significantly increased compared to the preoperative CSA ratio (122.0%) ($p < 0.005$). The last follow-up CSA ratio of the multifidus and erector spine muscles significantly decreased compared to the preoperative CSA ratio (all $p < 0.005$). The CSA ratio of the erector spine muscle was correlated with the CSA ratio of the psoas major (correlation coefficient = 0.546, $p < 0.001$). Therefore, minimizing the injury to the erector spine muscle is imperative to maintaining psoas major muscle development in AIS surgery by posterior approach.

Keywords: adolescent idiopathic scoliosis; paraspinal muscles; cross-sectional area; posterior approach; computed tomography

1. Introduction

Adolescent idiopathic scoliosis (AIS) comprises three-dimensional deformities of the spine, including structural, lateral, and rotated curvature, with unknown etiology, presenting at or around puberty [1]. From a radiological view, surgical management in AIS is indicated when the Cobb's angle >45° in the thoracolumbar or >50° in the thoracic curve preventing curve progression, achieving maximum permanent correction of the three-dimensional deformity, improve walking, in general functional aspects, and minimizing complications [1,2]. With the advent of the thoracic pedicle screw, pedicle screw instrumentation (PSI) has been widely applied to achieve three-dimensional correction and stable fixation in AIS [3].

Age-related structural change in paraspinal muscles has an important role for movement and stabilization of the spine [4,5]. Some studies suggest relationships between

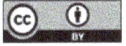

paraspinal muscles and global sagittal alignment in adult spinal deformity [6]. However, paraspinal muscle in AIS was observed in the asymmetric aspect in accordance with scoliotic curves. These curves showed a shortened muscle on the concave side and a lengthened muscle on the convex side of the curve [7,8]. Furthermore, asymmetric imbalances of the paraspinal muscles have been considered as contributing factors to scoliotic curve progression [9,10].

Although the impact on paraspinal muscle development in AIS has been studied in conservative treatment, there have been no reports of the long-term influence on paraspinal muscles in AIS following PSI with posterior approach [7,9]. Therefore, this study aimed to investigate long-term follow-up changes in paraspinal muscle volume for AIS following PSI with posterior approach.

2. Materials and Methods

This study was performed through a retrospective comparative analysis at a single institute where spinal deformity correction was performed routinely. The concept and procedures of the study were approved by our institutional review board. Informed consent was waived by the Institutional Review Board due to the retrospective design. The medical record data of 281 patients with AIS who underwent deformity correction using PSI by posterior approach were collected from 2002 to 2012. Among the 281 patients with AIS, the exclusion criteria of this study were (1) patients with non-idiopathic etiology (neuromuscular or congenital scoliosis), (2) patients with a history of revision surgery, (3) follow-up loss within 5 years, and (4) cases in which CT was not performed preoperatively or at last follow up. A total of 42 patients were included, and data from these patients were analyzed longitudinally.

All patients underwent posterior surgery using rod derotation (RD) and direct vertebral rotation (DVR) with PSI. Fusion levels were determined by Suk classification [3]. Pedicle screws were inserted segmentally on both sides of the lumbar curve, on the concave side, and in every other or every third vertebra on the convex side in the thoracic curve. A contoured rod to one-third exaggeration of the normal sagittal alignment was inserted into correction side and derotated 90° to transform scoliotic curve into thoracic kyphosis and/or lumbar lordosis. DVR was performed to correct rotational deformity after correcting the coronal and sagittal curves by RD [3]. All patients wore a thoracolumbosacral orthosis brace (TLSO) for three months after surgery without any specific rehabilitation.

All patient data were collected from the hospital database and retrospectively analyzed. Demographic and operative variables were gender, ages at surgery and at last follow-up, body mass index (BMI) at the time of surgery, Risser stage at the time of surgery, fused segments, thoracoplasty, and number of resected ribs. Radiological variables were coronal and sagittal spinopelvic parameters preoperatively, postoperatively, and at last follow up. Main curve and coronal balance were collected as coronal parameters and were measured by Cobb's angle. Sagittal vertical axis (SVA), thoracic kyphosis (TK), and lumbar lordosis (LL) were collected as radiological parameters.

The cross-sectional areas (CSAs) of individual paraspinal muscles (multifidus, erectus spine, and psoas major) and L4 vertebrae body (VB) were measured by assessment of axial CT images considering characteristics of motion segments and less affected vertebrae by deformity correction in included patients (Figure 1) [11]. The section from the upper endplate of the L4 vertebra was used. CSAs were measured bilaterally using the Picture Archiving and Communication Systems (PACS, INFINITT PACS, INFINITT Healthcare Company, Korea) to create a free line region of interest for each muscle. To minimize bias caused by individual relative body size and disk pathology, the CSA ratio was evaluated using the ratio of each muscle to VB (individual muscle CSA/L4 VB CSA), which was expressed as a percentage. The symmetry ratio of CSA between right and left paraspinal muscles was also evaluated. Measurement of the CSAs of the individual muscles and L4 vertebral body were carried out by two orthopedic surgeons to determine inter-examiner error. All parameters were measured 3 times with 2 week intervals to evaluate the intra-examiner reproducibility.

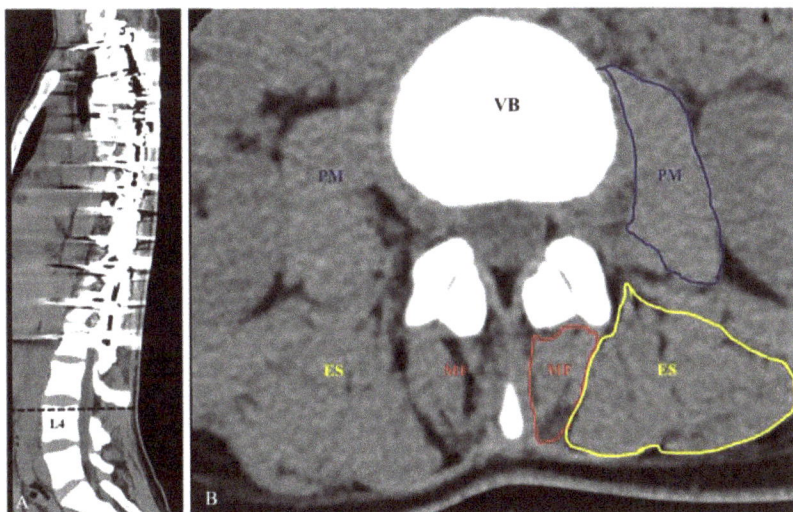

Figure 1. The cross-sectional areas (CSAs) of individual paraspinal muscles (multifidus (MF), erectus spine (ES), and psoas major (PM) muscles), and L4 vertebrae body (VB) were measured by assessment of axial computed tomography (CT) images. Measurements of the CSA of the paraspinal muscles were obtained at the level of the upper endplate of L4 by manual tracing (**A**,**B**).

Statistical analysis was performed using SPSS Statistics for Windows, version 21.0 (IBM Corp., Armonk, NY, USA). A normal distribution was confirmed by the Kolmogorov–Smirnov test. Regarding continuous variables, a Student's *t*-test (paired means) was used for parametric data. Longitudinal comparison of three groups used one-way repeated measures analysis of variance (ANOVA) and post hoc analysis used the Tukey honestly significant difference (HSD) test. Correlation of the CSA ratio with radiological parameters was analyzed using the Pearson correlation test. The intraclass coefficient (ICC) of individual CSA was measured to assess inter-examiner reliability with standardized agreement [12]. For variables having negative or positive values based on the measured reference point, such as coronal balance and SVA, statistical comparisons of groups required converting negative numbers to positive numbers because of the necessity to analyze differences from a reference point. Statistical significance was set at $p < 0.05$.

3. Results

3.1. Comparison of Patient Demographic Data

All demographic and operative data, including gender, age, body mass index (BMI), follow-up period, Risser stage at surgery, fused segments, thoracoplasty, and number of resected ribs are summarized in Table 1. A total of 42 patients (five males and 37 females) were enrolled in this study. The mean age at surgery and at last follow up was 14.6 years and 27.4 years, respectively, with a statistically significant difference ($p < 0.001$). The mean follow-up period was 9.9 years. For operative data, the mean number of fused segments was 11.1 and the mean number of resected ribs was 5.5 (Table 1).

Table 1. Demographic and operative data of this study.

Variables	Cases (n = 42)	p-Value
Gender (n (%))		
Male	5 (11.9%)	-
Female	37 (88.1%)	-
Age (years)		<0.001
At surgery	14.6 ± 2.4 *	
At last follow up	27.4 ± 3.6 *	
Follow-up period (years)	9.9 ± 2.4 *	-
BMI at surgery (kg/m^2)	18.1 ± 3.1 *	-
Risser stage at surgery	3.1 ± 0.9 *	-
Fused segments	11.1 ± 2.4 *	-
Thoracoplasty (Yes:No)	40:2	-
Number of resected ribs	5.5 ± 1.7 *	-

* All values are expressed as mean ± standard deviation. Significant differences were accepted for $p < 0.05$. N = number; M = male; F = female; BMI = body mass index.

The number of curve types by Suk's classification as follows: nineteen (45.2%) single thoracic curves, 10 (23.8%) double thoracic curves, 10 (23.8%) double major curves, and three (7.2%) thoracolumbar/lumbar curves.

3.2. Comparison of Radiological Parameters

Regarding parameters of radiological outcomes, the mean correction rate was 72.7% and the loss of correction was 1.3°. The mean values of CB and SVA were within normal limits preoperatively, postoperatively, and last-follow-up. Last follow-up TK (32.2°) was significantly higher than preoperative TK (25.3°) ($p < 0.001$). For post hoc analysis, there was no statistical significance between preoperative TK and postoperative TK ($p = 0.445$). Last follow-up LL (44.6°) was significantly higher than preoperative LL (37.3°) ($p < 0.001$). With post hoc analysis, there was no statistical significance between preoperative LL and postoperative LL ($p = 0.660$) (Table 2).

Table 2. Radiological parameters of this study.

Variables	Cases (n = 42)	p-Value
Coronal parameters		
Main curve		<0.001
Preoperative (°)	59.9 ± 15.1	* Pre vs. Post: <0.001
Postoperative (°)	16.4 ± 11.5	* Post vs. Last: 0.973
Last follow up (°)	15.7 ± 12.0	* Last vs. Pre: <0.001
Correction rate (%)	72.7 ± 12.6	
Loss of correction (°)	1.3 ± 16.4	
Coronal balance (mm)		<0.001
Preoperative	13.4 ± 8.3	* Pre vs. Post: 0.849
Postoperative	14.4 ± 10.9	* Post vs. Last: 0.005
Last follow up	8.3 ± 6.0	* Last vs. Pre: 0.024
Sagittal parameters		-
Sagittal vertical axis (mm)		0.319
Preoperative	18.2 ± 17.5	
Postoperative	22.1 ± 13.8	
Last follow up	18.1 ± 12.1	
Thoracic kyphosis (°)		<0.001
Preoperative	25.3 ± 10.2	* Pre vs. Post: 0.536
Postoperative	27.4 ± 6.7	* Post vs. Last: 0.002
Last follow up	32.2 ± 8.7	* Pre vs. Last: 0.001
Lumbar lordosis (°)		<0.001
Preoperative	37.3 ± 11.4	* Pre vs. Post: 0.660
Postoperative	39.5 ± 10.2	* Post vs. Last: 0.032
Last follow up	44.6 ± 12.6	* Last vs. Pre: 0.012

Data are presented as mean ± standard deviation values for each group. p-Values are calculated by one-way repeated measures ANOVA test. * Post hoc analysis was performed by the Tukey HSD test. Significant differences were accepted for $p < 0.05$. N = number; Pre = preoperative; Post = postoperative; Last = last follow up.

3.3. Comparison of CSAs of the Paraspinal Muscles

The mean last follow-up CSAs of the multifidus, erector spine, and psoas major were significantly higher than the corresponding preoperative CSAs (all p-values < 0.001). Last follow-up CSA of the L4 vertebra body was 1179.9 mm^2, which was significantly higher than the preoperative CSA of the L4 vertebra body (p < 0.001). The CSA ratio of the multifidus was 33.5% preoperatively and 30.4% at last follow up, a significant decrease (p = 0.001). The CSA ratio of the erector spine between preoperative and last follow up was 242.0% preoperatively and 235.0% at last follow up, a significant decrease (p < 0.001). Only the CSA ratio of the psoas major increased, from 122.0% to 124.5%, with statistical significance (p = 0.002) The symmetry ratio of multifidus was 1.3 preoperatively and 1.2 at last follow up (p = 0.209). The symmetry ratio of erector spine was 1.2 preoperatively and 1.1 at last follow up (p = 0.095). The symmetry ratio of psoas muscle was 1.2 preoperatively and 1.1 at last follow up, a significant improvement (p = 0.005) (Table 3) (Figure 2).

Table 3. Longitudinal comparison of paraspinal muscle cross-sectional areas between preoperative and last follow-up data.

Variables	Preoperative (n = 42)	Last Follow Up (n = 42)	p-Value
CSA (mm^2)			
Multifidus (mm^2)			
Right	173.9 ± 54.5	185.5 ± 61.1	0.001
Left	170.9 ± 76.1	170.4 ± 60.6	0.015
Mean	172.4 ± 59.3	177.9 ± 57.4	<0.001
Erector spine (mm^2)			
Right	1291.3 ± 280.6	1478.5 ± 343.1	0.001
Left	1229.1 ± 250.2	1261.5 ± 272.4	0.002
Mean	1260.2 ± 243.1	1370.0 ± 291.8	<0.001
Psoas major (mm^2)			
Right	609.3 ± 168.1	737.4 ± 197.2	<0.001
Left	656.4 ± 145.7	728.3 ± 201.2	0.001
Mean	632.8 ± 144.9	732.8 ± 193.3	<0.001
L4 vertebrae body (mm^2)	1046.3 ± 132.9	1179.9 ± 183.0	<0.001
Symmetry of CSA			
Multifidus	1.3 ± 0.3	1.2 ± 0.1	0.209
Erector spine	1.2 ± 0.1	1.1 ± 0.1	0.095
Psoas major	1.2 ± 0.2	1.1 ± 0.1	0.005
CSA ratio (%)			
Multifidus	33.5 ± 12.4	30.4 ± 10.1	0.001
Erector spine	242.0 ± 40.6	235.0 ± 41.0	<0.001
Psoas major	122.0 ± 26.6	124.5 ± 27.4	0.002

Data are presented as mean ± standard deviation values for each group. p-Values were calculated by paired t-tests. Significant differences were accepted for p < 0.05. Mean CSAs of paraspinal muscles were calculated as the average of right and left CSAs of paraspinal muscles. CSA ratios were evaluated as each muscle CSA to that of the L4 vertebra body expressed as a percentage. N = number; CSA = cross-sectional area.

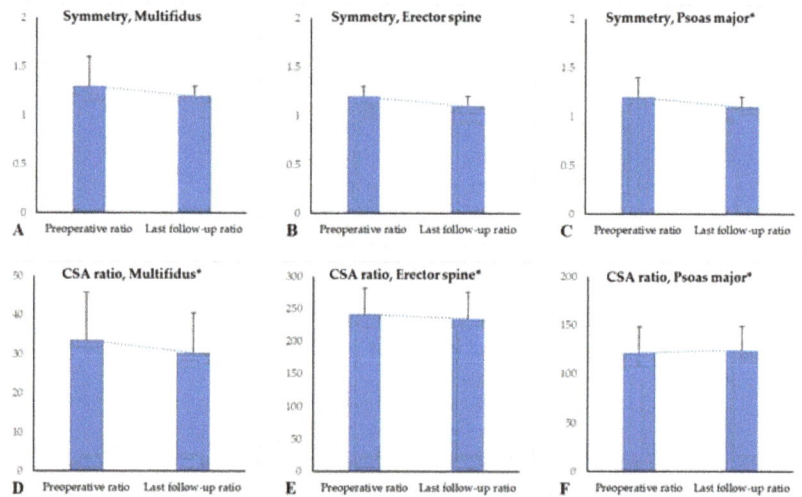

Figure 2. Symmetry difference between preoperative and last follow-up data. Symmetry was compared by ratio between large and small CSAs in the right and left paraspinal muscles. Only the symmetry of the psoas muscles showed statistical significance (**A–C**). The CSA ratio between preoperative and last follow-up data (**D–F**). Only the CSA ratio of the psoas muscle increased, from 122% to 124%, with statistical significance. * means statistical significance ($p < 0.05$).

3.4. Correlation Analysis for CSA Ratios of Paraspinal Muscles

Analysis of correlation was performed between the last follow-up CSA ratios of paraspinal muscles and between the last follow-up CSA ratios of paraspinal muscles and radiological parameters. Correlations between last follow-up CSA ratio of psoas major and erector spine were significant with a correlation coefficient of 0.546 ($p < 0.001$). Correlations between last follow-up CSA ratio of psoas major and coronal balance were significant with a correlation coefficient of 0.314 ($p = 0.043$) (Table 4).

All ICCs for the CSA ratio of multifidus, erector spine, and psoas major were greater than 0.75. Thus, all measurements of the CSA ratio showed excellent strength of agreement according to Fleiss guidelines (Table S1).

Table 4. Pearson's correlation analysis between last-follow-up paraspinal muscle and the measured parameters.

Parameters of CSA Ratio	Comparative Parameters	Correlation Coefficient	p-Value
Multifidus	Age	0.048	0.765
	Duration	0.193	0.221
	BMI	0.146	0.355
	Correction rate	−0.266	0.088
	Loss of correction	0.177	0.262
	CB (Last follow up)	0.023	0.886
	SVA (Last follow up)	0.046	0.770
	TK (Last follow up)	0.239	0.127
	LL (Last follow up)	0.081	0.611
Erector spine	Age	0.304	0.051
	Duration	0.179	0.257
	BMI	−0.280	0.073
	Correction rate	0.202	0.200
	Loss of correction	0.041	0.795
	CB (Last follow up)	0.160	0.312
	SVA (Last follow up)	−0.197	0.211
	TK (Last follow up)	0.281	0.072
	LL (Last follow up)	0.294	0.058
	Multifidus CSA ratio	0.039	0.808

Table 4. Cont.

Parameters of CSA Ratio	Comparative Parameters	Correlation Coefficient	p-Value
Psoas major	Age	0.095	0.549
	Duration	0.089	0.575
	BMI	−0.187	0.235
	Correction rate	0.268	0.087
	Loss of correction	0.029	0.855
	CB (Last follow up)	0.314	0.043
	SVA (Last follow up)	−0.127	0.423
	TK (Last follow up)	0.027	0.865
	LL (Last follow up)	0.035	0.827
	Multifidus CSA ratio	−0.116	0.465
	Erector spine CSA ratio	0.546	<0.001

Significant differences were accepted for $p < 0.05$. CSA = cross-sectional area; BMI = body mass index; CB = coronal balance; SVA = sagittal vertical axis; TK = thoracic kyphosis; LL = lumbar lordosis.

4. Discussion

Studies on the impact of paraspinal muscle quantity and quality on spinal diseases have been evaluated by CT and MRI [5,6,13]. The poor quantity and quality of paraspinal muscles resulted in degenerative lumbar kyphosis by quantitative analysis using CT [14–16]. However, there is no study of the changes in paraspinal muscles in the growth process after PSI by posterior approach in AIS. To the best of our knowledge, this is the first study investigating the long-term follow-up changes in paraspinal muscle volume in patients with AIS following deformity correction by posterior approach. Furthermore, our longitudinal study aimed to analyze the long-term follow-up changes in paraspinal muscles that are affected by injury during the growth process after deformity correction. AIS occurs more frequently in females and progress faster than in males. In our study, the enrolled patients were also mainly females.

Yeung et al. showed paraspinal muscle compositional change on the concave side by prolonged compression and reduced muscle activity in AIS, which illustrated that paraspinal muscle imbalances are associated with curve progression in AIS [10]. However, no studies have reported changes in paraspinal muscles after correction of scoliotic curve by surgery. In our study, correction rate and loss of correction showed no correlation with the CSA ratio of paraspinal muscles by Pearson's correlation analysis. Therefore, even if paraspinal muscle imbalances affect scoliotic curve progression, the degree of correction does not significantly affect the development of paraspinal muscles after deformity correction by posterior approach.

Even though PSI with posterior approach has been applied widely for AIS, surgery can lead to massive damage to the multifidus and erectus major muscles [2]. TK and LL were significantly increased to the normal range of an adult over the 9.9 year follow up of this study. From the post hoc analysis, last follow-up TK and LL significantly increased compared to preoperative values; this was thought to be the result of growth after deformity correction. Degeneration of the paraspinal muscles was related to sagittal imbalances in elderly groups [13,17]. Jun et al. illustrated that the quantity and quality of paraspinal muscles had greater influence on parameters of sagittal balance in elderly patients than in younger groups [6]. Our study showed that there were no correlations between paraspinal muscle and sagittal parameters in patients with AIS following deformity correction by posterior approach.

The psoas muscle of the deep back musculature plays a valuable role in the bolstering effect on the anterolateral aspect of the lumbar spine, stabilizing the spine in the upright position, and maintaining load-absorptive capacity [18]. Poor quantity and quality of the psoas muscle not only limit spinal movement, but also cause lower back pain [19]. In our study, the CSA ratios of paraspinal muscles significantly decreased during the 9.9 year follow-up period except for that of the psoas muscle. This was due to the fact of injury of the multifidus and erector spine muscles during deformity correction through posterior approach. The psoas muscle, as a deep muscle group, seems to have no significant restrictions on growth and development, because it is a less-damaged area during the deformity correction process. Furthermore, only the psoas muscle significantly improved for symmetry. It was also associated with deep muscle group, less-damaged area in deformity correction, and developed during growth process.

The role of the psoas muscle after PSI by posterior approach in AIS patients is important because of its effect on the load absorptive capacity. The psoas muscle strengthens adjacent spinal segments and reduces stress on the spinal fusion instrumentation segment [5,18,19]. For correlation analysis in our study, the CSA ratio of the psoas muscle correlated with that of the erector spine muscle. The degree of damage to the erector spine muscle could affect the development of the psoas muscle. Therefore, minimizing the injury to the erector spine muscle is imperative to maintaining psoas major muscle development after AIS surgery by posterior approach. Furthermore, last follow-up CB correlated with psoas muscle CSA ratio. In AIS patients, CB has a greater effect on the upright position than on sagittal parameters, which reflects the role of psoas muscle [9].

Minimal invasive scoliosis surgery (MISS) recently showed comparable radiological and clinical outcomes with fewer complications compared to conventional open scoliosis surgery [20,21]. The smaller incision in MISS has esthetic benefits in addition to preservation of paraspinal muscles [22,23]. Therefore, MISS could be an alternative procedure to COSS to preserve the paraspinal muscles. However, comparative studies of paraspinal muscle quantity between MISS and COSS are needed.

There were several limitations in our study. First, the number of patients was relatively small, and we utilized a retrospective design. Second, this study did not reflect the morphological quality of paraspinal muscles. Large multi-center comparative studies are needed to confirm our results. However, our study focused on paraspinal muscle quantity, which is associated with development of paraspinal muscles after deformity correction. Third, the evolution pattern of paraspinal muscle quantity could not be examined in this study because of radiation hazards by CT scan in especially young adolescents. Lastly, although various muscles can effect on growth process in AIS, this study only limited on paraspinal muscles by using spine CT. Further trials will be needed for influences of abdominal musculatures in AIS. Nonetheless, our study suggested that minimizing the injury to the erector spine muscle was important to maintain psoas major muscle development in AIS patients following deformity correction.

5. Conclusions

Minimizing the injury to the erector spine muscle is imperative to maintain psoas major muscle development in patients who underwent AIS surgery with posterior approach. A minimally invasive surgical technique with preservation of the erector spine muscle could be important for skeletally immature AIS patients.

Supplementary Materials: The following are available online at https://www.mdpi.com/article/10.3390/jcm10204790/s1, Table S1: Intra-examiner reproducibility and inter-examiner reliability by intraclass correlation coefficient.

Author Contributions: Conceptualization, H.J.K., J.H.Y. and D.-G.C.; methodology, H.J.K., J.H.Y., and S.W.S.; validation, H.J.K., J.H.Y., S.-I.K., K.-S.S. and Y.N.; investigation, H.J.K.; data curation, H.J.K.; writing—original draft preparation, H.J.K., J.H.Y. and D.-G.C.; writing—review and editing, H.J.K., J.H.Y., S.-I.S. and D.-G.C.; visualization, J.H.Y. and S.W.S.; supervision, D.-G.C.; project administration, D.-G.C. All authors have read and agreed to the published version of the manuscript.

Funding: This research was partially supported by KOREA UNITED PHARM.

Institutional Review Board Statement: The study was conducted according to the guidelines of the Declaration of Helsinki and approved by the Institutional Review Board of Inje University Sanggye Paik Hospital (IRB number: 2021-06-001).

Informed Consent Statement: Patient consent was waived due to the retrospective design.

Data Availability Statement: Data collected for this study, including individual patient data, will not be made available.

Conflicts of Interest: The authors declare no conflict of interest.

References

1. Weinstein, S.L.; Dolan, L.A.; Cheng, J.C.Y.; Danielsson, A.; Morcuende, J.A. Adolescent idiopathic scoliosis. *Lancet* **2008**, *371*, 1527–1537. [CrossRef]
2. Jada, A.; Mackel, C.E.; Hwang, S.W.; Samdani, A.F.; Stephen, J.H.; Bennett, J.T.; Baaj, A.A. Evaluation and management of adolescent idiopathic scoliosis: A review. *Neurosurg. Focus* **2017**, *43*, E2. [CrossRef]
3. Suk, S.I.; Kim, J.H.; Kim, S.S.; Lim, D.J. Pedicle screw instrumentation in adolescent idiopathic scoliosis (AIS). *Eur. Spine J.* **2012**, *21*, 13–22. [CrossRef]
4. Maki, T.; Oura, P.; Paananen, M.; Niinimaki, J.; Karppinen, J.; Junno, J.A. Longitudinal Analysis of Paraspinal Muscle Cross-Sectional Area During Early Adulthood—A 10-Year Follow-Up MRI Study. *Sci. Rep.* **2019**, *9*, 19497. [CrossRef] [PubMed]
5. Khan, A.B.; Weiss, E.H.; Khan, A.W.; Omeis, I.; Verla, T. Back Muscle Morphometry: Effects on Outcomes of Spine Surgery. *World Neurosurg.* **2017**, *103*, 174–179. [CrossRef] [PubMed]
6. Jun, H.S.; Kim, J.H.; Ahn, J.H.; Chang, I.B.; Song, J.H.; Kim, T.H.; Park, M.S.; Chan Kim, Y.; Kim, S.W.; Oh, J.K.; et al. The Effect of Lumbar Spinal Muscle on Spinal Sagittal Alignment: Evaluating Muscle Quantity and Quality. *Neurosurgery* **2016**, *79*, 847–855. [CrossRef] [PubMed]
7. Ohashi, M.; Watanabe, K.; Hirano, T.; Hasegawa, K.; Katsumi, K.; Shoji, H.; Mizouchi, T.; Endo, N. Long-term Impacts of Brace Treatment for Adolescent Idiopathic Scoliosis on Body Composition, Paraspinal Muscle Morphology, and Bone Mineral Density. *Spine* **2019**, *44*, E1075–E1082. [CrossRef]
8. Zapata, K.A.; Wang-Price, S.S.; Sucato, D.J.; Dempsey-Robertson, M. Ultrasonographic measurements of paraspinal muscle thickness in adolescent idiopathic scoliosis: A comparison and reliability study. *Pediatr. Phys.* **2015**, *27*, 119–125. [CrossRef] [PubMed]
9. Watanabe, K.; Ohashi, M.; Hirano, T.; Katsumi, K.; Shoji, H.; Mizouchi, T.; Endo, N.; Hasegawa, K. The Influence of Lumbar Muscle Volume on Curve Progression after Skeletal Maturity in Patients with Adolescent Idiopathic Scoliosis: A Long-Term Follow-up Study. *Spine Deform.* **2018**, *6*, 691–698. [CrossRef]
10. Yeung, K.H.; Man, G.C.W.; Shi, L.; Hui, S.C.N.; Chiyanika, C.; Lam, T.P.; Ng, B.K.W.; Cheng, J.C.Y.; Chu, W.C.W. Magnetic Resonance Imaging-Based Morphological Change of Paraspinal Muscles in Girls with Adolescent Idiopathic Scoliosis. *Spine* **2019**, *44*, 1356–1363. [CrossRef] [PubMed]
11. Hyun, S.J.; Bae, C.W.; Lee, S.H.; Rhim, S.C. Fatty Degeneration of the Paraspinal Muscle in Patients With Degenerative Lumbar Kyphosis: A New Evaluation Method of Quantitative Digital Analysis Using MRI and CT Scan. *Clin. Spine Surg.* **2016**, *29*, 441–447. [CrossRef]
12. Dang, N.R.; Moreau, M.J.; Hill, D.L.; Mahood, J.K.; Raso, J. Intra-observer reproducibility and interobserver reliability of the radiographic parameters in the Spinal Deformity Study Group's AIS Radiographic Measurement Manual. *Spine* **2005**, *30*, 1064–1069. [CrossRef] [PubMed]
13. Hiyama, A.; Katoh, H.; Sakai, D.; Tanaka, M.; Sato, M.; Watanabe, M. The correlation analysis between sagittal alignment and cross-sectional area of paraspinal muscle in patients with lumbar spinal stenosis and degenerative spondylolisthesis. *BMC Musculoskelet Disord* **2019**, *20*, 352. [CrossRef] [PubMed]
14. Kim, H.J.; Yang, J.H.; Chang, D.G.; Suk, S.I.; Suh, S.W.; Kim, S.I.; Song, K.S.; Park, J.B.; Cho, W. Proximal Junctional Kyphosis in Adult Spinal Deformity: Definition, Classification, Risk Factors, and Prevention Strategies. *Asian Spine J.* **2021**, in press. [CrossRef]
15. Kim, H.J.; Yang, J.H.; Chang, D.G.; Suk, S.I.; Suh, S.W.; Song, K.S.; Park, J.B.; Cho, W. Adult Spinal Deformity: Current Concepts and Decision-Making Strategies for Management. *Asian Spine J.* **2020**, *14*, 886–897. [CrossRef]
16. Danneels, L.A.; Vanderstraeten, G.G.; Cambier, D.C.; Witvrouw, E.E.; De Cuyper, H.J. CT imaging of trunk muscles in chronic low back pain patients and healthy control subjects. *Eur. Spine J.* **2000**, *9*, 266–272. [CrossRef]
17. Tamai, K.; Chen, J.; Stone, M.; Arakelyan, A.; Paholpak, P.; Nakamura, H.; Buser, Z.; Wang, J.C. The evaluation of lumbar paraspinal muscle quantity and quality using the Goutallier classification and lumbar indentation value. *Eur. Spine J.* **2018**, *27*, 1005–1012. [CrossRef]
18. Penning, L. Psoas muscle and lumbar spine stability: A concept uniting existing controversies. Critical review and hypothesis. *Eur. Spine J.* **2000**, *9*, 577–585. [CrossRef]
19. Verla, T.; Adogwa, O.; Elsamadicy, A.; Moreno, J.R.; Farber, H.; Cheng, J.; Bagley, C.A. Effects of Psoas Muscle Thickness on Outcomes of Lumbar Fusion Surgery. *World Neurosurg.* **2016**, *87*, 283–289. [CrossRef]
20. Yang, J.H.; Kim, H.J.; Chang, D.G.; Suh, S.W. Comparative Analysis of Radiologic and Clinical Outcomes between Conventional Open and Minimally Invasive Scoliosis Surgery for Adolescent Idiopathic Scoliosis. *World Neurosurg.* **2021**, *151*, e234–e240. [CrossRef]
21. Yang, J.H.; Kim, H.J.; Chang, D.G.; Suh, S.W. Minimally invasive scoliosis surgery for adolescent idiopathic scoliosis using posterior mini-open technique. *J. Clin. Neurosci.* **2021**, *89*, 199–205. [CrossRef]

22. Yang, J.H.; Chang, D.G.; Suh, S.W.; Damani, N.; Lee, H.N.; Lim, J.; Mun, F. Safety and effectiveness of minimally invasive scoliosis surgery for adolescent idiopathic scoliosis: A retrospective case series of 84 patients. *Eur. Spine J.* **2020**, *29*, 761–769. [CrossRef] [PubMed]
23. Neradi, D.; Kumar, V.; Kumar, S.; Sodavarapu, P.; Goni, V.; Dhatt, S.S. Minimally Invasive Surgery versus Open Surgery for Adolescent Idiopathic Scoliosis: A Systematic Review and Meta-Analysis. *Asian Spin J.* **2021**, in press. [CrossRef] [PubMed]

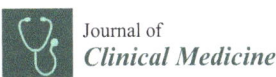

Article

The Measurement of Health-Related Quality of Life of Girls with Mild to Moderate Idiopathic Scoliosis—Comparison of ISYQOL versus SRS-22 Questionnaire

Edyta Kinel [1,*], Krzysztof Korbel [2], Mateusz Kozinoga [3], Dariusz Czaprowski [2,4], Łukasz Stępniak [3] and Tomasz Kotwicki [3]

1. Department of Rehabilitation, University of Medical Sciences in Poznan, 61-545 Poznan, Poland
2. Department of Physiotherapy, University of Medical Sciences in Poznan, 61-545 Poznan, Poland; kkorbel@ump.edu.pl (K.K.); dariusz.czaprowski@interia.pl (D.C.)
3. Department of Spine Disorders and Pediatric Orthopedics, University of Medical Sciences in Poznan, 61-545 Poznan, Poland; mkozinoga@hotmail.com (M.K.); lstepniak@ump.edu.pl (Ł.S.); kotwicki@ump.edu.pl (T.K.)
4. Department of Health Sciences, Olsztyn University, 10-243 Olsztyn, Poland
* Correspondence: ekinel@ump.edu.pl; Tel.: +48-61-831-0217

Abstract: This study aimed to compare the Italian Spine Youth Quality of Life Questionnaire (ISYQOL-PL) versus the Scoliosis Research Society-22 (SRS-22) questionnaire scores evaluating the validity of the concurrent and known-groups. Eighty-one girls (mean age 13.5 ± 1.8 years) with idiopathic scoliosis (IS) with a mean Cobb angle of 31.0 (±10.0) degrees were examined, all treated with a corrective TLSO brace for an average duration of 2.6 (±1.9) years. The patients' scores were compared as follows: (1) age: ≤13 years vs. >13 years); (2) scoliosis severity: mild (Cobb angle 10–30°) vs. moderate (Cobb angle > 30°); (3) single curve pattern vs. double curve pattern. Lin's concordance correlation coefficient was used to evaluate the strength of the association between ISYQOL-PL and SRS-22 scores. *t*-tests were applied to assess if the ISYQOL-PL measure and SRS-22 total score were significantly different in the different groups of patients. The concurrent validity analysis showed a moderate correlation (Lin p_{ccc} = 0.47). The ISYQOL-PL showed a significantly better quality of life in mild than moderate scoliosis. The severity of scoliosis but not the age or the curve pattern demonstrated a direct statistically significant effect on patients' quality of life only when evaluated using the ISYQOL-PL.

Keywords: idiopathic scoliosis; health-related quality of life; Italian spine youth quality of life questionnaire; SRS-22

1. Introduction

Currently, specialists in various medical disciplines include assessing patients' health-related quality of life (HRQoL) into routine clinical practice. Considering the HRQoL, girls with idiopathic scoliosis (IS) due to visible deformation of the trunk and exposure to long-term stress related to disease and therapy seem to constitute a particular group [1,2]. Their treatment is complex, long-lasting, often occurs in a challenging period in adolescents' lives, and requires both patients' and parents'/legal guardians' approval [3]. The specificity of the 20/24 h brace treatment and its influence on aesthetics, school activities, and sports activities, such as cycling, can significantly affect IS girls' stress levels' perception [4–6]. In severe scoliosis, an additional stressor may be the fear of possible surgery. In patients after surgery, both mental and physical discomfort due to spinal fusion or a large scar can appear [7]. To summarize, the need to monitor the HRQoL of patients with IS is justified. It allows for, at the right moment, the decision of implementing appropriate psychological therapy to support the treatment. The HRQoL of patients with IS is studied with specific standardized questionnaires. Vasiliadis et al. [8] developed the

Brace Questionnaire (BrQ) for adolescents with IS treated by wearing a corrective brace. There are questionnaires that measure the level of stress induced by the deformity (Bad Sobernheim Stress Questionnaire Deformity, BSSQ—Deformity) and the stress caused by the treatment with a brace (Bad Sobernheim Stress Questionnaire Brace, BSSQ—Brace) for patients with IS [9]. The BSSQ questionnaires, however, do not evaluate the overall HRQoL. The Scoliosis Research Society-22 (SRS-22) questionnaire is the most commonly used [10–12]; however, new tools are being developed. The Italian Spine Youth Quality of Life (ISYQOL) questionnaire, translated and culturally validated into English, Spanish, and Polish (ISYQOL-PL), is the first questionnaire developed using Rasch analysis to measure the HRQoL in spine deformity during growth [13–17]. Rasch analysis is a statistical technique for evaluating questionnaires and developing questionnaires' ordinal scores into interval measures [13,14]. According to Caronni et al., Rasch analysis showed that the SRS-22 suffers poor metric properties, which prevents it from adequately measuring patients' quality of life [13]. Caronni et al. [14] demonstrated the superiority of the ISYQOL over the SRS-22 questionnaire in the Rasch analysis framework. The aim of this study was to compare the performance of the ISYQOL-PL versus the SRS-22 questionnaire (Polish version) to evaluate HRQoL in patients with IS. The comparison was carried out analyzing the concurrent and known-groups validity of both questionnaires. The a priori hypothesis was proposed as follows: The ISYQOL-PL questionnaire provides additional information compared to SRS-22 in evaluating HRQoL in IS girls undergoing conservative treatment.

The results of the present study led to the conclusion that ISYQOL-PL seems to offer advantageous capacities of analysis comparing to the SRS-22 when applied to adolescent girls undergoing non-surgical treatment for mild or moderate idiopathic scoliosis.

2. Materials and Methods

2.1. Study Population

The sample included eighty-one girls with IS diagnosis treated by the same specialist in orthopedics. The following criteria for inclusion were applied: (1) girls with diagnosed IS at the age of 10–18 years; (2) with a Cobb angle > 10°; (3) under brace treatment (TLSO, at least three months for at least 12h per day); (4) who completed both the ISYQOL-PL and the SRS-22 questionnaires. Exclusion criteria: (1) history of spine surgery; (2) combined spinal deformities (e.g., scoliosis plus spondylolisthesis); (3) history of relevant diseases, surgery, or trauma, including a positive neurologic examination.

All the invited girls with IS selected through the inclusion criteria participated in the study. Table 1 reports the participants' demographic and clinical data.

Table 1. Participants' demographic and clinical data.

Number of Participants	Gender	Mean Age (SD) Years	Mean Cobb Angle (SD) Degrees	Mean TLSO Brace Wear (SD) Years
81	females	13.5 (1.8)	31.0° (10.0)	2.6 (1.9)

SD—Standard deviation.

After a brief explanation about the aim of questionnaires, the participants were left to fill in the questionnaires alone, in a separate space, to minimize any influence from parents or medical staff. They completed both questionnaires before clinical evaluation.

The Institutional Review Board of Poznan University of Medical Sciences approved the study (5 November 2019).

Data from the ISYQOL-PL and SRS-22 were collected from March to May 2020.

Before inclusion in the study, the parents and the patients signed their informed consent.

2.2. Polish Version of the Italian Spine Youth Quality of Life (ISYQOL-PL) Questionnaire

The ISYQOL is a 20 items questionnaire. Each item is scored 0, 1, or 2. Items investigating the presence of spine-related problems (questions 1–4, 7–9, 11–12, and 14–20) are coded 0-1-2 ((0): never; (1): sometimes; (2): often). Conversely, questions 5, 6, 10, and 13, investigating positive reactions, are coded 2-1-0 ((2): never; (1): sometimes; (0): often). The questionnaire provides a total score, with lower scores representing a higher quality of life. The ordinal ISYQOL total score is subsequently converted to an interval measure, expressed on a 0–100% scale, where 100% indicates the highest quality of life. The ISYQOL questionnaire has two domains: Spine health (13 items) and Brace (7 items) specifically devoted to brace wearers. The Rasch method used in the analysis allows for comparing the ISYQOL result of non-brace wearers (who answer only 13 of the 20 items) with brace wearers (who complete the entire questionnaire). In the present study, only the brace wearer IS girls were included. The questionnaire is developmentally appropriate for ages 10–18 years and is designed to be self-administered [13,14]. The recently validated Polish language version (ISYQOL-PL) of the ISYQOL questionnaire was used in the study [13,17].

2.3. Polish Version of the Scoliosis Research Society-22 (SRS-22) Questionnaire

SRS-22 is the criterion standard for measuring the HRQoL in IS. The SRS-22 questionnaire was developed according to the classical test theory and, in this framework, presents satisfactory psychometric properties such as concurrent validity and reliability [11]. It includes 22 items scored on five ordinal categories: Intensity of Pain—5 items (items 1, 2, 8, 11, and 17); Self-image—5 items (items 4, 6, 10, 14, and 19); Function/activity—5 items (items 5, 9, 12, 15, and 18); Mental health—5 items (items 3, 7, 13, 16, and 20); Satisfaction from treatment—2 items (items 21 and 22). The scores for each answer range from 1–5 points. In each category, the recipient can score from 5–25 points, except for the satisfaction from the treatment category, where they can score from 2–10 points. The overall score can range from 22 to 110 points. A total score is obtained by adding individual item scores so that the higher the total score, the better the HRQoL [10–12]. A previously validated Polish version of the SRS-22 questionnaire was used in the study [18].

2.4. Statistical Analyses

Statistical analysis was applied and managed at various levels beginning with general descriptive statistics for the entire sample. Thus, when applicable, tests for normality were carried out (Shapiro–Wilk Test), followed by tests for homogeneity of variance (Fisher Test).

All statistical analyses were carried out using the Real Statistics Resource Pack software with a significance level of $\alpha < 0.05$ (Real Statistics Resource Pack software (Release 7.6). Copyright (2013–2021) Charles Zaiontz. www.real-statistics.com) accessed on 17 October 2021.

2.5. Known-Groups Validity

There could exist a variety of factors negatively affecting adolescents' HRQoL. We subdivided patients into different known-groups considering: perception at different ages, pathological severity, and curve pattern.

A measure has high known-groups validity (a type of construct validity) if it discriminates across groups of patients believed to be different on theoretical or clinical grounds [19].

For the known-groups' validity analysis, the patients' scores were compared as follows: (1) age: ≤ 13 years vs. >13 years; (2) scoliosis severity: mild (Cobb angle 10–30°) vs. moderate (Cobb angle > 30°); (3) single curve pattern vs. double curve pattern, Figure 1.

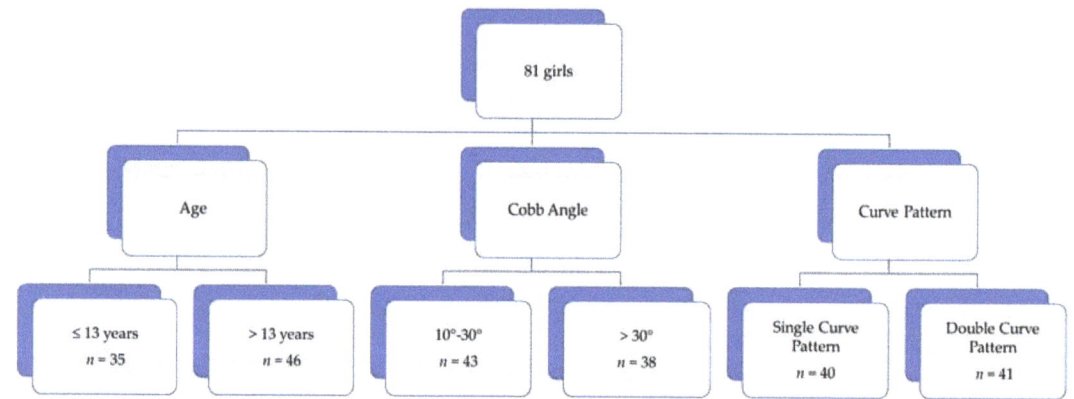

Figure 1. Patients' distribution according to age, Cobb angle, and curve pattern.

Depending on normality and homogeneity of variance conditions, parametric or non-parametric comparison tests (t-test, Mann–Whitney Test, Welch's Test) were applied to assess if the ISYQOL-PL measure and the SRS-22 total scores were significantly different in the different groups of patients.

2.6. Concurrent Validity

The concurrent validity of the ISYQOL-PL was checked using the SRS-22 questionnaire considered the standard measure criterion of HRQol in patients with IS. We used Lin's concordance correlation coefficient (CCC) as a measure of agreement, which, unlike the intraclass correlation (ICC), does not present the limitation of assuming a common mean for compared ratings at the outset, so it can be used to assess both the level of agreement and the level of disagreement [20,21]. In addition, to compare our results with the reference literature, the Spearman non-parametric correlation test was applied to evaluate the strength of the association between the two questionnaires.

2.7. Factors Influencing the HRQoL

Further investigation was carried out to study the influence on the HRQoL given by selected pairs of factors. Such an analysis was performed using a battery of two-way ANOVA tests ($\alpha = 5\%$) examining the following pairs of factors, respectively: (1) age and Cobb angle; (2) number of curves and Cobb angle; (3) years of treatment and Cobb angle.

3. Results

3.1. Known-Groups Validity

The data were revealed to be normally distributed in both questionnaires, as verified with Shapiro–Wilk test for normality. Therefore, parametric tests were used. The known-groups validity analysis was performed by applying an Independent Two-sample t-test. In addition, analysis with a non-parametric approach always confirmed the results obtained with a parametric one.

Both the ISYQOL-PL and the SRS-22 tools showed no difference (1) between the two age groups: ≤13 years vs. >13 years; and (2) between the groups of single vs. double curves. Conversely, the ISYQOL-PL was the only questionnaire showing significantly better HRQoL in mild than moderate scoliosis.

The values for the ISYQOL-PL and the SRS-22 questionnaires for (1) ≤13 years vs. >13 years, (2) Cobb angle 10–30° vs. Cobb angle > 30, and (3) single vs. double curves, are reported in Table 2.

Table 2. The known-groups validity analysis of the ISYQOL-PL and the SRS-22 questionnaires.

Questionnaire	Number of Participants	Mean of Score Points (%) (SD)	p-Value
ISYQOL-PL ≤13 years vs. >13 years	35 vs. 46	48.1% (6.6%) vs. 49.2% (7.8%)	NS
SRS-22 ≤13 years vs. >13 years	35 vs. 46	48.2% (4.3%) vs. 49.6% (5.3%)	NS
ISYQOL-PL Cobb angle 10–30° vs. Cobb angle > 30°	43 vs. 38	48.9 (7.4%) vs. 44.8% (8.1%)	0.019
SRS-22 Cobb angle 10–30° vs. Cobb angle > 30°	43 vs. 38	48.4% (4.6%) vs. 49.6% (5.4%)	NS
ISYQOL-PL single vs. double curves	41 vs. 40	46.9% (8.6%) vs. 47.0% (7.3%)	NS
SRS-22 single vs. double curves	41 vs. 40	48.1% (4.7%) vs. 49.9% (5.2%)	NS

SD—Standard deviation; NS—Not Statistically Significant.

3.2. Concurrent Validity

The agreement measured through the Lin's CCC (p_{ccc} = 0.47) demonstrated a moderate/low concordance. The Spearman correlation coefficient value rho = 0.53, showed a moderate correlation [22] between the two questionnaires.

3.3. Factors Influencing the HRQoL

As the data were normally distributed in both questionnaires, we used a two-way ANOVA test. Results confirmed no interactions between: (1) age and Cobb angle; (2) number of curves and Cobb angle; (3) years of treatment and Cobb angle; for the ISYQOL-PL questionnaire, while moderate (<30° Cobb) vs. severe (>30° Cobb) scoliosis is a statistically significant factor influencing HRQoL perception measured through ISYQOL. Conversely, the SRS-22 two-way ANOVA tests highlighted a significant interaction between age and Cobb angle. In particular, the combination of levels of these two factors inhibit each other's effects, showing a so-called "interference" [23], as shown in Table 3.

Table 3. Two-way ANOVA analysis to study the interaction of scoliosis severity level and age and years of treatment on patients' perceived HRQoL measured with the ISYQOL-PL and the SRS-22 questionnaires.

		Two Factor ANOVA (via Regression) ISYQOL-PL					Two Factor ANOVA (via Regression) SRS-22				
	ANOVA				Alpha	0.050	ANOVA			Alpha	0.050
Interaction Cobb Angle–Age		SS	df	MS	F	p-Value		SS	df	MS	F	p-Value
	Cobb Angle	342.875	1	342.875	5.578	0.021 *	Cobb Angle	39.554	1	39.554	1.674	0.200
	Age	0.007	1	0.007	0.000	0.992	Age	19.054	1	19.054	0.807	0.372
	Interaction	12.701	1	12.701	0.207	0.651	Interaction	110.054	1	110.054	4.658	0.034 *
	Within	4733.231	77	61.471			Within	1819.138	77	23.625		
	Total	5091.482	80	63.644			Total	1987.777	80	24.847		
Interaction Cobb Angle –Number of Curves	ANOVA				Alpha	0.050	ANOVA			Alpha	0.050
		SS	df	MS	F	p-Value		SS	df	MS	F	p-Value
	Cobb Angle	342.875	1	342.875	5.578	0.021 *	Cobb Angle	33.074	1	33.074	1.349	0.249
	Number of Curves	0.007	1	0.007	0.000	0.992	Number of Curves	69.984	1	69.984	2.855	0.095
	Interaction	12.701	1	12.701	0.207	0.651	Interaction	2.509	1	2.509	0.102	0.750
	Within	4733.231	77	61.471			Within	1887.346	77	24.511		
	Total	5091.482	80	63.644			Total	1987.777	80	24.847		

Table 3. *Cont.*

		Two Factor ANOVA (via Regression) ISYQOL-PL					Two Factor ANOVA (via Regression) SRS-22				
	ANOVA				Alpha	0.050	ANOVA			Alpha	0.050
		SS	df	MS	F	*p*-Value		SS	df	MS	F	*p*-Value
Interaction Cobb Angle–Years of Treatment	Cobb Angle	342.444	1	342.444	5.579	0.021 *	Cobb Angle	34.503	1	34.503	1.371	0.245
	Years of Treatment	18.904	1	18.904	0.308	0.581	Years of Treatment	13.359	1	13.359	0.531	0.468
	Interaction	0.446	1	0.446	0.007	0.932	Interaction	6.211	1	6.211	0.247	0.621
	Within	4726.246	77	61.380			Within	1937.882	77	25.167		
	Total	5091.482	80	63.644			Total	1987.777	80	24.847		

SS—sum of squares; F—statistic; df—degrees of freedom; MS—mean square; * (bold)—significant values.

4. Discussion

The currently published SOSORT (International Scientific Society on Scoliosis Orthopaedic and Rehabilitation Treatment) guidelines for conservative scoliosis treatment promote the HRQoL as one of the essential aims of therapy [24]. This study included girls with IS treated by a corrective TLSO brace, for at least three months for at least 12h per day. It is worth underlining that the treatment's usefulness has been shown to depend on the patients' treatment compliance [25,26] and the quality of brace usage [26]. Furthermore, in the recently presented consensus on the best practice guidelines for bracing in adolescent idiopathic scoliosis, some emphasis was put on the patient's emotional/psychological health as a factor in making bracing decisions [27]. Brace-based treatment, gender, and severity of the disease can significantly interfere with several aspects of patients' lives, resulting in high levels of stress and a negative impact on daily life [7]. Therefore, using HRQoL questionnaire outcomes is very important in monitoring and assessing the results of treatment.

In this study, we compared for the first time the Polish language version of the ISYQOL-PL with the Polish language version of the SRS-22 questionnaire (considered as a standard criterion for measuring HRQoL in IS). Both questionnaires were culturally adapted and validated as reliable tools for HRQoL evaluation in the Polish language for patients with spinal deformity.

Caronni et al. [14] found that the newly developed ISYQOL questionnaire to measure the HRQoL of adolescents with spinal deformities performs better than the SRS-22 questionnaire when used in the Italian language. The authors claimed that the ISYQOL questionnaire was the first questionnaire developed by using Rasch analysis. Questionnaires built up with Rasch analysis have several advantages compared to questionnaires created according to classical test theory [14]. The same group of authors in a different study using Rasch analysis showed that the SRS-22 questionnaire suffers from poor metric properties, preventing it from adequately measuring patients' quality of life [28]. Given such limitations, statistical analysis using the SRS-22 should be applied with caution [28]. However, the SRS-22 questionnaire, developed according to the classical test theory, presented satisfactory psychometric properties such as concurrent validity and reliability [11].

Debate is still open on how to statistically treat Likert scale and Likert-type scale data. Indeed, an important and often underestimated limitation of questionnaires comes from their ordinal nature, which does not support proper arithmetic operations assuming linear interval properties (e.g., addition and subtraction) [29–31]. Due to the lack of additivity of rating scale data [30], questionnaire scores should be formally excluded from parametric statistics [32].

Some experts view Likert scales as being strictly ordinal in nature; thus, parametric analysis approaches assuming quantitative, or at least interval-level measurements, are not appropriate [33–35]. These "ordinalist" views seem to stem from overlooking the difference between individual items and overall Likert scales, as pointed out by those holding the contrasting "intervalist" viewpoint [33,36–38].

However, Likert scales can be included in a larger group of measures that are sometimes referred to as summated (or aggregated) rating scales. The reason is because they are based on the idea that some underlying phenomenon can be measured by aggregating an individual's rating of his/her feelings, attitudes, or perceptions related to a series of individual statements or items [33].

In particular, a restriction should hold for the SRS-22 questionnaire, for which Rasch analysis showed it to suffer from poor metric properties [13]. However, such a position has been criticized as an overly restrictive approach, in practice, since numerous studies have suggested that parametric approaches are acceptable when the data are not strictly on the interval level of measurement [33,39–43].

A very informative review by Harpe on this topic suggests several recommendations to follow in such a case [33]. In particular, in the present study, we considered the first two recommendations when approaching the statistical analysis. Recommendation 1: "Scales that have been developed to be used as a group must be analyzed as a group, and only as a group." Recommendation 2: "Aggregated rating scales can be treated as continuous data." Thus, to analyze the ISYQOL-PL and SRS-22 scales' behaviors (considered as a group), we decided to use parametric statistics [33]. The same approach was applied by Caronni et al. [14], in which they compared the Italian language versions of the ISYQOL and SRS-22 questionnaires using parametric analysis, stating that despite being "aware that parametric statistics should be avoided on ordinal data, however, because it is a common practice to use parametric statistics for SRS-22 analysis, they preferred to compare ISYQOL with the current practice".

Moreover, in the present study, the non-parametric statistics for the SRS-22 questionnaire confirmed all the findings obtained through parametric statistics.

The known-groups validity analysis demonstrated that both the ISYQOL-PL and the SRS-22 tools showed no difference (1) between the two age groups: ≤ 13 years vs. >13 years; and (2) between the groups of single vs. double curves.

Conversely, the ISYQOL-PL showed significantly better HRQoL in mild rather than moderate scoliosis, as was found by Caronni et al. [14]. This result supports the idea that the ISYQOL-PL questionnaire depicts better what is perceived in clinical observations.

In Caronni et al. [14], the concurrent validity analysis was approached using correlation and the Spearman rho coefficient. Agreement and correlation are widely used concepts in the medical literature. Both are used to indicate the strength of association between variables of interest, but they are conceptually distinct, and, thus, require the use of different statistics [20,21]. In our results, Lin's CCC $p_{CCC} = 0.47$ showed low/moderate agreement between the two questionnaires [21]. Additionally, using the Spearman rho = 0.53, the concurrent validity analysis showed a moderate validity [22] of the ISYQOL-PL measure vs. SRS-22. A questionnaire has good concurrent validity if it shows a good agreement with an accepted standard measure [44]. The found correlation is lower than the one found by Caronni et al. for scoliotic patients (Spearman r = 0.71). Conversely, our value appears to be closer to the results (Spearman r = 0.56), which Caronni et al. found for the concurrent validity of the two questionnaires when hyperkyphosis patients were considered [14]. The lack of agreement/correlation could be explained concerning the structure of the questionnaires: SRS-22 is a multidimensional questionnaire (with its five domains) while ISYQOL is unidimensional.

The two-way ANOVA confirmed no interactions between severity of pathology and age, or years of treatment, or number of scoliotic curves. This substantially confirms that only severity of pathology in our sample has a direct statistically significant effect on the HRQoL of patients when evaluated via the ISYQOL-PL tool. Such a result complies with what it is commonly observed in clinical practice. Conversely, the statistically significant interaction (interference) found for SRS-22 shows some limitations of this questionnaire, introducing some unclear outcomes. Indeed, while in the ISYQOL-PL the value of Cobb angle was always a significant factor, showing its importance in the perceived HRQoL level in the SRS-22, the age and Cobb angle values interfere, masking which of the two factors has a direct influence on the perceived HRQoL.

The study's clinical relevance is related to the need to use tools with high metric properties in daily clinical practice to measure patients' HRQoL by specialists involved in the treatment process. It is important to underline that the monitoring of the HRQoL is one of the essential recommendations in the treatment of patients with spinal deformities. The ISYQOL-PL will simplify collecting individual results and interpret them adequately and objectively for Polish language clinicians and patients. Health professionals could produce an important practical clinical impact by using such as tool as a basis to discuss with the patient their disease, to support them, clarify common myths and fears associated with the deformity, or help them concerning the brace experience. In addition, the clinician can use the outcomes of the questionnaire to tune the treatment process.

Given that the data collection was during the first wave of the COVID-19 pandemic in Europe, we strongly considered eventual influence impacting the patients' perceived HRQoL, so we asked the patients to focus on their scoliosis-related issues strictly. The questions refer to spine diseases, and the patients, when answering the questions, understood them in this way. None of the patients presented and reported malaise in connection with the COVID-19 pandemic. In addition, parents or legal guardians did not raise any objections to the behavior and well-being of their children. There were no circumstances that affected the quality of the answers provided.

As a limitation, our study analyzed only girls with IS under brace treatment. Ongoing research aims to compare groups with and without brace treatment, including gender differences and per-spinal deformities differences.

5. Conclusions

Both questionnaires adequately measure HRQoL. ISYQOL-PL seems to offer advantageous analytical capacities compared to SRS-22 when applied to adolescent girls undergoing non-surgical treatment for mild or moderate idiopathic scoliosis. The severity of scoliosis but neither the age nor the curve pattern demonstrated a direct statistically significant effect on HRQoL in girls with IS when evaluated using the ISYQOL-PL tool. Such an effect could not be detected using the SRS-22 questionnaire. Using the HRQoL questionnaire, with high metric properties, in different languages, could constitute the basis for creating a multicenter study to better understand the changes in the quality of life of girls with IS during treatment of a larger population with different cultural backgrounds and environments.

Author Contributions: Conceptualization, E.K. and K.K.; methodology, E.K.; software, E.K.; validation, E.K. and K.K.; formal analysis, E.K., K.K., M.K., D.C., Ł.S. and T.K.; investigation, E.K., K.K., M.K., D.C. and Ł.S.; resources, K.K., M.K. and D.C.; data curation, K.K.; writing—original draft preparation, E.K.; writing—review and editing, E.K. and T.K.; visualization, E.K.; supervision, T.K.; project administration, K.K.; funding acquisition, K.K. All authors have read and agreed to the published version of the manuscript.

Funding: This research received no external funding. The publication cost was partly covered by the Poznan University of Medical Sciences.

Institutional Review Board Statement: All subjects gave their informed consent for inclusion before they participated in the study. The study was conducted in accordance with the Declaration of Helsinki, and the Institutional Review Board of Poznan University of Medical Sciences approved the study (5 November 2019).

Informed Consent Statement: Informed consent was obtained from the parents and the patients involved in the study.

Data Availability Statement: The data presented in this study are available on request from the corresponding author.

Acknowledgments: We would like to express deep gratitude to Moreno D'Amico and Piero Roncoletta from SMART Lab (Skeleton Movement Analysis and Advanced Rehabilitation Technologies)—Bioengineering & Biomedicine Company, Pescara, Italy, for their valuable and constructive suggestions during the methodological data analysis.

Conflicts of Interest: The authors declare no conflict of interest.

References

1. Vasiliadis, E.; Grivas, T.B. Quality of Life after Conservative Treatment of Adolescent Idiopathic Scoliosis. *Stud. Health Technol. Inform.* **2008**, *135*, 409–413.
2. Aulisa, A.G.; Guzzanti, V.; Perisano, C.; Marzetti, E.; Specchia, A.; Galli, M.; Giordano, M.; Aulisa, L. Determination of Quality of Life in Adolescents with Idiopathic Scoliosis Subjected to Conservative Treatment. *Scoliosis* **2010**, *5*, 21. [CrossRef]
3. Wang, H.; Tetteroo, D.; Arts, J.J.C.; Markopoulos, P.; Ito, K. Quality of Life of Adolescent Idiopathic Scoliosis Patients under Brace Treatment: A Brief Communication of Literature Review. *Qual. Life Res.* **2021**, *30*, 703–711. [CrossRef]
4. Kinel, E.; Kotwicki, T.; Podolska, A.; Białek, M.; Stryła, W. Quality of Life and Stress Level in Adolescents with Idiopathic Scoliosis Subjected to Conservative Treatment. *Stud. Health Technol. Inform.* **2012**, *176*, 419–422. [CrossRef]
5. Leszczewska, J.; Czaprowski, D.; Pawłowska, P.; Kolwicz, A.; Kotwicki, T. Evaluation of the Stress Level of Children with Idiopathic Scoliosis in Relation to the Method of Treatment and Parameters of the Deformity. *Sci. World J.* **2012**, *2012*, 538409. [CrossRef] [PubMed]
6. Negrini, S.; Minozzi, S.; Bettany-Saltikov, J.; Chockalingam, N.; Grivas, T.B.; Kotwicki, T.; Maruyama, T.; Romano, M.; Zaina, F. Braces for Idiopathic Scoliosis in Adolescents. *Cochrane Database Syst. Rev.* **2015**, *18*, CD006850. [CrossRef]
7. Tomaszewski, R.; Janowska, M. *Psychological Aspects of Scoliosis Treatment in Children*; IntechOpen: Rijeka, Croatia, 2012; ISBN 978-953-51-0595-4.
8. Vasiliadis, E.; Grivas, T.B.; Gkoltsiou, K. Development and Preliminary Validation of Brace Questionnaire (BrQ): A New Instrument for Measuring Quality of Life of Brace Treated Scoliotics. *Scoliosis* **2006**, *1*, 7. [CrossRef] [PubMed]
9. Botens-Helmus, C.; Klein, R.; Stephan, C. The Reliability of the Bad Sobernheim Stress Questionnaire (BSSQbrace) in Adolescents with Scoliosis during Brace Treatment. *Scoliosis* **2006**, *1*, 22. [CrossRef] [PubMed]
10. Asher, M.; Min Lai, S.; Burton, D.; Manna, B. Discrimination Validity of the Scoliosis Research Society-22 Patient Questionnaire: Relationship to Idiopathic Scoliosis Curve Pattern and Curve Size. *Spine* **2003**, *28*, 74–78. [CrossRef] [PubMed]
11. Asher, M.; Min Lai, S.; Burton, D.; Manna, B. The Reliability and Concurrent Validity of the Scoliosis Research Society-22 Patient Questionnaire for Idiopathic Scoliosis. *Spine* **2003**, *28*, 63–69. [CrossRef] [PubMed]
12. Asher, M.; Lai, S.M.; Burton, D.; Manna, B. The Influence of Spine and Trunk Deformity on Preoperative Idiopathic Scoliosis Patients' Health-Related Quality of Life Questionnaire Responses. *Spine* **2004**, *29*, 861–868. [CrossRef] [PubMed]
13. Caronni, A.; Sciumè, L.; Donzelli, S.; Zaina, F.; Negrini, S. ISYQOL: A Rasch-Consistent Questionnaire for Measuring Health-Related Quality of Life in Adolescents with Spinal Deformities. *Spine J.* **2017**, *17*, 1364–1372. [CrossRef] [PubMed]
14. Caronni, A.; Donzelli, S.; Zaina, F.; Negrini, S. The Italian Spine Youth Quality of Life Questionnaire Measures Health-Related Quality of Life of Adolescents with Spinal Deformities Better Than the Reference Standard, the Scoliosis Research Society 22 Questionnaire. *Clin. Rehabil.* **2019**, *33*, 1404–1415. [CrossRef]
15. ISYQOL. Available online: https://www.isyqol.org/ (accessed on 3 February 2021).
16. Sánchez-Raya, J.; D'Agata, E.; Donzelli, S.; Caronni, A.; Bagó, J.; Rigo, M.; Figueras, C.; Negrini, S. Spanish Validation Of Italian Spine Youth Quality of Life (ISYQOL) Questionnaire. *J. Phys. Med. Rehabil.* **2020**, *2*, 1–4. [CrossRef]
17. Kinel, E.; Korbel, K.; Janusz, P.; Kozinoga, M.; Czaprowski, D.; Kotwicki, T. Polish Adaptation of the Italian Spine Youth Quality of Life Questionnaire. *J. Clin. Med.* **2021**, *10*, 2081. [CrossRef] [PubMed]
18. Glowacki, M.; Misterska, E.; Laurentowska, M.; Mankowski, P. Polish Adaptation of Scoliosis Research Society-22 Questionnaire. *Spine* **2009**, *34*, 1060–1065. [CrossRef]
19. Hattie, J.; Cooksey, R.W. Procedures for Assessing the Validities of Tests Using the "Known-Groups" Method. *Appl. Psychol. Meas.* **1984**, *8*, 295–305. [CrossRef]
20. Liu, J.; Tang, W.; Chen, G.; Lu, Y.; Feng, C.; Tu, X.M. Correlation and Agreement: Overview and Clarification of Competing Concepts and Measures. *Shanghai Arch. Psychiatry* **2016**, *28*, 115–120. [CrossRef] [PubMed]
21. Berchtold, A. Test–Retest: Agreement or Reliability? *Methodol. Innov.* **2016**, *9*, 205979911667287. [CrossRef]
22. Schober, P.; Boer, C.; Schwarte, L.A. Correlation Coefficients: Appropriate Use and Interpretation. *Anesth. Analg.* **2018**, *126*, 1763–1768. [CrossRef] [PubMed]
23. Sokal, R.R.; Rohlf, F.J. *Biometry: Principles and Practice of Statistics in Biological Research*; W H Freeman & Co: New York, NY, USA, 1994; ISBN 978-0-7167-2411-7.
24. Negrini, S.; Donzelli, S.; Aulisa, A.G.; Czaprowski, D.; Schreiber, S.; de Mauroy, J.C.; Diers, H.; Grivas, T.B.; Knott, P.; Kotwicki, T.; et al. 2016 SOSORT Guidelines: Orthopaedic and Rehabilitation Treatment of Idiopathic Scoliosis during Growth. *Scoliosis Spinal Disord.* **2018**, *13*, 3. [CrossRef] [PubMed]
25. Bunge, E.M.; Habbema, J.D.F.; de Koning, H.J. A Randomised Controlled Trial on the Effectiveness of Bracing Patients with Idiopathic Scoliosis: Failure to Include Patients and Lessons to Be Learnt. *Eur. Spine J.* **2010**, *19*, 747–753. [CrossRef]

26. Lou, E.H.M.; Hill, D.L.; Raso, J.V.; Moreau, M.; Hedden, D. How Quantity and Quality of Brace Wear Affect the Brace Treatment Outcomes for AIS. *Eur. Spine J.* **2016**, *25*, 495–499. [CrossRef] [PubMed]
27. Roye, B.D.; Simhon, M.E.; Matsumoto, H.; Bakarania, P.; Berdishevsky, H.; Dolan, L.A.; Grimes, K.; Grivas, T.B.; Hresko, M.T.; Karol, L.A.; et al. Establishing Consensus on the Best Practice Guidelines for the Use of Bracing in Adolescent Idiopathic Scoliosis. *Spine Deform.* **2020**, *8*, 597–604. [CrossRef]
28. Caronni, A.; Zaina, F.; Negrini, S. Improving the Measurement of Health-Related Quality of Life in Adolescent with Idiopathic Scoliosis: The SRS-7, a Rasch-Developed Short Form of the SRS-22 Questionnaire. *Res. Dev. Disabil.* **2014**, *35*, 784–799. [CrossRef] [PubMed]
29. Penta, M.; Arnould, C.; Decruynaere, C. *Développer et Interpréter Une Échelle de Mesure. Applications Du Modèle de Rasch*; Editions Mardaga: Sprimont, Belgium, 2005; ISBN 978-2-87009-897-4.
30. Prieto, L.; Alonso, J.; Lamarca, R. Classical Test Theory versus Rasch Analysis for Quality of Life Questionnaire Reduction. *Health Qual. Life Outcomes* **2003**, *1*, 27. [CrossRef] [PubMed]
31. Stevens, S.S. On the Theory of Scales of Measurement. *Science* **1946**, *103*, 677–680. [CrossRef] [PubMed]
32. da Rocha, N.S.; Chachamovich, E.; de Almeida Fleck, M.P.; Tennant, A. An Introduction to Rasch Analysis for Psychiatric Practice and Research. *J. Psychiatr. Res.* **2013**, *47*, 141–148. [CrossRef]
33. Harpe, S.E. How to Analyze Likert and Other Rating Scale Data. *Curr. Pharm. Teach. Learn.* **2015**, *7*, 836–850. [CrossRef]
34. Kuzon, W.M.; Urbanchek, M.G.; McCabe, S. The Seven Deadly Sins of Statistical Analysis. *Ann. Plast. Surg.* **1996**, *37*, 265–272. [CrossRef]
35. Jamieson, S. Likert Scales: How to (Ab)Use Them. *Med. Educ.* **2004**, *38*, 1217–1218. [CrossRef] [PubMed]
36. Carifio, J.; Perla, R. Resolving the 50-Year Debate around Using and Misusing Likert Scales. *Med. Educ.* **2008**, *42*, 1150–1152. [CrossRef]
37. Carifio, J.; Perla, R.J. Ten Common Misunderstandings, Misconceptions, Persistent Myths and Urban Legends about Likert Scales and Likert Response Formats and Their Antidotes. *J. Soc. Sci.* **2007**, *3*, 106–116. [CrossRef]
38. Norman, G. Likert Scales, Levels of Measurement and the "Laws" of Statistics. *Adv. Health Sci. Educ. Theory Pract.* **2010**, *15*, 625–632. [CrossRef]
39. Baker, B.O.; Hardyck, C.D.; Petrinovich, L.F. Weak Measurements vs. Strong Statistics: An Empirical Critique of S. S. Stevens' Proscriptions Nn Statistics. *Educ. Psychol. Meas.* **1966**, *26*, 291–309. [CrossRef]
40. Labovitz, S. The Assignment of Numbers to Rank Order Categories. *Am. Sociol. Rev.* **1970**, *35*, 515–524. [CrossRef]
41. Labovitz, S. Some Observations on Measurement and Statistics. *Soc. Forces* **1967**, *46*, 151–160. [CrossRef]
42. Glass, G.V.; Peckham, P.D.; Sanders, J.R. Consequences of Failure to Meet Assumptions Underlying the Fixed Effects Analyses of Variance and Covariance. *Rev. Educ. Res.* **1972**, *42*, 237–288. [CrossRef]
43. Baggaley, A.R.; Hull, A.L. The Effect of Nonlinear Transformations on a Likert Scale. *Eval. Health Prof.* **1983**, *6*, 483–491. [CrossRef]
44. de Vet, H.; Terwee, C.; Mokkink, L.; Knol, D. *Measurement in Medicine: A Practical Guide (Practical Guides to Biostatistics and Epidemiology)*; Cambridge University Press: Cambridge, UK, 2011.

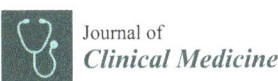

Article

22q11.2 Deletion Syndrome as a Human Model for Idiopathic Scoliosis

Steven de Reuver [1], Jelle F. Homans [1], Tom P. C. Schlösser [1], Michiel L. Houben [2], Vincent F. X. Deeney [3,4], Terrence B. Crowley [5], Ralf Stücker [6,7], Saba Pasha [3,4], Moyo C. Kruyt [1], Donna M. McDonald-McGinn [4,5] and René M. Castelein [1,*]

1. Department of Orthopaedic Surgery, University Medical Center Utrecht, 3584CX Utrecht, The Netherlands; s.dereuver-4@umcutrecht.nl (S.d.R.); J.F.Homans-3@umcutrecht.nl (J.F.H.); t.p.c.schlosser@umcutrecht.nl (T.P.C.S.); m.c.kruyt@umcutrecht.nl (M.C.K.)
2. Department of Pediatrics, Wilhelmina Children's Hospital, University Medical Center Utrecht, 3584CX Utrecht, The Netherlands; M.L.Houben@umcutrecht.nl
3. Department of Orthopaedic Surgery, The Children's Hospital of Philadelphia (CHOP), Philadelphia, PA 19104, USA; Vincent.deeney@chp.edu (V.F.X.D.); PashaS@email.chop.edu (S.P.)
4. The Perelman School of Medicine, University of Pennsylvania, Philadelphia, PA 19104, USA; MCGINN@chop.edu
5. Division of Human Genetics and 22q and You Center, The Children's Hospital of Philadelphia (CHOP), Philadelphia, PA 19104, USA; CrowleyT@email.chop.edu
6. Department of Pediatric Orthopedics, Altona Children's Hospital, 22763 Hamburg, Germany; ralf.stuecker@kinderkrankenhaus.net
7. Department of Orthopedics, University Medical Center Hamburg-Eppendorf (UKE), 22763 Hamburg, Germany
* Correspondence: r.m.castelein-3@umcutrecht.nl; Tel.: +31-88-75-5555

Citation: de Reuver, S.; Homans, J.F.; Schlösser, T.P.C.; Houben, M.L.; Deeney, V.F.X.; Crowley, T.B.; Stücker, R.; Pasha, S.; Kruyt, M.C.; McDonald-McGinn, D.M.; et al. 22q11.2 Deletion Syndrome as a Human Model for Idiopathic Scoliosis. *J. Clin. Med.* **2021**, *10*, 4823. https://doi.org/10.3390/jcm10214823

Academic Editor: Theodoros B. Grivas

Received: 1 October 2021
Accepted: 18 October 2021
Published: 20 October 2021

Publisher's Note: MDPI stays neutral with regard to jurisdictional claims in published maps and institutional affiliations.

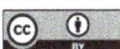

Copyright: © 2021 by the authors. Licensee MDPI, Basel, Switzerland. This article is an open access article distributed under the terms and conditions of the Creative Commons Attribution (CC BY) license (https://creativecommons.org/licenses/by/4.0/).

Abstract: To better understand the etiology of idiopathic scoliosis, prospective research into the pre-scoliotic state is required, but this research is practically impossible to carry out in the general population. The use of 'models', such as idiopathic-like scoliosis established in genetically modified animals, may elucidate certain elements, but their translatability to the human situation is questionable. The 22q11.2 deletion syndrome (22q11.2DS), with a 20-fold increased risk of developing scoliosis, may be a valuable and more relevant alternative and serve as a human 'model' for idiopathic scoliosis. This multicenter study investigates the morphology, dynamic behavior, and presence of intraspinal anomalies in patients with 22q11.2DS and scoliosis compared to idiopathic scoliosis. Scoliosis patients with 22q11.2DS and spinal radiography (n = 185) or MRI (n = 38) were included (mean age 11.6 ± 4.2; median Cobb angle 16°) and compared to idiopathic scoliosis patients from recent literature. Radiographic analysis revealed that 98.4% of 22q11.2DS patients with scoliosis had a curve morphology following predefined criteria for idiopathic curves: eight or fewer vertebrae, an S-shape and no inclusion of the lowest lumbar vertebrae. Furthermore, curve progression was present in 54.2%, with a mean progression rate of 2.5°/year, similar to reports on idiopathic scoliosis with 49% and 2.2–9.6°/year. The prevalence of intraspinal anomalies on MRI was 10.5% in 22q11.2DS, which is also comparable to 11.4% reported for idiopathic scoliosis. This indicates that 22q11.2DS may be a good model for prospective studies to better understand the etiology of idiopathic scoliosis.

Keywords: idiopathic scoliosis; 22q11.2 deletion syndrome; human model; neuromuscular scoliosis; radiography; MRI; curve morphology; intraspinal anomaly

1. Introduction

Scoliosis is a deformity of the spine and trunk that can have a clear cause, such as neuromuscular disease or congenital spinal malformation; however, the majority of cases are referred to as 'idiopathic' and occur in otherwise healthy adolescents [1]. Idiopathic scoliosis is quite common, with a prevalence of 2–4% in the general population, but its exact etiology remains clouded, despite important recent discoveries about genetics and the role of human upright spinal biomechanics [1–6]. Knowing the exact cause(s) is of utmost importance for potential scoliosis prevention and optimal treatment. The problem with current human etiology research is that, by necessity, only patients with an already established idiopathic scoliosis are studied; therefore, it is impossible to distinguish cause from effect [1,3].

Prospective cohort research, which follows the development of scoliosis starting in the pre-scoliotic spine, is practically impossible in the general population due to practical and ethical obstacles: the prevalence of idiopathic scoliosis would require thousands of children to be included for sufficient statistical power, and there would have to be periodic follow-ups with full spine radiographs, raising ionizing radiation concerns. The next best option is to use a 'model' with better availability or a higher idiopathic scoliosis prevalence—for instance, an animal model. Unfortunately, idiopathic scoliosis is a disease unique to humans, mainly due to our unique upright spinal biomechanics [7]. Earlier studies demonstrated that the computation of spinal biomechanics, for instance, with finite element models, can help understand idiopathic scoliosis [8]. Additionally, idiopathic-like scoliosis can be established in genetically modified animals such as zebrafish, pinealectomized chickens, or bipedal-forced mice; however, the translatability of this model to the human situation is questionable [9–12].

To prospectively study the etiology of idiopathic scoliosis, a human model is therefore preferred but has not yet been described. In other fields of medicine, such as psychiatry, the innovative use of a subset of the population with a high risk of a certain disease has been used and validated to serve as a 'model' for the disease in the general population [13]. This approach obviously also has scientific limitations, but if the model sufficiently resembles the condition in the general population, it can yield important information on specific aspects of the earliest phases of the disorder that cannot otherwise be studied prospectively.

The 22q11.2 deletion syndrome (22q11.2DS), the most common cause of DiGeorge syndrome, is the most common microdeletion syndrome in humans, with an incidence of 1 in 992 unselected pregnancies and 1 in 2148 live births [14–16]. Compared to the general population, these children have a 20-fold increased risk of developing scoliosis during their growing years, with a prevalence of around 50% [17]. Children with 22q11.2DS are often identified before or shortly after birth, well before potential scoliosis onset, are usually known in the pediatric circuit, and could therefore be studied prospectively [18,19]. It is currently unknown if scoliosis in 22q11.2DS sufficiently resembles idiopathic scoliosis in the general population, which is a prerequisite to be used as a 'model'. This study focused on the morphology, dynamic behavior, and presence of intraspinal anomalies, all of which are quantifiable features relevant to idiopathic scoliosis development. These were studied in 22q11.2DS and scoliosis patient cohorts from multiple centers and compared to what is reported in the literature for idiopathic scoliosis in the general population.

2. Materials and Methods

2.1. Study Population

The local Ethical Review Boards of the three hospitals involved approved this study and waived the necessity of explicit (parental) informed consent since data were collected as part of standard care and were handled anonymously. In all participating centers, spinal radiographs are made of each patient at two-year intervals as part of a global standard 22q11.2DS follow-up protocol [20].

From databases of two specialized 22q11.2DS centers, patients with an available full spine radiograph were extracted. All patients that were ambulant, had a genetically confirmed 22q11.2 deletion (via FISH, 22q11.2 specific MLPA, CGH, or SNP micro-array), were aged >4, and had scoliosis defined as a Cobb angle >10° were included [21]. Patients with congenital spinal anomalies (based on spinal radiography review) that induced congenital scoliosis were excluded since the pathoetiology varies greatly from the development of idiopathic scoliosis [22]. Additionally, non-ambulant patients (based on the patient's chart review) were excluded. Sex, age at the time of radiography, and data on comorbidities were collected. For the further analysis of curve progression, all included patients with at least one year of radiographic follow-up were analyzed.

Additionally, patients were included from a database of a third specialized 22q11.2DS center, where patients with scoliosis frequently receive an MRI of the spine for indications such as pain, fast progression, or pre-operative screening. Patients with congenital spinal anomalies or with only post-operative MRIs were excluded. These MRIs were analyzed for intraspinal anomalies.

2.2. Radiographic Analysis

One trained and experienced observer (JH), blinded for all other clinical parameters, analyzed all radiographs in chronological order. First, the Cobb angle was measured of all scoliotic curve(s), and the location of the major curve (i.e., the largest) was noted as either thoracic (apex at T2 – disc T11/T12), thoracolumbar (apex at T12 – L1), or lumbar (apex at disc L1/L2 – L4), according to the Scoliosis Research Society guidelines [21]. Next, curve morphology was determined based on the first available radiograph of each patient, according to the criteria determined by Abul-Kasim et al. in 2010 [23]. Curves were classified as non-idiopathic if three conditions were met: (1) the Cobb-to-Cobb segment exceeded eight vertebrae, (2) the curve was C-shaped, and (3) the curve included the lowest or second-lowest lumbar vertebra (Figure 1). The findings in the 22q11.2DS patients in this study were compared to reference observations in idiopathic and non-idiopathic scoliosis patients in the general population [23].

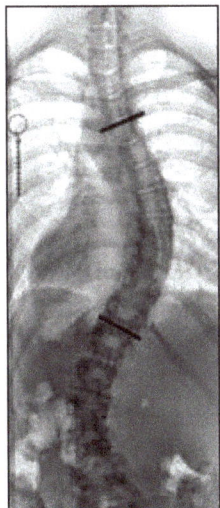 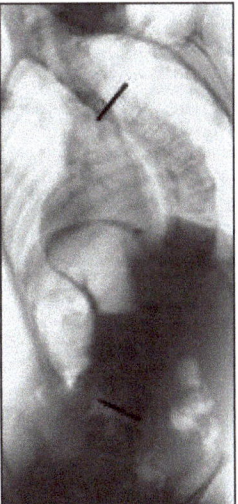

Figure 1. Two examples of different scoliosis curve types. On the left is an idiopathic-like curve, which is S-shaped with the apex of the major curve located at vertebral level T9 and a curve length of 8 vertebrae. On the right is a non-idiopathic neuromuscular-like curve, which is C-shaped with a curve length of 12 vertebrae, and a lower-end vertebra located at level L4.

Furthermore, the progression of scoliosis curve severity was analyzed by measuring the Cobb angle on the first and last radiograph available for each patient with at least one year of follow-up. A progressive curve was defined as at least a 5° increase over the follow-up period [24]. Additionally, if a patient had received brace treatment or surgery, the curve was considered progressive. Of all 22q11.2DS patients with progressive scoliosis, the curve progression rate in degrees of Cobb angle per year was calculated and compared to reference values of idiopathic scoliosis in the general population, as described in a meta-analysis by Di Felice et al. in 2018 [24].

2.3. MRI Analysis

Of the spinal MRIs made of 22q11.2DS patients with scoliosis, all reports were screened for the presence of intraspinal anomalies and annotated as described by the clinically involved radiologist at the time of investigation. The rate of intraspinal anomalies in 22q11.2DS patients with scoliosis was compared to that reported in idiopathic scoliosis in the general population, as described in a meta-analysis by Heemskerk et al. in 2018 [25].

2.4. Statistical Analysis

The age at diagnosis, sex, curve progression (< or >5°), and presence of spinal anomalies in the 22q11.2DS patients in this study were compared to data on idiopathic scoliosis in the general population from literature. Normality of distribution was tested with Q–Q plots, the means ± standard deviations were calculated for normally distributed variables, and medians and interquartile ranges (IQR) were calculated for not normally distributed variables. Since data were compiled from multiple cohorts with different criteria, no comparative statistics were performed to produce irrelevant p-values. The descriptive statistical analyses were performed with SPSS 25.0 for Windows (IBM, Armonk, NY, USA).

3. Results

3.1. Study Population

From two databases, 206 patients with 22q11.2DS, scoliosis, and a full spine radiograph were retrieved; after 21 exclusions, 185 patients were included for radiographic analysis (Figure 2). From these 185 patients, a further 48 had at least one year of radiographic follow-up and were included for analysis of their scoliosis curve progression. Finally, for the MRI analysis, after nine exclusions, 38 patients were included for analysis of the rate of intraspinal anomalies (Figure 2).

The mean age at diagnosis of scoliosis in 22q11.2DS patients was 11.6 ± 4.2, and 92 (49.7%) were female (Figure 3). In literature, the mean age at idiopathic scoliosis diagnosis in the general population varies due to different screening and diagnosis protocols but is reported 9.5–13.6 [26–28]. Furthermore, the ratio of females to males in idiopathic scoliosis is reported as 1.44 to 1, corresponding to 59% females [26].

3.2. Radiographic Analysis

Of the 185 patients with 22q11.2DS and scoliosis, the median Cobb angle was 16° (IQR: 13–25°). A total of 182 patients (98.4%) had an idiopathic-like curve based on Abul-Kasim's criteria (Table 1) [23]. The other three patients (1.6%) fitted the criteria for neuromuscular-like scoliosis. Remarkably, the proportion of S-shaped curves was 69%, much higher than the 18% reported earlier for idiopathic scoliosis (Table 1) [23]. Of the 48 patients with at least one year of radiographic follow-up, the mean age at scoliosis diagnosis was 9.8 ± 2.7, and the median follow-up was 3.4 years (IQR: 2.3–5.1). There was a curve progression of at least 5° in 26 patients (54.2%), at an average progression rate of 2.5° per year, ranging from 1.4° to 5.0°. This is very comparable to idiopathic scoliosis, which has a reported proportion of 49% and a similar rate of 2.2–9.6° per year in the general population [24].

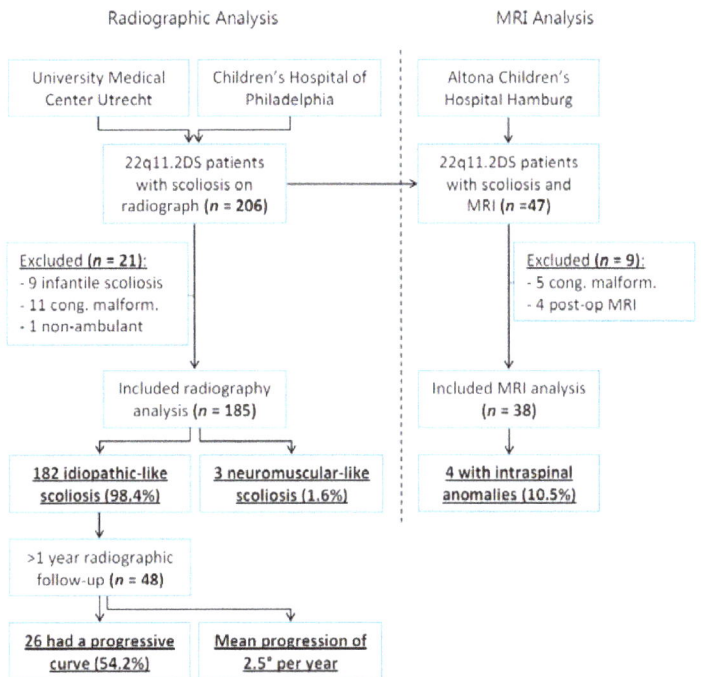

Figure 2. Flowchart shows the inclusion and exclusion of patients in the current study. Furthermore, the results of both the radiographic and MRI analysis are displayed.

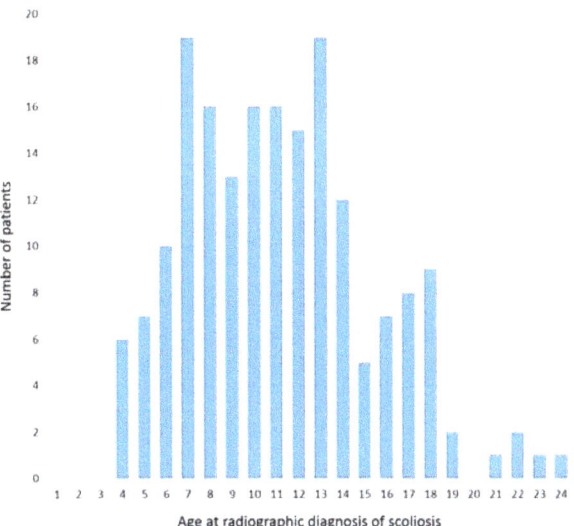

Figure 3. The age distribution at the moment of initial radiographic diagnosis of scoliosis. In the 185 included 22q11.2 deletion syndrome patients in this study, the mean age at diagnosis was 11.6 ± 4.2.

Table 1. Curve characteristics of the 185 ambulant 22q11.2 deletion syndrome patients with scoliosis next to references values of the idiopathic and neuromuscular scoliosis. From Abul-Kasim et al. (2010).

	Current Study	Abul-Kasim et al. (2010) [1]	
	22q11.2DS	Idiopathic Scoliosis	Neuro. Scoliosis
n	185	77	21
Major curve location			
- Thoracic	79 (43%)	52 (68%)	5 (24%)
- Thoracolumbar	54 (29%)	13 (17%)	12 (57%)
- Lumbar	52 (28%)	12 (16%)	4 (19%)
Median curve length in № vertebrae (IQR)	6 (5–7)	7 (7–8)	10 (9–11)
>8 vertebrae in curve	18 (10%)	3 (4%)	19 (90%)
Curve morphology			
- S-shape	127 (69%)	14 (18%)	0 (0%)
- C-shape	58 (31%)	63 (82%)	21 (100%)
Lower-end vertebra			
- L3+	114 (62%)	62 (81%)	5 (24%)
- L4	67 (36%)	15 (19%)	8 (38%)
- L5	4 (2%)	0 (0%)	8 (38%)
Fulfilled criteria for [2]			
- Neuro. scoliosis	3 (2%)	0 (0%)	16 (76%)
- Idiopathic scoliosis	183 (98%)	77 (100%)	5 (24%)

[1] Reprinted by Permission of SAGE Publications, Ltd. [23]. [2] The combination of a Cobb-to-Cobb curve length > 8 vertebrae, a C-shaped curve, and the location of the lower-end vertebrae at the lowest or second-lowest lumbar vertebrae is determined as a non-idiopathic (neuromuscular) curve pattern [23].

3.3. MRI Analysis

Out of 38 scoliosis patients with 22q11.2DS and an available MRI of the complete spine, four patients (10.5%) had a total of five intraspinal anomalies. The different anomalies were one tonsillar herniation, one extradural cyst, one intraspinal lipoma, and two vertebral body abnormalities. This is comparable to a prevalence of 11.4% in idiopathic scoliosis in the general population (Table 2) [25].

Table 2. Intraspinal anomalies in 38 patients with 22q11.22 deletion syndrome and scoliosis compared to idiopathic scoliosis in the general population, as described by Heemskerk et al. (2018).

	Current Study	Heemskerk et al. (2018) [1]
	22q11.2DS	Idiopathic Scoliosis
n	38	8622
Spinal anomaly:		
-Isolated syrinx		318 (3.7%)
-Isolated Arnold-Chiari malf.		259 (3.0%)
-Arnold-Chiari malf. with syrinx		218 (2.5%)
-Tethered cord		49 (0.57%)
-Dural ectasia		33 (0.38%)
-Cerabral or intra/paraspinal tumors		22 (0.26%)
-Tonsilar herniation	1 (3%)	20 (0.23%)
-Diastematomyelia		19 (0.22%)
-Abnormal position of conus		10 (0.12%)
-Extra- or intradural cysts	1 (3%)	6 (0.07%)
-Intraspinal lipoma	1 (3%)	5 (0.06%)
-Discopathy		4 (0.05%)
-Hydrocephalus		3 (0.03%)
-Vertebral body abnormality	2 (5%) [2]	3 (0.03%) [3]
-Hydromyelia		2 (0.02%)

Table 2. *Cont.*

	Current Study	Heemskerk et al. (2018) [1]
	22q11.2DS	Idiopathic Scoliosis
-Craniocervical junctional narrowing		1 (0.01%)
-Cerebellar angioma		1 (0.01%)
-Dandy-Walker syndrome		1 (0.01%)
-Arteriovenous fistula		1 (0.01%)
-Not specified		88 (1%)

[1] Compiled from the systematic review and meta-analysis as performed by Heemskerk et al. [25]. [2] Patient 1: Mild osteophytic ridging at T10-T11 and T11-T12 with Schmorl's nodes and decreased disc height at these levels. Patient 2: Vertical cleft in the midline of the T7 vertebral body. [3] Hemangioma or lipoma in vertebral body.

4. Discussion

The problem with the current etiology research on idiopathic scoliosis is that only established cases can be studied, and prospective research before the onset of the deformity is unfeasible in the general population [1,3]. The solution is the use of a 'model'; however, currently, for idiopathic scoliosis, only 'models' of genetically or anatomically modified small animals exist [7,9–12]. This study investigated the relevance of a human 'model' for idiopathic scoliosis by using a subset of the population with a high risk for the disease. Children with 22q11.2DS have a 20-fold increased prevalence of scoliosis at around 50% and are usually prospectively followed from birth [14,17,18]. The purpose of this multicenter study was to analyze the morphology, dynamic behavior, and presence of intraspinal anomalies in scoliosis patients from 22q11.2DS cohorts in comparison to idiopathic scoliosis.

Over two hundred patients with 22q11.2DS and scoliosis were compared to thousands of patients with idiopathic scoliosis from the recent literature. The mean age at diagnosis of scoliosis in patients with 22q11.2DS was 11.6, and 49.7% were females. In idiopathic scoliosis, this is reported as 9.5–13.6 years old and 59% females [26–28]. This broad range of reported age at diagnosis is caused by the many different scoliosis screening protocols in different countries. However, if scoliosis in 22q11.2DS onsets at the same age as idiopathic scoliosis, the mean age at diagnosis in patients with 22q11.2DS is likely to be lower since spinal radiography is part of the standard follow-up, promoting early diagnosis. The vast majority of included patients with 22q11.2DS and scoliosis (98.4%) had a curve morphology that was consistent with predefined criteria for an idiopathic curve [23]. Additionally, the proportion of progressive curves (54.2%) and the rate of curve progression (2.5° per year) was similar to reports on idiopathic scoliosis, with 49% being progressive at a rate of 2.2–9.6° per year [24]. Finally, the prevalence of intraspinal anomalies in 22q11.2DS patients with scoliosis was 10.5%, which was similar to the 11.4% prevalence in idiopathic scoliosis in the general population [25].

There are multiple classification systems that describe the curve morphology pattern in scoliosis. The well-known King and Lenke classifications were created mainly for surgical planning by distinguishing stiffer/structural curves from non-structural curves rather than distinguishing between idiopathic and non-idiopathic scoliosis [29,30]. Abul-Kasim et al. showed that non-idiopathic curves display distinct morphologic characteristics on upright standing spinal radiographs, including the scoliosis shape, the curve length, and the contribution of the lowest lumbar vertebrae to the curve (Figure 1). These characteristics were translated into three criteria to distinguish idiopathic from non-idiopathic curves, which were used in this study of 22q11.2DS scoliosis [23]. While these three criteria are all assessed from anterior–posterior standing spinal radiographs, idiopathic scoliosis is a 3D deformation of the spine and trunk, including vertebral rotation and sagittal plane deformation. However, since lateral radiographs were not routinely made in all participating centers, these were not analyzed in this study. Furthermore, accurate assessment of the sagittal spinal profile is notoriously unreliable on lateral radiographs, especially in more severe curves with a larger Cobb angle, due to coupling of the spinal curvature in all three planes [31,32].

Besides the global curve morphology criteria for idiopathic scoliosis, the curve behavior over time was also reckoned as relevant. Although similar values for the proportion and rate of curve progression were observed in 22q11.2DS scoliosis in comparison to idiopathic scoliosis, this should be interpreted with caution since scoliosis progression is heavily influenced by age, sex, curve location, and curve magnitude, all parameters that were not normalized or matched in this study [24,33]. Additionally, in the 22q11.2DS cohort, there was a median follow-up difference between the progressive curves (4.4 years) and non-progressive curves (2.5 years); therefore, the number of progressive curves in 22q11.2DS might be underestimated by this study. Future studies, with, for instance, an age- and sex-matched design, could aim to confirm the similarities in curve behavior between 22q11.2DS and idiopathic scoliosis. The addition of an MRI-based analysis to this study was mainly to exclude intraspinal anomalies as an important cause of scoliosis in 22q11.2DS. Indeed, the intraspinal anomaly prevalence was comparable to idiopathic scoliosis [25].

Although this study demonstrated similarities in curve morphology and behavior between scoliosis in 22q11.2DS and idiopathic scoliosis, the validity of 22q11.2DS as a 'model' has obvious limitations. First, the absence of typical non-idiopathic features that were identified for neuromuscular scoliosis does not imply that the curve is similar to idiopathic scoliosis. On the contrary, more subtle differences could be observed, such as the distribution between thoracic, thoracolumbar, and lumbar curves, as well as the contribution of L4 to the curve. Second, in this study, patients with congenital spinal anomalies that induced congenital scoliosis were excluded. This was because in the general population, and most likely also in 22q11.2DS, the pathoetiology of congenital scoliosis varies greatly from the development of idiopathic scoliosis [22]. It is known that in 22q11.2DS, the rate of congenital spinal malformations, especially in the cervical spine, is higher than the general population; therefore, if 22q11.2DS scoliosis were to be used as a 'model' to study idiopathic scoliosis, the congenital curves should be excluded [34]. Third, 22q11.2DS is a multisystem syndrome with many phenotypes resulting, for example, in hypocalcemia and a lower bone mineral density in half of the patients [14,35]. Interestingly, a proportion of patients with idiopathic scoliosis in the general population have lower bone mineral density [36–39]. Irrespective of a 22q11.2 deletion, a lower bone mineral density might be an independent risk factor for idiopathic-like scoliosis. Additionally, congenital heart disease is prevalent in 22q11.2DS, and for many decades, congenital heart disease has been linked to scoliosis in the general population [40,41]. Recent observations in different cohorts demonstrate that the 22q11.2 deletion itself is a confounder in this relationship and that in both the general population and in 22q11.2DS, congenital heart disease itself is not a large scoliosis risk factor [42]. Finally, children with 22q11.2DS differ from the general population in frequent phenotypes such as slow maturation, short stature, and articular laxity, which could all influence scoliosis development, but their exact effects are currently unknown. Future studies using 22q11.2DS scoliosis as a model should aim to normalize these as much as possible, for instance, by determining the individual offset from maturity, i.e., the difference between chronological age and biological maturity [43].

For a scientific 'model' to be valid, the disease of the 'model' must sufficiently resemble the condition in the general population before it can be used to study etiological aspects of the disorder. Of course, any 'model' is at best an approximation of the true disease; this holds true for the often-used animal model as well. Scoliosis in 22q11.2DS does have differences from true idiopathic scoliosis in the general population, but this study demonstrated many important similarities in curve morphology and behavior. A future goal could be to utilize this 'human model' in prospective studies on idiopathic scoliosis etiology—for example, to study the spinal sagittal profile before scoliosis onset and its influence on scoliosis development [8,44]. Another option is to examine whole-genome sequencing in patients with scoliosis and 22q11.2DS, and those in the general population, as a clue to identifying the genomic etiology. Studying psychotic, 'schizophrenia-like' disorders in the 22q11.2DS population has yielded important information on idiopathic schizophrenia, a disorder that also seems exclusive to humans in the general population [13]. We propose to use the same approach in idiopathic scoliosis research.

5. Conclusions

To better understand idiopathic scoliosis etiology, prospective research on the pre-scoliotic spine is needed but is practically impossible in the general population. Animal models can help, but a validated human model would be superior. This study explored scoliosis in patients with 22q11.2DS as a possible human 'model' for idiopathic scoliosis. These patients have a 20-fold increased scoliosis risk and a curve morphology that resembles idiopathic scoliosis. Additionally, the curve dynamic behavior, in terms of prevalence and rate of curve progression and the prevalence of intraspinal anomalies, closely mimicked idiopathic scoliosis. This suggests that 22q11.2DS scoliosis may be a very relevant 'model' to prospectively study and help better understand certain aspects of idiopathic scoliosis etiology in the general population.

Author Contributions: Conceptualization, S.d.R., J.F.H., T.P.C.S., M.C.K., D.M.M.-M. and R.M.C.; methodology, S.d.R., J.F.H., T.P.C.S., M.C.K., D.M.M.-M. and R.M.C.; formal analysis, J.F.H.; resources, J.F.H., T.B.C., D.M.M.-M. and R.S.; data curation, J.F.H., T.B.C. and R.S.; writing—original draft preparation, S.d.R., J.F.H., T.P.C.S., M.C.K. and R.M.C.; writing—review and editing, S.d.R., J.F.H., T.P.C.S., M.L.H., V.F.X.D., T.B.C., R.S., S.P., M.C.K., D.M.M.-M. and R.M.C.; supervision, T.P.C.S., M.L.H., V.F.X.D., R.S., S.P., M.C.K., D.M.M.-M. and R.M.C.; funding acquisition, S.d.R., J.F.H., T.P.C.S., M.C.K. and R.M.C. All authors have read and agreed to the published version of the manuscript.

Funding: This research was funded by the Scoliosis Research Society and the Fondation Yves-Cotrel.

Institutional Review Board Statement: The study was conducted according to the guidelines of the Declaration of Helsinki. The local Ethical Review Boards of the three hospitals involved approved this study and waived the necessity of explicit (parental) informed consent since data were collected as part of standard care and were handled anonymously.

Informed Consent Statement: Patient consent was waived since data were collected as part of standard care and were handled anonymously.

Data Availability Statement: The data presented in this study are available on request from the corresponding author. The data are not publicly available due to local ethical guidelines.

Conflicts of Interest: The authors declare no conflict of interest. The funders had no role in the design of the study; in the collection, analyses, or interpretation of data; in the writing of the manuscript, or in the decision to publish the results.

References

1. Cheng, J.C.; Castelein, R.M.; Chu, W.C.; Danielsson, A.J.; Dobbs, M.B.; Grivas, T.B.; Gurnett, C.A.; Luk, K.D.; Moreau, A.; Newton, P.O.; et al. Adolescent idiopathic scoliosis. *Nat. Rev. Dis. Prim.* **2015**, *1*, 15–30. [CrossRef]
2. Kouwenhoven, J.-W.M.; Castelein, R.M. The pathogenesis of adolescent idiopathic scoliosis: Review of the literature. *Spine* **2008**, *33*, 2898–2908. [CrossRef]
3. Schlösser, T.P.C.; van der Heijden, G.J.M.G.; Versteeg, A.L.; Castelein, R.M. How "idiopathic" is adolescent idiopathic scoliosis? A systematic review on associated abnormalities. *PLoS ONE* **2014**, *9*, e97461. [CrossRef]
4. Gorman, K.F.; Julien, C.; Moreau, A. The genetic epidemiology of idiopathic scoliosis. *Eur. Spine J.* **2012**, *21*, 1905–1919. [CrossRef]
5. Kesling, K.L.; Reinker, K.A. Scoliosis in twins: A meta-analysis of the literature and report of six cases. *Spine* **1997**, *22*, 2009–2015. [CrossRef]
6. Kouwenhoven, J.W.; Smit, T.H.; van der Veen, A.J.; Kingma, I.; van Dieen, J.H.; Castelein, R.M. Effects of dorsal versus ventral shear loads on the rotational stability of the thoracic spine: A biomechanical porcine and human cadaveric study. *Spine* **2007**, *32*, 2545–2550. [CrossRef]
7. Castelein, R.M.; Pasha, S.; Cheng, J.C.Y.C.; Dubousset, J. Idiopathic Scoliosis as a Rotatory Decompensation of the Spine. *J. Bone Miner. Res.* **2020**, *35*, 1850–1857. [CrossRef] [PubMed]
8. Pasha, S.; de Reuver, S.; Homans, J.F.; Castelein, R.M. Sagittal curvature of the spine as a predictor of the pediatric spinal deformity development. *Spine Deform.* **2021**, *9*, 923–932. [CrossRef]
9. Janssen, M.M.A.; de Wilde, R.F.; Kouwenhoven, J.-W.M.; Castelein, R.M. Experimental animal models in scoliosis research: A review of the literature. *Spine J.* **2011**, *11*, 347–358. [CrossRef]

10. Boswell, C.W.; Ciruna, B. Understanding Idiopathic Scoliosis: A New Zebrafish School of Thought. *Trends Genet.* **2017**, *33*, 183–196. [CrossRef] [PubMed]
11. Machida, M.; Dubousset, J.; Imamura, Y.; Iwaya, T.; Yamada, T.; Kimura, J. An experimental study in chickens for the pathogenesis of idiopathic scoliosis. *Spine* **1993**, *18*, 1609–1615. [CrossRef] [PubMed]
12. Bobyn, J.D.; Little, D.G.; Gray, R.; Schindeler, A. Animal models of scoliosis. *J. Orthop. Res.* **2015**, *33*, 458–467. [CrossRef] [PubMed]
13. Gur, R.E.; Bassett, A.S.; McDonald-McGinn, D.M.; Bearden, C.E.; Chow, E.; Emanuel, B.S.; Owen, M.; Swillen, A.; Van den Bree, M.; Vermeesch, J.; et al. A neurogenetic model for the study of schizophrenia spectrum disorders: The International 22q11.2 Deletion Syndrome Brain Behavior Consortium. *Mol. Psychiatry* **2017**, *22*, 1664–1672. [CrossRef]
14. McDonald-McGinn, D.M.; Sullivan, K.E.; Marino, B.; Philip, N.; Swillen, A.; Vorstman, J.A.S.; Zackai, E.H.; Emanuel, B.S.; Vermeesch, J.R.; Morrow, B.E.; et al. 22Q11.2 Deletion Syndrome. *Nat. Rev. Dis. Prim.* **2015**, *1*, 1–19. [CrossRef]
15. Grati, F.R.; Molina Gomes, D.; Ferreira, J.C.P.B.; Dupont, C.; Alesi, V.; Gouas, L.; Horelli-Kuitunen, N.; Choy, K.W.; García-Herrero, S.; de la Vega, A.G.; et al. Prevalence of recurrent pathogenic microdeletions and microduplications in over 9500 pregnancies. *Prenat. Diagn.* **2015**, *35*, 801–809. [CrossRef]
16. Blagojevic, C.; Heung, T.; Theriault, M.; Tomita-Mitchell, A.; Chakraborty, P.; Kernohan, K.; Bulman, D.E.; Bassett, A.S. Estimate of the contemporary live-birth prevalence of recurrent 22q11.2 deletions: A cross-sectional analysis from population-based newborn screening. *Can. Med Assoc. Open Access J.* **2021**, *9*, E802–E809.
17. Homans, J.F.; Baldew, V.G.M.; Brink, R.C.; Kruyt, M.C.; Schlösser, T.P.C.; Houben, M.L.; Deeney, V.F.X.; Crowley, T.B.; Castelein, R.M.; McDonald-McGinn, D.M. Scoliosis in association with the 22q11.2 deletion syndrome: An observational study. *Arch. Dis. Child.* **2019**, *104*, 19–24. [CrossRef]
18. Homans, J.F.; de Reuver, S.; Breetvelt, E.J.; Vorstman, J.A.S.; Deeney, V.F.X.; Flynn, J.M.; McDonald-McGinn, D.M.; Kruyt, M.C.; Castelein, R.M. The 22q11.2 deletion syndrome as a model for idiopathic scoliosis—A hypothesis. *Med. Hypotheses* **2019**, *127*, 57–62. [CrossRef]
19. Campbell, I.M.; Sheppard, S.E.; Crowley, T.B.; McGinn, D.E.; Bailey, A.; McGinn, M.J.; Unolt, M.; Homans, J.F.; Chen, E.Y.; Salmons, H.I.; et al. What is new with 22q? An update from the 22q and You Center at the Children's Hospital of Philadelphia. *Am. J. Med. Genet. Part. A* **2018**, *176*, 2058–2069. [CrossRef]
20. Bassett, A.S.; McDonald-McGinn, D.M.; Devriendt, K.; Digilio, M.C.; Goldenberg, P.; Habel, A.; Marino, B.; Oskarsdottir, S.; Philip, N.; Sullivan, K.; et al. Practical Guidelines for Managing Patients with 22q11.2 Deletion Syndrome. *J. Pediatr.* **2011**, *159*, 332–339. [CrossRef]
21. O'Brien, M.; Kulklo, T.; Blanke, K.; Lenke, L. *Spinal Deformity Study Group Radiographic Measurement Manual*; Medtronic Sofamor Danek USA, Inc.: Memphis, TN, USA, 2008.
22. McMaster, M.J.; Ohtsuka, K. The natural history of congenital scoliosis. A study of two hundred and fifty-one patients. *J. Bone Jt. Surg. Am.* **1982**, *64*, 1128–1147. [CrossRef]
23. Abul-Kasim, K.; Ohlin, A. Curve Length, Curve Form, and Location of Lower-End Vertebra as a Means of Identifying the Type of Scoliosis. *J. Orthop. Surg.* **2010**, *18*, 1–5. [CrossRef] [PubMed]
24. Di Felice, F.; Zaina, F.; Donzelli, S.; Negrini, S. The Natural History of Idiopathic Scoliosis during Growth: A Meta-Analysis. *Am. J. Phys. Med. Rehabil.* **2018**, *97*, 346–356. [CrossRef] [PubMed]
25. Heemskerk, J.L.; Kruyt, M.C.; Colo, D.; Castelein, R.M.; Kempen, D.H.R. Prevalence and risk factors for neural axis anomalies in idiopathic scoliosis: A systematic review. *Spine J.* **2018**, *18*, 1261–1271. [CrossRef] [PubMed]
26. Sung, S.; Chae, H.-W.; Lee, H.S.; Kim, S.; Kwon, J.-W.; Lee, S.-B.; Moon, S.-H.; Lee, B.H. Incidence and Surgery Rate of Idiopathic Scoliosis: A Nationwide Database Study. *Int. J. Environ. Res. Public Health* **2021**, *18*, 8152. [CrossRef] [PubMed]
27. Strahle, J.; Smith, B.W.; Martinez, M.; Bapuraj, J.R.; Muraszko, K.M.; Garton, H.J.L.; Maher, C.O. The association between Chiari malformation Type I, spinal syrinx, and scoliosis. *J. Neurosurg. Pediatr.* **2015**, *15*, 607–611. [CrossRef] [PubMed]
28. Yılmaz, H.; Zateri, C.; Kusvuran Ozkan, A.; Kayalar, G.; Berk, H. Prevalence of adolescent idiopathic scoliosis in Turkey: An epidemiological study. *Spine J.* **2020**, *20*, 947–955. [CrossRef]
29. King, H.A.; Moe, J.H.; Bradford, D.S.; Winter, R.B. The selection of fusion levels in thoracic idiopathic scoliosis. *J. Bone Jt. Surg. Am. Vol.* **1983**, *65*, 1302–1313. [CrossRef]
30. Lenke, L.G.; Betz, R.R.; Harms, J.; Bridwell, K.H.; Clements, D.H.; Lowe, T.G.; Blanke, K. Adolescent idiopathic scoliosis. A new classification to determine extent of spinal arthrodesis. *J. Bone Jt. Surg.-Ser. A* **2001**, *83*, 1169–1181. [CrossRef]
31. Schlösser, T.P.C.; Shah, S.A.; Reichard, S.J.; Rogers, K.; Vincken, K.L.; Castelein, R.M. Differences in early sagittal plane alignment between thoracic and lumbar adolescent idiopathic scoliosis. *Spine J.* **2014**, *14*, 282–290. [CrossRef]
32. Sullivan, T.B.; Reighard, F.G.; Osborn, E.J.; Parvaresh, K.C.; Newton, P.O. Thoracic Idiopathic Scoliosis Severity Is Highly Correlated with 3D Measures of Thoracic Kyphosis. *J. Bone Jt. Surg.* **2017**, *99*, e54. [CrossRef]
33. Lonstein, J.; Carlson, J. The prediction of curve progression in untreated idiopathic scoliosis during growth Untreated of Curve Scoliosis in Growth. *J. Bone Jt. Surg.* **1984**, *66*, 1061–1071. [CrossRef]
34. Homans, J.F.; Tromp, I.N.; Colo, D.; Schlösser, T.P.C.; Kruyt, M.C.; Deeney, V.F.X.; Crowley, T.B.; McDonald-McGinn, D.M.; Castelein, R.M. Orthopaedic manifestations within the 22q11.2 Deletion syndrome: A systematic review. *Am. J. Med. Genet. Part. A* **2018**, *176*, 2104–2120. [CrossRef] [PubMed]

35. Stagi, S.; Lapi, E.; Gambineri, E.; Salti, R.; Genuardi, M.; Colarusso, G.; Conti, C.; Jenuso, R.; Chiarelli, F.; Azzari, C.; et al. Thyroid function and morphology in subjects with microdeletion of chromosome 22q11 (del(22)(q11)). *Clin. Endocrinol.* **2010**, *72*, 839–844. [CrossRef] [PubMed]
36. Cheng, J.C.; Qin, L.; Cheung, C.S.; Sher, A.H.; Lee, K.M.; Ng, S.W.; Guo, X. Generalized low areal and volumetric bone mineral density in adolescent idiopathic scoliosis. *J. Bone Miner. Res.* **2000**, *15*, 1587–1595. [CrossRef]
37. Cook, S.D.; Harding, A.F.; Morgan, E.L.; Nicholson, R.J.; Thomas, K.A.; Whitecloud, T.S.; Ratner, E.S. Trabecular bone mineral density in idiopathic scoliosis. *J. Pediatr. Orthop.* **1987**, *7*, 168–174. [CrossRef]
38. Sadat-Ali, M.; Al-Othman, A.; Bubshait, D.; Al-Dakheel, D. Does scoliosis causes low bone mass? A comparative study between siblings. *Eur. Spine J.* **2008**, *17*, 944–947. [CrossRef]
39. Burner, W.L.; Badger, V.M.; Sherman, F.C. Osteoporosis and acquired back deformities. *J. Pediatr. Orthop.* **1982**, *2*, 383–385. [CrossRef]
40. Beals, R.K.; Haglund Kenny, K.; Lees, M.H. Congenital heart disease and idiopathic scoliosis. *Clin. Orthop. Relat. Res.* **1972**, *89*, 112–116. [CrossRef]
41. Jordan, C.E.; White, R.I.; Fischer, K.C.; Neill, C.; Dorst, J.P. The scoliosis of congenital heart disease. *Am. Heart J.* **1972**, *84*, 463–469. [CrossRef]
42. Homans, J.F.; de Reuver, S.; Heung, T.; Silversides, C.K.; Oechslin, E.N.; Houben, M.L.; McDonald-McGinn, D.M.; Kruyt, M.C.; Castelein, R.M.; Bassett, A.S. The role of 22q11.2 deletion syndrome in the relationship between congenital heart disease and scoliosis. *Spine J.* **2020**, *20*, 956–963. [CrossRef] [PubMed]
43. Mirwald, R.L.; Baxter-Jones, A.D.G.; Bailey, D.A.; Beunen, G.P. An assessment of maturity from anthropometric measurements. *Med. Sci. Sports Exerc.* **2002**, *34*, 689–694. [PubMed]
44. Homans, J.F.; Schlosser, T.P.C.; Pasha, S.; Kruyt, M.; Castelein, R. Variations in the sagittal spinal profile precede the development of scoliosis: A pilot study of a new approach. *Spine J.* **2021**, *21*, 638–641. [CrossRef] [PubMed]

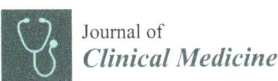

Article

Spirometry Examination of Adolescents with Thoracic Idiopathic Scoliosis: Is Correction for Height Loss Useful?

Katarzyna Politarczyk [1,*], Mateusz Kozinoga [1], Łukasz Stępniak [1], Paweł Panieński [2] and Tomasz Kotwicki [1]

1 Department of Spine Disorders and Pediatric Orthopaedics, University of Medical Sciences, 61-545 Poznan, Poland; mkozinoga@hotmail.com (M.K.); lukaszstepniak22@gmail.com (Ł.S.); kotwicki@ump.edu.pl (T.K.)
2 Department of Emergency Medicine, University of Medical Sciences, 60-355 Poznan, Poland; ppanienski@ump.edu.pl
* Correspondence: k.politarczyk@gmail.com; Tel.: +48-661-078-278

Abstract: Loss of body height is observed in patients with idiopathic scoliosis (IS) due to spine curvatures. The study compared pulmonary parameters obtained from spirometry examination considering the measured versus the corrected body height. One hundred and twenty adolescents with Lenke type 1 or 3 IS who underwent preoperative spirometry examination and radiographic evaluation were enrolled. The mean thoracic Cobb angle was 68° ± 12.6, range 48–102°. The difference between the measured and the corrected body height increased with the greater Cobb angle. Using the corrected body height instead of the measured body height significantly changed the predicted values of pulmonary parameters and influenced the interpretation of the pulmonary testing results.

Keywords: idiopathic scoliosis; body height; pulmonary function test; Cobb angle

1. Introduction

Spine and trunk alignment can be altered due to idiopathic scoliosis (IS), and this can impair pulmonary function in the case of spinal curvatures developing in the thoracic region [1]. Previous publications regarding possible factors contributing to pulmonary function impairment revealed that radiological parameters such as thoracic Cobb angle, thoracic kyphosis angle, the number of vertebrae involved and the limitation of rib cage mobility might correlate with the pulmonary parameters [2–6]. Due to spine deformity, a loss of body height is observed in patients with idiopathic scoliosis, which can be considered another factor which may impact pulmonary testing results. In previous studies, several mathematical formulas for calculating scoliosis-induced body height loss were proposed, but none are considered a gold standard [7–11]. No study comparing the impact of the application of the measured body height versus the corrected body height (defined as the sum of the measured body height and the body height loss caused by the spinal deformity) on the interpretation of the spirometry testing results was identified.

The aim of the study was to compare the pulmonary parameters revealed during spirometry examination in adolescents with thoracic idiopathic scoliosis in relation to measured versus corrected body height. The hypothesis is that using the patients' measured body height introduces a bias in the interpretation of the spirometry examination in patients with thoracic idiopathic scoliosis.

2. Materials and Methods

2.1. Study Population

Retrospective analysis of preoperative radiographs and preoperative pulmonary testing was performed in 120 adolescents (88 females and 32 males) aged 15.0 ± 1.8 years (range 12–18), who were admitted for surgical IS treatment and met the inclusion criteria:

diagnosis of IS, Lenke 1 or 3 type curve, surgical treatment, spirometry evaluation. The exclusion criteria comprised non-idiopathic scoliosis and previous surgical treatment. The Lenke 1 group consisted of 73 patients (53 girls and 20 boys), the Lenke 3 group of 47 patients (35 girls and 12 boys).

The patients' charts were analyzed according to the Lenke curve type (Lenke 1 vs. Lenke 3) and according to the thoracic Cobb angle: subgroup I. of 84 patients with thoracic Cobb angle less than 75° vs. subgroup II. of 36 patients with thoracic Cobb angle of 75° or more.

2.2. Radiological Examination

In accordance with the Cobb method [12], the thoracic and lumbar curve measurements were taken from the standing anteroposterior radiograph of the whole spine.

2.3. Corrected Body Height Calculation

The loss of body height was calculated on the basis of Stokes' formula [10]. The corrected body height was calculated as the sum of the measured body height and the loss of body height. In the case of single scoliosis (Lenke 1), the formula for calculating the loss of body height was $1.55 - 0.0471 Cobb + 0.009 Cobb^2$, while in the case of double curves (Lenke 3) the formula was $1.0 + 0.066 Cobb + 0.0084 Cobb^2$ [10].

2.4. Pulmonary Testing

Pulmonary testing (PT) was performed in a sitting position using a LungTest LT 250 spirometer (MES, Kraków, Poland). Forced Vital Capacity (FVC) and Forced Expiratory Volume in one second (FEV1) were measured 3 times. The single best effort was taken for analysis [5,13–16]. The predicted values of the pulmonary parameters, the lower limit of normal (LLN), the upper limit of normal (ULN), z-scores and percentages of the predicted values of the pulmonary parameters were calculated according to the Global Lung Function Initiative (GLI 2012) reference values, independently for the measured and the corrected body height [17].

2.5. Statistical Analysis

The mean value, standard deviation and range of the parameters were calculated using Microsoft Excel Software (Microsoft, Redmond, WA, USA). The Kolmogorov–Smirnov test was used to analyze normal data distribution. Since the parameters revealed normal distribution, Student's t-test was used to determine the significance of the differences for predicted values LLN, ULN, z-scores and percentages of the predicted values of the pulmonary parameters calculated according to the measured and the corrected body height. The correlation between the thoracic Cobb angle magnitude versus the loss of body height was calculated using Pearson's correlation coefficient.

The statistical significance level was set at $p = 0.05$. The analysis was performed with Statistica Software (TIBCO Software Inc., Palo Alto, CA, USA).

3. Results

3.1. Cobb Angle Analysis

The mean thoracic Cobb angle was 68° ± 12.6 (48–102°) for all patients. For Lenke 1 subgroup I, the thoracic Cobb angle was 60.2° ± 6.6 (48–74°); for Lenke 1 subgroup II, the thoracic Cobb angle was 82.6° ± 6.7 (75–102°). In Lenke 3 subgroup I, the thoracic Cobb angle was 63.8° ± 6.0 (50–74°); in Lenke 3 subgroup II, the thoracic Cobb angle was 87.3° ± 6.2 (76–95°).

3.2. Measured versus Corrected Body Height

The values of the measured body height, the calculated corrected body height and the calculated loss of body height are presented in Table 1.

Table 1. Comparison of the measured body height versus the calculated corrected body height.

	Thoracic Cobb Angle Range [°]	Measured Body Height [cm]	Calculated Height Loss [cm] (Stokes)	Calculated Corrected Body Height [cm]	Measured versus Corrected Body Height
		Lenke 1 and 3 types			
Subgroup I and II N = 120	48–102	164.9 ± 7.9 (145.0–185.0)	3.9 ± 1.4 (1.5–9.0)	168.8 ± 8.0 (151.3–188.5)	$p < 0.01$ *
Subgroup I N = 84	48–74	164.9 ± 7.9 (148.0–184.0)	3.1 ± 0.7 (1.5–4.7)	168.0 ± 7.8 (151.2–187.5)	$p = 0.01$ *
Subgroup II N = 36	75–102	165.0 ± 8.1 (145.0–185.0)	5.7 ± 1.2 (3.5–9.0)	170.7 ± 8.2 (151.3–188.5)	$p = 0.004$ *
		Lenke 1 type			
Subgroup I and II N = 73	48–102	165.1 ± 7.7 (145–184)	3.9 ± 1.4 (2.0–9.0)	169.0 ± 7.7 (151.2–188.0)	$p < 0.01$ *
Subgroup I N = 54	48–74	165.57 ± 9 (151.0–184.0)	3.2 ± 0.7 (2.0–4.7)	168.6 ± 7.8 (153.3–187.2)	$p < 0.01$ *
Subgroup II N = 19	75–102	163.9 ± 7.2 (145.0–182.0)	5.9 ± 1.0 (4.8–9.0)	169.9 ± 7.2 (151.2–188.0)	$p < 0.01$ *
		Lenke 3 type			
Subgroup I and II N = 47	50–95	164.7 ± 8.3 (148.0–185.0)	3.9 ± 1.4 (1.5–7.9)	168.6 ± 8.6 (151.5–188.5)	$p < 0.01$ *
Subgroup I N = 30	50–74	163.8 ± 7.8 (148.0–184.0)	3.1 ± 0.7 (1.46–4.1)	166.9 ± 7.8 (151.5–187.5)	$p < 0.01$ *
Subgroup II N = 17	76–95	166.3 ± 9.0 (149.0–185)	5.3 ± 1.2 (3.5–7.9)	171.6 ± 9.3 (152.5–189.6)	$p < 0.01$ *

All values are presented as a mean ± standard deviation, minimum and maximum in brackets. * difference statistically significant.

The body height loss was significantly higher in subgroup II patients than in subgroup I (5.7 cm vs. 3.1 cm, $p < 0.01$). For the Lenke 1 and Lenke 3 type considered separately, body height loss was also higher in subgroup II than in subgroup I (5.9 cm vs. 3.2 cm, $p < 0.01$; 5.3 cm vs. 3.1 cm, $p < 0.01$, respectively).

With the increasing Cobb angle, increased body height loss was observed, as presented in Figure 1.

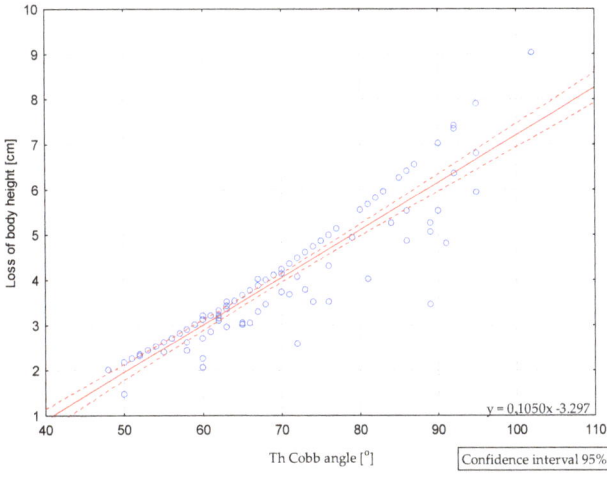

Figure 1. Thoracic Cobb angle magnitude versus loss of body height, Pearson's correlation coefficient r = 0.93, $p < 0.01$, N = 120.

3.3. Predicted Pulmonary Parameters Calculated for the Measured versus the Corrected Body Height

The predicted absolute value of FVC and FEV1, as well as the values of the LLN and ULN for each of the two pulmonary parameters (FVC and FEV1), were calculated according to the GLI 2012 reference values [17], using the measured body height and using the corrected body height, separately (Table 2), as well as within the Lenke types and the subgroups (Appendix A). All the corresponding values—the predicted values of the FVC and FEV1, LLN and ULN calculated for the FVC and FEV1—proved significantly different.

Table 2. Predicted values of the pulmonary parameters calculated (GLI 2012, [17]) for the measured versus the corrected body height, N = 120.

Parameter	FVC_m Measured Body Height	FVC_c Corrected Body Height	FVC_m vs. FVC_c p-Value
Predicted value [L]	3.83 ± 0.6	4.04 ± 0.7	$p < 0.01$ *
LLN [L]	3.09 ± 0.5	3.26 ± 0.5	$p < 0.01$ *
ULN [L]	4.59 ± 0.7	4.84 ± 0.8	$p < 0.01$ *
	$FEV1_m$ Measured Body Height	$FEV1_c$ Corrected Body Height	$FEV1_m$ vs. $FEV1_c$ p-Value
Predicted value [L]	3.36 ± 0.51	3.53 ± 0.53	$p < 0.01$ *
LLN [L]	2.70 ± 0.41	2.84 ± 0.42	$p < 0.01$ *
ULN [L]	4.00 ± 0.6	4.20 ± 0.6	$p < 0.01$ *

All values are presented as a mean ± standard deviation. FVC_m—forced vital capacity calculated for the measured body height; FVC_c—forced vital capacity calculated for the corrected body height; $FEV1_m$—forced expiratory volume in 1s calculated for the measured body height; $FEV1_c$—forced expiratory volume in 1s calculated for the corrected body height; LLN—lower limit of normal; ULN—upper limit of normal. * difference statistically significant.

3.4. Pulmonary Parameters Values Registered at Spirometry Examination

The absolute FVC and FEV1 values, followed by z-score and the percentage of the predicted normal value for FVC and FEV1, are presented in Table 3. Z-score and the percentage of the predicted normal value for FVC and FEV1 were calculated for the measured versus the corrected body height.

Table 3. The absolute FVC and FEV1 values, and values calculated for the measured vs. the corrected body height, N = 120.

Parameter	FVC 3.00 ± 0.8 L		
	FVC_m Measured Body Height	FVC_c Corrected Body Height	FVC_m vs. FVC_c p-Value
z-score	−1.83 ± 1.4	−2.19 ± 1.4	$p < 0.01$ *
%FVC	78.67 ± 16.7	74.62 ± 16.1	$p < 0.01$ *
	FEV1 2.59 ± 0.7 L		
	$FEV1_m$ Measured Body Height	$FEV1_c$ Corrected Body Height	$FEV1_m$ vs. $FEV1_c$ p-Value
z-score	−1.84 ± 1.6	−2.15 ± 1.5	$p < 0.01$ *
%FEV1	77.78 ± 18.7	74.03 ± 18.2	$p < 0.01$ *

All values are presented as a mean ± standard deviation. FVCm—forced vital capacity for the measured body height; FVCc—forced vital capacity for the corrected body height; %FVC—percentage of the predicted FVC value; FEV1m—forced expiratory volume in 1s for the measured body height; FEV1c—forced expiratory volume in 1s for the corrected body height, %FEV1—percentage of the predicted FEV1 value. * difference statistically significant.

3.5. Comparison of the Pulmonary Parameters in Subgroup I versus Subgroup II

The predicted absolute value of FVC and FEV1, as well as the values of LLN and ULN for each of the pulmonary parameters (FVC, FEV1), were calculated using the measured body height and using the corrected body height in subgroup I and subgroup II in Lenke 1 and Lenke 3 types, separately (Table A1), in Lenke 1 type (Table A2) and in Lenke 3 type (Table A3). All the corresponding values- the predicted values of the FVC and FEV1, LLN, and ULN calculated for the FVC and FEV1- proved significantly different.

The absolute FVC and FEV1 values, followed by z-score and the percentage of the predicated value of FVC and FEV1 for both subgroups calculated for the measured versus corrected body height, are presented in Table A4.

The FVC absolute values were not significantly different in both subgroups ($p = 0.14$); however, the absolute value of FEV1 was significantly lower in patients with a greater Cobb angle ($p = 0.04$).

The %FVC calculated for the corrected body height and %FEV1 values calculated for the measured and the corrected body height were significantly lower in subgroup II than in subgroup I ($p = 0.02; p = 0.04, p = 0.01$, respectively). Additionally, the FVC and FEV1 z-score values calculated for the corrected body height were significantly lower in subgroup II than subgroup I ($p = 0.01; p = 0.01$, respectively).

The absolute FVC and FEV1 values, as well as the z-score values and the percentages of the predicted values of both parameters calculated in subgroup I and subgroup II using the measured versus corrected body height in Lenke 1 type patients are presented in Table A5.

The absolute values of FVC and FEV1 were lower in subgroup II than in subgroup I patients, but the difference was not significant ($p = 0.58; p = 0.82$, respectively).

Significantly lower values of %FVC and %FEV1 were observed in subgroup II patients than in subgroup I when calculated for both the measured and the corrected body height values ($p = 0.04; p = 0.009; p = 0.02; p = 0.006$, respectively). Additionally, FVC and FEV1 z-score values proved significantly lower in patients with a greater Cobb angle when calculated using the measured and the corrected body height ($p = 0.04; p = 0.008; p = 0.03; p = 0.008$, respectively).

The absolute FVC and FEV1 values, as well as the z-score values and the percentages of the predicted values of both parameters calculated in subgroup I and subgroup II using the measured versus corrected body height in Lenke 3 type patients are presented in Table A6.

In Lenke 3 type, the differences in absolute FVC, FEV1 values were not significant in subgroup II versus subgroup I ($p = 0.20; p = 0.13$, respectively).

Additionally, in Lenke 3 type, the values of the %FVC and %FEV1 parameters were lower in subgroup II than in subgroup I when calculated for the measured and the corrected body height; however, the differences were not significant ($p = 0.89; p = 0.56; p = 0.81; p = 0.52$, respectively). Additionally, the FVC and FEV1 z-score values proved not significantly different when comparing subgroup I versus subgroup II ($p = 0.84; p = 0.51; p = 0.85; p = 0.85$, respectively).

An example of a different interpretation of the result of spirometry testing is shown in Figure A1.

4. Discussion

Spirometry is an examination that allows us to assess pulmonary function in patients with IS. Regular pulmonary testing allows to recognize pulmonary impairment, even though it may not be clinically evident until severe or irreversible changes have occur [18]. Even though spirometry cannot replace body plethysmography for diagnosing the restrictive patterns that occur in patients with idiopathic scoliosis, it may indicate their presence and suggest a need for further examination [19,20]. On the other hand, spirometry is recommended for diagnosing the obturation patterns which are less common in IS [19–22]. Loss of body height is observed in all patients with moderate or severe idiopathic scoliosis—the greater the Cobb angle, the higher the body height loss. Several methods have been proposed to replace the misleadingly low measured body height during pulmonary function testing.

Hepper et al. [23] observed that body height is correlated with arm span. The authors evaluated pulmonary parameters in patients with kyphoscoliosis using body height calculated from arm span. Using arm span instead of measured body height was recommended for calculating pulmonary parameters in patients with spinal deformities [24]. However, the arm span: body height ratio depends on age and gender [24–26]. Furthermore, arm span may be lower than predicted due to the trunk asymmetry caused by spinal deformity [27].

Several factors were previously identified as determinants contributing to body height loss due to idiopathic scoliosis: Cobb angle magnitude, curvature length and the number of vertebrae involved in the curve [7–10]. In previous studies, authors presented regression equations based on the Cobb angle values that may be used to calculate body height loss [7–10,28].

Tyrakowski et al. [11] compared four methods—Bjure, Stokes, Kono and Ylikoski—and concluded that none of them could be recommended as most valid. On the other hand, Gardner et al. [29], comparing five methods—Bjure, Stokes, Kono, Ylikoski and Hwang—concluded that the Kono and Stokes methods were the most valid in determining height loss in patients with idiopathic scoliosis.

Our preliminary study in 39 IS patients (29 girls and 10 boys) aged 12–17 with the mean thoracic Cobb angle 69.8° ± 12.4° (50–104°) showed that corrected body height was significantly higher than measured body height ($p = 0.01$) [30]. The impact of body height loss on the interpretation of the spirometry testing is based on the fact that the predicted reference values are calculated for every individual patient considering age, gender, body height and ethnicity. From these data, the predicted values are generated by means of the GLI 2012 regression equations using spirometry equipment software or the GLI 2012 software. Changing one component value—body height—the predicted values of the pulmonary parameters change accordingly. For example, in a 13-year-old girl, the application of the corrected body height (172.2 cm) instead of the measured one (168.0 cm) into the regression equation results in a 5.46% difference in the FVC predicted value (3.89 L vs. 3.67 L) and 5.26% difference in the FEV1 predicted value (3.40 L vs. 3.23 L; Appendix B).

Weinstein et al. [2] concluded that pulmonary parameters—FVC and FEV1—significantly correlate with the thoracic Cobb angle magnitude. The pulmonary parameters decreased when the thoracic Cobb angle value got close to 100°–120°. However, later observations suggested that pulmonary impairment was observed in patients with smaller curves [3,5,31]. In our study, the absolute value of FEV1 ($p = 0.04$) but not FVC ($p = 0.16$) was significantly lower in patients with a greater Cobb angle (Cobb > 75°). Meanwhile, when the spirometry absolute values are transformed into percentages of the predicted values, the impact of the body height correction appears evident. In adolescents with a Cobb angle > 75°, the %FVC$_c$, %FEV1$_m$ and %FEV1$_c$ values were lower than in those with a Cobb angle < 75° ($p = 0.02$; $p = 0.04$, $p = 0.01$, respectively).

In clinical practice, the absolute values of spirometry parameters are less useful for evaluating the patient's pulmonary status, so clinicians rely more on the percentages of the values predicted for a given gender, age and height. The calculation of the predicted values is automatically offered by spirometry equipment software. The modification of one component—body height—does impact the calculation of the predicted values. In consequence, one absolute value measured in liters may be interpreted differently due to different reference values. This study confirmed the discrepancy of the predicted FVC and FEV1 values depending on the height parameter introduced for calculation (measured vs. corrected). As body height loss increases with the Cobb angle, the discrepancy becomes significant in severe curves, over 75 Cobb degrees.

In previous studies of IS patients, the pulmonary parameters used to be interpreted using the threshold of 80% as the lower limit of normal predicted value, in accordance with the recommendation made by Bates and Christie [32]. The American Thoracic Society and European Respiratory Society recommend the 5th percentile as an LLN (z-score −1.64) [21,33,34]. The z-score value indicates by how many standard deviations a particular measurement is situated from the predicted value. Contrary to the percentage of the predicted value, the z-score parameter is not biased due to age, gender or ethnic group, and seems more useful for defining the LLN [17]. In Lenke 1 type subgroup I, the z-score values of FVC and FEV1 calculated for the measured body height indicated that the results were within the normal limits. However, when the z-score values of FVC and FEV1 were calculated for the corrected body height, the results were below the normal limits (−1.54 vs. −1.84; −1.51 vs. −1.78, respectively). Replacing the measured body height with the corrected body height can also change the classification of the severity of the pulmonary impairment. In subgroup II, the %FVC and %FEV1 calculated from the measured body height indicated a mild pulmonary impairment, but when the corrected body height was used, the interpretation changed to a moderate impairment [20].

A limitation of the study was that the study group consisted solely of patients with Lenke 1 or 3 type scoliosis. Another limitation is that the group contained both girls and boys.

5. Conclusions

Increasing height loss is observed with an increasing Cobb angle in adolescents with thoracic idiopathic scoliosis. Predicted spirometry reference values change significantly in proportion to a change in body height. At spirometry examination, the interpretation of the results of the pulmonary functional testing is affected by body height loss. Use of the corrected body height instead of the measured one can be seriously considered in severe thoracic curvatures over a 75 degree Cobb angle.

Author Contributions: Conceptualization, K.P., M.K. and T.K.; methodology, K.P., M.K., Ł.S. and T.K.; software, K.P. and Ł.S.; formal analysis, K.P., M.K., Ł.S., P.P. and T.K.; investigation, K.P. and Ł.S.; data curation, K.P., M.K. and Ł.S.; resources K.P., M.K. and P.P., writing—original draft preparation, K.P., M.K., Ł.S.; writing—review and editing, K.P., M.K., Ł.S., P.P. and T.K.; supervision, T.K. All authors have read and agreed to the published version of the manuscript.

Funding: This research received no external funding.

Institutional Review Board Statement: Not applicable.

Informed Consent Statement: Not applicable.

Data Availability Statement: The data presented in the study are available on request from the corresponding author.

Conflicts of Interest: The authors declare no conflict of interest.

Appendix A

Table A1. Comparison of the predicted values of the pulmonary parameters calculated (GLI 2012, [17]) for the measured versus the corrected body height in subgroup I, N = 84, and subgroup II, N = 36.

Parameter	Subgroup I			Subgroup II		
	FVC_m Measured Body Height	FVC_c Corrected Body Height	FVC_m vs. FVC_c p-Value	FVC_m Measured Body Height	FVC_c Corrected Body Height	FVC_m vs. FVC_c p-Value
Predicted value (L)	3.83 ± 0.6	4.00 ± 0.6	$p < 0.01$ *	3.82 ± 0.6	4.13 ± 0.7	$p < 0.01$ *
LLN (L)	3.09 ± 0.5	3.23 ± 0.5	$p < 0.01$ *	3.08 ± 0.5	3.34 ± 0.6	$p < 0.01$ *
ULN (L)	4.59 ± 0.7	4.80 ± 0.7	$p < 0.01$ *	4.57 ± 0.7	4.95 ± 0.8	$p < 0.01$ *
	$FEV1_m$ Measured Body Height	$FEV1_c$ Corrected Body Height	$FEV1_m$ vs. $FEV1_c$ p-Value	$FEV1_m$ Measured Body Height	$FEV1_c$ Corrected Body Height	$FEV1_m$ vs. $FEV1_c$ p-Value
Predicted value (L)	3.36 ± 0.6	3.50 ± 0.5	$p < 0.01$ *	3.34 ± 0.5	3.59 ± 0.5	$p < 0.01$ *
LLN (L)	2.70 ± 0.4	2.82 ± 0.5	$p < 0.01$ *	2.69 ± 0.4	2.89 ± 0.4	$p < 0.01$ *
ULN (L)	4.00 ± 0.7	4.17 ± 0.6	$p < 0.01$ *	3.98 ± 0.6	4.28 ± 0.6	$p < 0.01$ *

All values are presented as a mean ± standard deviation. FVCm—forced vital capacity for the measured body height; FVCc—forced vital capacity for the corrected body height; FEV1m—forced expiratory volume in 1 s for the measured body height; FEV1c—forced expiratory volume in 1s for the corrected body height; LLN—lower limit of normal; ULN—upper limit of normal. * difference statistically significant.

Table A2. Comparison of the predicted values of the pulmonary parameters calculated (GLI 2012, [17]) for the measured versus the corrected body height in subgroup I, N = 54, and subgroup II, N = 19, Lenke 1 type.

Parameter	Subgroup I			Subgroup II		
	FVC_m Measured Body Height	FVC_c Corrected Body Height	FVC_m vs. FVC_c p-Value	FVC_m Measured Body Height	FVC_c Corrected Body Height	FVC_m vs. FVC_c p-Value
Predicted value (L)	3.88 ± 0.6	4.05 ± 0.6	$p < 0.01$ *	3.74 ± 0.5	4.06 ± 0.6	$p < 0.01$ *
LLN (L)	3.13 ± 0.5	3.27 ± 0.5	$p < 0.01$ *	3.02 ± 0.4	3.27 ± 0.5	$p < 0.01$ *
ULN (L)	4.65 ± 0.7	4.86 ± 0.7	$p < 0.01$ *	4.49 ± 0.6	4.87 ± 0.7	$p < 0.01$ *
	$FEV1_m$ Measured Body Height	$FEV1_c$ Corrected Body Height	$FEV1_m$ vs. $FEV1_c$ p-Value	$FEV1_m$ Measured Body Height	$FEV1_c$ Corrected Body Height	$FEV1_m$ vs. $FEV1_c$ p-Value
Predicted value (L)	3.40 ± 0.5	3.54 ± 0.5	$p < 0.01$ *	3.29 ± 0.4	3.55 ± 0.5	$p < 0.01$ *
LLN (L)	2.73 ± 0.4	2.85 ± 0.4	$p < 0.01$ *	2.65 ± 0.4	2.86 ± 0.4	$p < 0.01$ *
ULN (L)	4.05 ± 0.6	4.21 ± 0.6	$p < 0.01$ *	3.91 ± 0.5	4.22 ± 0.6	$p < 0.01$ *

All values are presented as a mean ± standard deviation. FVCm—forced vital capacity for the measured body height; FVCc—forced vital capacity for the corrected body height; FEV1m—forced expiratory volume in 1 s for the measured body height; FEV1c—forced expiratory volume in 1s for the corrected body height; LLN—lower limit of normal; ULN—upper limit of normal. * difference statistically significant.

Table A3. Comparison of the predicted values of the pulmonary parameters calculated (GLI 2012, [17]) for the measured versus the corrected body height in subgroup I, N = 30, and subgroup II, N = 17, in Lenke 3 type patients.

Parameter	Subgroup I			Subgroup II		
	FVC_m Measured Body Height	FVC_c Corrected Body Height	FVC_m vs. FVC_c p-Value	FVC_m Measured Body Height	FVC_c Corrected Body Height	FVC_m vs. FVC_c p-Value
Predicted value (L)	3.75 ± 0.7	3.91 ± 0.7	$p < 0.01$ *	3.92 ± 0.7	4.22 ± 0.8	$p < 0.01$ *
LLN (L)	3.02 ± 0.5	3.15 ± 0.6	$p < 0.01$ *	3.17 ± 0.6	3.41 ± 0.6	$p < 0.01$ *
ULN (L)	4.50 ± 0.8	4.69 ± 0.8	$p < 0.01$ *	4.68 ± 0.8	5.04 ± 0.9	$p < 0.01$ *
	$FEV1_m$ Measured Body Height	$Fev1_c$ Corrected Body Height	$FEV1_m$ vs. $FEV1_c$ p-Value	$FEV1_m$ Measured Body Height	$FEV1_c$ Corrected Body Height	$FEV1_m$ vs. $FEV1_c$ p-Value
Predicted value (L)	3.30 ± 0.5	3.43 ± 0.6	$p < 0.01$ *	3.40 ± 0.6	3.64 ± 0.6	$p < 0.01$ *
LLN (L)	2.66 ± 0.4	2.76 ± 0.4	$p < 0.01$ *	2.73 ± 0.5	2.92 ± 0.5	$p < 0.01$ *
ULN (L)	3.92 ± 0.6	4.09 ± 0.7	$p < 0.01$ *	4.05 ± 0.7	4.34 ± 0.7	$p < 0.01$ *

All values are presented as a mean ± standard deviation. FVCm—forced vital capacity for the measured body height; FVCc—forced vital capacity for the corrected body height; FEV1m—forced expiratory volume in 1 s for the measured body height; FEV1c—forced expiratory volume in 1s for the corrected body height; LLN—lower limit of normal; ULN—upper limit of normal. * difference statistically significant.

Table A4. Comparison of the pulmonary parameters calculated for the measured versus the corrected body height in subgroup I, N = 84 and subgroup II, N = 36.

Parameter	Subgroup I			Subgroup II		
	FVC 3.07 ± 0.7 L			FVC 2.85 ± 0.8 L		
	FVC_m Measured Body Height	FVC_c Corrected Body Height	FVC_m vs. FVC_c p−Value	FVC_m Measured Body Height	FVC_c Corrected Body Height	FVC_m vs. FVC_c p−Value
z-score	−1.69 ± 1.4	−1.98 ± 1.3	$p < 0.01$ *	−2.18 ± 1.6	−2.67 ± 1.4	$p < 0.01$ *
%FVC	80.30 ± 16.0	76.89 ± 15.4	$p < 0.01$ *	74.87 ± 17.8	69.31 ± 16.8	$p < 0.01$ *
	FEV1 2.67 ± 0.7 L			FEV1 2.41 ± 0.6 L		
	$FEV1_m$ Measured Body Height	$FEV1_c$ Corrected Body Height	$FEV1_m$ vs. $FEV1_c$ p-Value	$FEV1_m$ Measured Body Height	$FEV1_c$ Corrected Body Height	$FEV1_m$ vs. $FEV1_c$ p-Value
z-score	−1.66 ± 1.8	−1.92 ± 1.5	$p < 0.01$ *	−2.26 ± 1.5	−2.67 ± 1.4	$p < 0.01$ *
%FEV1	79.90 ± 22.1	76.81 ± 17.7	$p < 0.01$ *	72.61 ± 18.9	67.56 ± 17.7	$p < 0.01$ *

All values are presented as a mean ± standard deviation. FVCm—forced vital capacity for the measured body height; FVCc—forced vital capacity for the corrected body height; %FVC—percentage of the predicted FVC value; FEV1m—forced expiratory volume in 1s for the measured body height; FEV1c—forced expiratory volume in 1 s for the corrected body height, %FEV1—percentage of the predicted FEV1 value. * difference statistically significant.

Table A5. Comparison of the pulmonary parameters calculated for the measured versus the corrected body height in subgroup I, N = 54 and subgroup II, N = 19, Lenke 1 type.

	Subgroup I			Subgroup II		
Parameter	FVC 3.07 ± 0.8 L			FVC 2.95 ± 0.7 L		
	FVC_m Measured Body Height	FVC_c Corrected Body Height	FVC_m vs. FVC_c p-Value	FVC_m Measured Body Height	FVC_c Corrected Body Height	FVC_m vs. FVC_c p-Value
z-score	−1.54 ± 1.3	−1.84 ± 1.2	$p < 0.01$ *	−2.30 ± 1.7	−2.80 ± 1.6	$p < 0.01$ *
%FVC	82.01 ± 14.6	78.49 ± 14.0	$p < 0.01$ *	73.41 ± 19.4	67.73 ± 18.2	$p < 0.01$ *
	FEV1 2.66 ± 0.7 L			FEV1 2.62 ± 0.6 L		
	$FEV1_m$ Measured Body Height	$FEV1_c$ Corrected Body Height	$FEV1_m$ vs. $FEV1_c$ p-Value	$FEV1_m$ Measured Body Height	$FEV1_c$ Corrected Body Height	$FEV1_m$ vs. $FEV1_c$ p-Value
z-score	−1.51 ± 1.6	−1.78 ± 1.2	$p < 0.01$ *	−2.48 ± 1.5	−2.89 ± 1.4	$p < 0.01$ *
%FEV1	81.79 ± 19.3	78.51 ± 18.5	$p < 0.01$ *	70.02 ± 18.6	64.93 ± 17.6	$p < 0.01$ *

All values are presented as a mean ± standard deviation. FVCm—forced vital capacity for the measured body height; FVCc—forced vital capacity for the corrected body height; %FVC—percentage of the predicted FVC value; FEV1m—forced expiratory volume in 1s for the measured body height; FEV1c—forced expiratory volume in 1 s for the corrected body height, %FEV1—percentage of the predicted FEV1 value. * difference statistically significant.

Table A6. Comparison of the pulmonary parameters calculated for the measured versus the corrected body height in subgroup I, N = 30 and subgroup II, N = 17 in Lenke 3 type patients.

	Subgroup I			Subgroup II		
Parameter	FVC 3.07 ± 0.7 L			FVC 2.78 ± 0.7 L		
	FVC_m Measured Body Height	FVC_c Corrected Body Height	FVC_m vs. FVC_c p-Value	FVC_m Measured Body Height	FVC_c Corrected Body Height	FVC_m vs. FVC_c p-Value
z-score	−1.96 ± 1.5	−2.23 ± 1.5	$p < 0.01$ *	−2.05 ± 1.4	−2.5 ± 1.4	$p < 0.01$ *
%FVC	77.23 ± 18.2	74.02 ± 17.5	$p < 0.01$ *	76.5 ± 16.3	71.09 ± 15.3	$p < 0.01$ *
	FEV1 2.59 ± 0.6 L			FEV1 2.32 ± 0.6 L		
	$FEV1_m$ Measured Body Height	$FEV1_c$ Corrected Body Height	$FEV1_m$ vs. $FEV1_c$ p-Value	$FEV1_m$ Measured Body Height	$FEV1_c$ Corrected body height	$FEV1_m$ vs. $FEV1_c$ p-value
z-score	−1.94 ± 1.4	−2.18 ± 1.3	$p < 0.01$ *	−2.02 ± 1.6	−2.43 ± 1.5	$p < 0.01$ *
%FEV1	76.77 ± 16.8	73.76 ± 16.1	$p < 0.01$ *	75.5 ± 19.3	70.49 ± 18.0	$p < 0.01$ *

All values are presented as a mean ± standard deviation. FVCm—forced vital capacity for the measured body height; FVCc—forced vital capacity for the corrected body height; %FVC—percentage of the predicted FVC value; FEV1m—forced expiratory volume in 1s for the measured body height; FEV1c—forced expiratory volume in 1 s for the corrected body height, %FEV1—percentage of the predicted FEV1 value. * difference statistically significant.

Appendix B

Example of a patient presenting a discrepancy in the interpretation of spirometry testing due to body height.

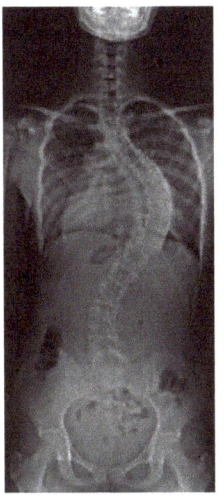

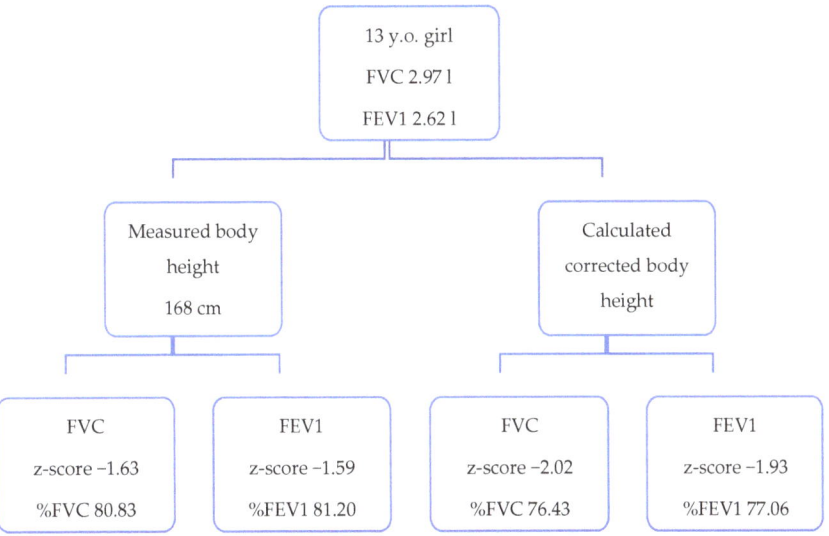

Figure A1. Example of a patient presenting a discrepancy in the interpretation of spirometry testing. A case of a 13-year-old girl with right idiopathic thoracic scoliosis, Cobb angle 70°. The pulmonary parameters are within the norm when the normal values are calculated for the measured body height. The parameters suggest a mild impairment of pulmonary function when calculated using the corrected body height.

References

1. Weinstein, S.L. Natural history. *Spine* **1999**, *24*, 2592–2600. [CrossRef] [PubMed]
2. Weinstein, S.L.; Zavala, D.C.; Ponseti, I.V. Idiopathic scoliosis: Long-term follow-up and prognosis in untreated patients. *J. Bone Jt. Surg. Am.* **1981**, *63*, 702–712. [CrossRef]

3. Johnston, C.E.; Richards, B.S.; Sucato, D.J.; Bridwell, K.H.; Lenke, L.G.; Erickson, M.; Spinal Deformity Study Group. Correlation of preoperative deformity magnitude and pulmonary function tests in adolescent idiopathic scoliosis. *Spine* **2011**, *36*, 1096–1102. [CrossRef] [PubMed]
4. Kearon, C.; Viviani, G.R.; Kirkley, A.; Killian, K.J. Factors determining pulmonary function in adolescent idiopathic thoracic scoliosis. *Am. Rev. Respir. Dis.* **1993**, *148*, 288–294. [CrossRef]
5. Newton, P.O.; Faro, F.D.; Gollogly, S.; Betz, R.R.; Lenke, L.G.; Lowe, T.G. Results of preoperative pulmonary function testing of adolescents with idiopathic scoliosis. A study of six hundred and thirty-one patients. *J. Bone Jt. Surg. Am.* **2005**, *87*, 1937–1946. [CrossRef]
6. Kotani, T.; Minami, S.; Takahashi, K.; Isobe, K.; Nakata, Y.; Takaso, M.; Inoue, M.; Maruta, T.; Akazawa, T.; Ueda, T.; et al. An analysis of chest wall and diaphragm motions in patients with idiopathic scoliosis using dynamic breathing MRI. *Spine* **2004**, *29*, 298–302. [CrossRef] [PubMed]
7. Bjure, J.; Grimby, G.; Nachemson, A. Correction of body height in predicting spirometric values in scoliotic patients. *Scand. J. Clin. Lab. Investig.* **1968**, *21*, 191–192. [CrossRef]
8. Kono, K.; Asazuma, T.; Suzuki, N.; Ono, T. Body height correction in scoliosis patients for pulmonary function test. *J. Orthop. Surg.* **2000**, *8*, 19–26. [CrossRef] [PubMed]
9. Ylikoski, M. Height of girls with adolescent idiopathic scoliosis. *Eur. Spine J.* **2003**, *12*, 288–291. [CrossRef]
10. Stokes, I.A. Stature and growth compensation for spinal curvature. *Stud. Health Technol. Inform.* **2008**, *140*, 48–51.
11. Tyrakowski, M.; Kotwicki, T.; Czubak, J.; Siemionow, K. Calculation of corrected body height in idiopathic scoliosis: Comparison of four methods. *Eur. Spine J* **2014**, *23*, 1244–1250. [CrossRef] [PubMed]
12. Cobb, J.R. Outline for the study of scoliosis. *Instr. Course Lect.* **1948**, *5*, 261–275.
13. Miller, M.R.; Hankinson, J.; Brusasco, V.; Burgos, F.; Casaburi, R.; Coates, A.; Crapo, R.; Enright, P.; van der Grinten, C.P.; Gustafsson, P.; et al. Standardisation of spirometry. *Eur. Respir. J.* **2005**, *26*, 319–338. [CrossRef] [PubMed]
14. Kim, Y.J.; Lenke, L.G.; Bridwell, K.H.; Kim, K.L.; Steger-May, K. Pulmonary function in adolescent idiopathic scoliosis relative to the surgical procedure. *J. Bone Jt. Surg. Am.* **2005**, *87*, 1534–1541.
15. Kim, Y.J.; Lenke, L.G.; Bridwell, K.H.; Cheh, G.; Whorton, J.; Sides, B. Prospective pulmonary function comparison following posterior segmental spinal instrumentation and fusion of adolescent idiopathic scoliosis: Is there a relationship between major thoracic curve correction and pulmonary function test improvement? *Spine* **2007**, *32*, 2685–2693. [CrossRef] [PubMed]
16. Vedantam, R.; Lenke, L.G.; Bridwell, K.H.; Haas, J.; Linville, D.A. A prospective evaluation of pulmonary function in patients with adolescent idiopathic scoliosis relative to the surgical approach used for spinal arthrodesis. *Spine* **2000**, *25*, 82–90. [CrossRef]
17. Quanjer, P.H.; Stanojevic, S.; Cole, T.J.; Baur, X.; Hall, G.L.; Culver, B.H.; Enright, P.L.; Hankinson, J.L.; Ip, M.S.M.; Zheng, J.; et al. Multi-ethnic reference values for spirometry for the 3–95-yr age range: The global lung function 2012 equations. *Eur. Res. J.* **2012**, *40*, 1324–1343. [CrossRef]
18. Tsiligiannis, T.; Grivas, T. Pulmonary function in children with idiopathic scoliosis. *Scoliosis* **2012**, *7*, 7. [CrossRef]
19. McMaster, M.J.; Glasby, M.A.; Singh, H.; Cunningham, S. Lung function in congenital kyphosis and kyphoscoliosis. *J. Spinal Disord. Tech.* **2007**, *20*, 203–208. [CrossRef]
20. American Thoracic Society. Lung function testing: Selection of reference values and interpretative strategies. *Am. Rev. Respir. Dis.* **1991**, *144*, 1202–1218. [CrossRef]
21. Borowitz, D.; Armstrong, D.; Cerny, F. Relief of central airways obstruction following spinal release in a patient with idiopathic scoliosis. *Pediatr. Pulmonol.* **2001**, *31*, 86–88. [CrossRef]
22. Bartlett, W.; Garrido, E.; Wallis, C.; Tucker, S.K.; Noordeen, H. Lordoscoliosis and large intrathoracic airway obstruction. *Spine* **2009**, *34*, 59–65. [CrossRef] [PubMed]
23. Hepper, N.G.; Black, L.F.; Fowler, W.S. Relationships of lung volume to height and arm span in normal subjects and in patients with spinal deformity. *Am. Rev. Respir. Dis.* **1965**, *91*, 356–362. [CrossRef] [PubMed]
24. Miller, M.R.; Crapo, R.; Hankinson, J.; Brusasco, V.; Burgos, F.; Casaburi, R.; Coates, A.; Enright, P.; van der Grinten, C.P.M.; Gustafsson, P.; et al. General considerations for lung function testing. *Eur. Respir. J.* **2005**, *26*, 153–161. [CrossRef] [PubMed]
25. Golshan, M.; Crapo, R.O.; Jensen, R.L.; Golshan, R. Arm span as an independent predictor of pulmonary function parameters: Validation and reference values. *Respirology* **2007**, *12*, 361–366. [CrossRef]
26. Johnson, B.E.; Westgate, H.D. Methods of predicting vital capacity in patients with thoracic scoliosis. *J. Bone Jt. Surg. Am.* **1970**, *52*, 1433–1439. [CrossRef]
27. Linderholm, H.; Lindgren, U. Prediction of spirometric values in patients with scoliosis. *Acta Orthop. Scand.* **1978**, *49*, 469–474. [CrossRef]
28. Shi, B.; Mao, S.; Xu, L.; Sun, X.; Liu, Z.; Cheng, J.C.Y.; Zhu, Z.; Qiu, Y. Accurate prediction of height loss in adolescent idiopathic scoliosis: Cobb angle alone is insufficient. *Eur. Spine J.* **2016**, *25*, 3341–3346. [CrossRef]
29. Gardner, A.; Price, A.; Berryman, F.; Pynsent, P. The use of growth standards and corrective formulae to calculate the height loss caused by idiopathic scoliosis. *Scoliosis Spinal Disord.* **2016**, *26*, 6. [CrossRef]
30. Politarczyk, K.; Stępniak, Ł.; Kozinoga, M.; Czaprowski, D.; Kotwicki, T. Loss of the body height due to severe thoracic curvature does impact pulmonary testing results in adolescents with idiopathic scoliosis. *Stud. Health Technol. Inform.* **2021**, *280*, 231–234.

31. Politarczyk, K.; Janusz, P.; Stępniak, Ł.; Kozinoga, M.; Kotwicki, T. Relationship between radiological parameters and preoperative pulmonary function in adolescents with idiopathic scoliosis—Preliminary study. *Issue Rehabil. Orthop. Neurophysiol. Sport Promot.* **2019**, *28*, 7–14.
32. Bates, D.V.; Christie, R.V. *Respiratory Function in Disease*; Saunders: Philadelphia, PA, USA, 1964; p. 9.
33. Quanjer, P.H.; Tammeling, G.J.; Cotes, J.E.; Pedersen, O.F.; Peslin, R.; Yernault, J.C. Lung volumes and forced ventilatory flows. *Eur. Respir. J.* **1993**, *6*, 5–40. [CrossRef] [PubMed]
34. Pellegrino, R.; Viegi, G.; Brusasco, V.; Crapo, R.O.; Burgos, F.; Casaburi, R.; Coates, A.; van der Grinten, C.P.M.; Gustafsson, P.; Hankinson, J.; et al. Interpretative strategies for lung function tests. *Eur. Respir. J.* **2005**, *26*, 948–968. [CrossRef] [PubMed]

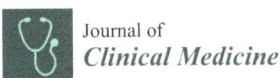

Article

Potential Muscle-Related Biomarkers in Predicting Curve Progression to the Surgical Threshold in Adolescent Idiopathic Scoliosis—A Pilot Proteomic Study Comparing Four Non-Progressive vs. Four Progressive Patients vs. A Control Cohort

Yujia Wang [1,2], Huanxiong Chen [1,3], Jiajun Zhang [1], Tsz-ping Lam [1], A.L.H. Hung [1], J.C.Y. Cheng [1,*] and W.Y.W. Lee [1,2,*]

1 Department of Orthopaedics and Traumatology, SH Ho Scoliosis Research Laboratory, Joint Scoliosis Research Center of the Chinese University of Hong Kong and Nanjing University, The Chinese University of Hong Kong, Hong Kong 999077, China; wangyujia716@foxmail.com (Y.W.); chenhuanxiong@hainmc.edu.cn (H.C.); zhangjiajun1@genomics.cn (J.Z.); tplam@cuhk.edu.hk (T.-p.L.); lhhung@ort.cuhk.edu.hk (A.H.)
2 Li Ka Shing Institute of Health Sciences, The Chinese University of Hong Kong, Hong Kong 999077, China
3 Department of Spine and Osteopathic Surgery, The First Affiliated Hospital of Hainan Medical University, Haikou 570102, China
* Correspondence: jackcheng@cuhk.edu.hk (J.C.); waynelee@cuhk.edu.hk (W.L.); Tel.: +852-24716706 (W.L.)

Abstract: Previous studies have reported abnormal muscle morphology and functions in patients with adolescent idiopathic scoliosis (AIS). To answer whether such abnormalities could be reflected in their circulation and their clinical implication for predicting curve progression to the surgical threshold, this preliminary study explored the presence of baseline muscle-related proteins and their association with curve progression. Plasma samples were collected at the first clinical visit for AIS, with patients divided into non-progressive or progressive groups (N = four and four) according to their Cobb angle in six-year follow-ups, with age- and sex-matched healthy subjects (N = 50). Then, the samples were subjected to isobaric tags for relative and absolute quantitation (iTRAQ) for global comparison of untargeted protein expression. Seventy-one differentially expressed proteins (DEPs) were found elevated in progressive AIS. Functional analysis showed that 18 of these are expressed in muscles and play an essential role in muscle activities. Among the muscle-related DEPs, α-actin had the highest fold change in progressive/non-progressive groups. This preliminary study firstly suggested higher circulating levels of muscle structural proteins in progressive AIS, indicating the likelihood of structural damage at the microscopic level and its association with progression to the surgical threshold. Further studies with larger sample sizes are warranted to validate these novel candidates for early diagnosis and predicting progression.

Keywords: scoliosis; iTRAQ; α-actin; progressive; differentially expressed proteins

Citation: Wang, Y.; Chen, H.; Zhang, J.; Lam, T.-p.; Hung, A.L.H.; Cheng, J.C.Y.; Lee, W.Y.W. Potential Muscle-Related Biomarkers in Predicting Curve Progression to the Surgical Threshold in Adolescent Idiopathic Scoliosis—A Pilot Proteomic Study Comparing Four Non-Progressive vs. Four Progressive Patients vs. A Control Cohort. *J. Clin. Med.* **2021**, *10*, 4927. https://doi.org/10.3390/jcm10214927

Academic Editors: Han Jo Kim and Hiroyuki Katoh

Received: 22 August 2021
Accepted: 17 October 2021
Published: 25 October 2021

Publisher's Note: MDPI stays neutral with regard to jurisdictional claims in published maps and institutional affiliations.

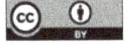

Copyright: © 2021 by the authors. Licensee MDPI, Basel, Switzerland. This article is an open access article distributed under the terms and conditions of the Creative Commons Attribution (CC BY) license (https://creativecommons.org/licenses/by/4.0/).

1. Introduction

Adolescent idiopathic scoliosis (AIS) is the most common type of three-dimensional structural deformity occurring during the puberty growth period, with a prevalence of 1~4% worldwide. AIS is more prevalent in girls than in boys [1]. For example, a five-year idiopathic scoliosis screening program of 255,875 children aged 11~14 years old in Japan reported that the prevalent ratio of girls to boys was 11:1 [2]. Our local scoliosis study on 115,190 fifth grade children indicated that the prevalence ratio of girls to boys with a Cobb angle ≥10° was 2.7 by the age of 19 years, and the ratio increased to 4.5 and 8.1 with a Cobb angle ≥20° and ≥40°, respectively [3]. Unlike congenital, neuromuscular, and other types of scoliosis, the etiopathogenesis of AIS is largely unknown [1]. Bracing is an evidence-based effective treatment for patients with a Cobb angle ≥20° by means of preventing curve progression [4]. However, wearing braces could cause a negative cosmetic appearance, poor self-esteem, and functional discomfort [5], resulting in insufficient wearing time and thus affecting the effectiveness of this treatment. Those that develop a Cobb angle of major curve >40~45° in the thoracolumbar region, or >50° in the thoracic region, might accept invasive surgery to correct the anatomical deformation and to reduce the risk of further progression during adulthood. However, the potential complications of surgery, including partial or complete loss of neurological function, infection, implant failure or pseudoarthrosis, recurrence, or additional deformity, should be carefully taken into consideration [1]. Current understanding of the etiopathogenesis is limited. Investigation on unexplored areas is worthwhile to develop more effective prognostication and treatment.

AIS patients have been reported to have weaker muscle strength than healthy subjects of a similar age and sex [6,7]. Decreased respiratory muscle strength in patients with AIS has been described in pulmonary function studies [6,8]. The posterior paraspinal muscles, including the multifidus and erector spinal muscle, provide dynamic stability to the spinal column [9], and its imbalance has been postulated to contribute to the initiation and/or progression of spinal deformity in AIS [10,11]. Previous studies have reported abnormal and asymmetric muscle phenotypes in concave and convex side paraspinal muscles of AIS patients, including electromyography (EMG) activities, muscle volume, muscle fiber types, and fatty and fibrosis infiltration [12–16]. Additionally, one recent study demonstrated a significantly lower density of activated satellite cells for fiber type I in AIS patients when compared to non-scoliosis controls, and the curve severity appeared to be associated with the density of satellite cells and other histological parameters such as cross-sectional areas of muscle fiber and myonuclear density [17]. Collectively, these findings suggest that patients with AIS have generalized muscle dysfunction, which is potentially associated with the curve severity. Until now, whether muscle abnormalities could be a predictive value for AIS onset or curve progression remained unexplored.

In AIS, the current studies on paraspinal muscles rely heavily on muscle biopsies, which is a major research hurdle due to ethical concerns and the scarcity of muscle biopsies from healthy control subjects or AIS patients with mild curvature for fair comparison. Thus, less invasive tests are widely used to reveal muscle-related changes at earlier time points and for longitudinal study. Blood samples are a surrogate for systemic phenotype research, which allows for biomarker discovery. Currently, the advancement in "omics" research enables researchers to quantify a large amount of proteins/peptides and metabolites in the circulation in a non-targeted and unbiased manner, resulting in identification of numerous AIS-related predictive and prognostic biomarkers [18]. A recent metabolomics study that performed UPLC/QTOF-MS (ultra-high-performance liquid chromatography coupled with quadrupole time-of-flight mass spectrometry) analysis revealed differential serum lipid metabolism profiles in patients with AIS [19]. This study suggested disrupted glycerophospholipid, glycerolipid, and fatty acid metabolism in AIS patients when compared to age-matched healthy controls, and provided a list of metabolites for diagnostic biomarkers. Another two proteomic studies described the differential circulating proteomes in AIS. Shen et al. [20] compared the plasma samples derived from four AIS patients and four healthy controls using 10-plex tandem mass tag (TMT)-based quantitative MS analysis. They identified several proteins correlating with the differential gut microbiota species in AIS patients. Makino et al. [21] employed two-dimensional fluorescence difference gel electrophoresis (2D-DIGE) quantitation followed by an MS-based proteins identification strategy to compare pooled plasma samples from five severe AIS and five non-AIS control subjects, revealing the association between vitamin D binding protein and coagulation-related proteins with AIS pathogenesis. However, these studies did not step further to explore the link between the acquired proteomic data and the risk of curve progression in AIS, specifically exploring biomarkers with respect to muscles. Therefore, the current study aimed to compare proteomic profiles among healthy girls and AIS subjects with either remaining curvature or progressing into severe cases, further providing a candidate list of muscle-related DEPs for functional and clinical validation.

In this study, we aimed to (1) conduct a quantitative proteomic study screening the plasma samples from healthy controls and AIS patients, who were further divided into non-progressive and progressive subgroups regarding their curve progression in a longitudinal follow-up; (2) compare the proteomic profiles among these three groups and filter out a list of candidate muscle-related proteins.

2. Materials and Methods

2.1. Subjects Recruitment and Blood Taking

As referred by the local population-based School Scoliosis Screening Service, students of the fifth grade or above with a maximal Cobb angle of $\geq 20°$ were referred to our scoliosis special clinic [3]. As the prevalence of AIS is likely linked to sex and there is a higher risk of curve progression in girls, female subjects with AIS with a maximal Cobb angle of <30° at their first clinical visit were recruited from our scoliosis clinic. Patients with other types of scoliosis with known causes or with congenital deformities, neuromuscular diseases, autoimmune disorders, endocrine disturbances, or medical conditions that affect the bone metabolism were excluded, as previously reported [22]. Non-progressive subjects prescribed with bracing or any other treatment that might interfere with curve progression during the follow-up were excluded.

Blood samples and clinical data from the CAL cohort (NCT01103115) were used. The Cobb angle of a major curve was measured via standard standing posterior–anterior radiography of the whole spine at the first visit and at six-month intervals for six years (reaching skeletal maturity). All of the subjects were regularly followed, observed, and/or treated with bracing or surgical correction according to standard clinical practice (CREC Reference Number: 2009.491-T). Four subjects with curve progression that increased less than 6° in the follow-up period were defined as the non-progressive (NP) group [23], and four subjects that had reached the surgical threshold ($\geq 45°$) at any time point within the follow-up period were defined as the progressive (P) group. The classification criteria for the NP and P groups are illustrated in Figure 1a. Basic anthropometric data were measured with standardized methodology. Tanner staging and age at menarche were recorded. The body composition parameters were determined via bioelectrical impedance analysis (BIA, InBody 720, Biospace, Seoul, Korea). Handgrip strength was assessed with portable dynamometers (Nakamura Scientific Co., Ltd., Tokyo, Japan) three times using the dominant and non-dominant hands, and the mean of the three measurements was calculated.

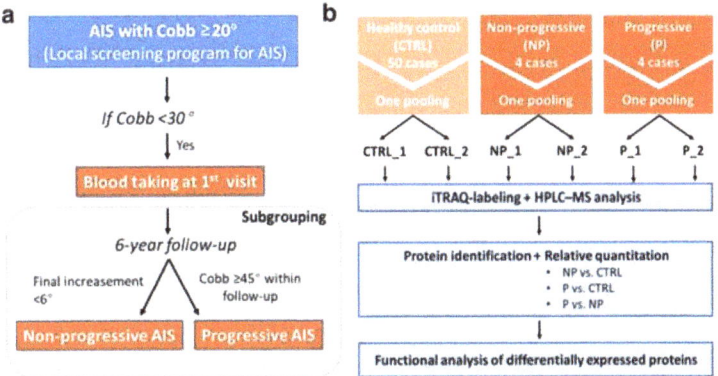

Figure 1. Proteomic analysis of the plasma in the healthy control (CTRL) vs. non-progressive (NP) vs. progressive (P) AIS groups. (**a**) Illustration of the selection criteria for the AIS groups. (**b**) Main procedures of sample pooling, iTRAQ labeling, HPLC–MS analysis, and bioinformatic analysis.

A total of 50 age-matched healthy Chinese girls were recruited randomly from local secondary schools to serve as the control (CTRL) group. Clinical examination was carried out by experienced orthopedic surgeons to exclude spinal deformities. The basic information for the CTRL, AIS NP, and AIS P groups is described in Table 1.

Table 1. Basic information for the three groups.

Groups	CTRL (N = 50)	NP (N = 4)	P (N = 4)	p-Value [1]
Age (years)	13.1 ± 0.5	13.4 ± 0.5	12.6 ± 0.9	0.155
Body Weight (kg)	49.6 ± 9.8	42.2 ± 3.2	34.3 ± 3.8 *	0.002
Body Height (cm)	157.4 ± 6.1	154.0 ± 10.6	145.8 ± 3.4 *	0.014
Arm Span (cm)	156.1 ± 6.9	152.4 ± 12.2	146.9 ± 8.1	0.090
BMI (kg/m^2)	20.23 ± 3.0	18.3 ± 2.3	15.9 ± 0.5 *	0.005

Abbreviations: CTRL, healthy control; NP, non-progressive AIS; P, progressive AIS. Data are shown as mean ± SD. [1] Kruskal–Wallis test was used. * $p < 0.05$ when compared to the CTRL group using a post hoc test.

Peripheral venous blood samples (2 mL) were collected from the participants' arms at their first visit to our scoliosis special clinic. The blood was centrifuged at 4 °C, 3000× g for 10 min. The plasma were aliquoted to minimize the freeze–thaw cycle and stored at −80 °C for further analysis.

2.2. Sample Preparation for iTRAQ-Based Proteomic Analysis

Isobaric tags for relative and absolute quantitation (iTRAQ)-based [24] proteomic analysis allows relative quantitation, comparing the proteomic profiles of plasma from three groups. Considering the limitation of the maximal eight samples for one 8-plex analysis and the sample sizes of the designed comparison groups (CTRL: N = 50; NP: N = 4; P: N = 4), the strategy of groupwise pooling followed by technical duplicates was adopted (Figure 1b). An equal volume (300 μL) of each plasma sample within each group was pooled into one mixture and further divided into two duplicates, resulting in six plasma samples (CTRL_1, CTRL_2, NP_1, NP_2, P_1, and P_2). The duplicates in this study allowed for a decrease in the variance due to the technical error of the experimental technique.

High abundance protein depletion was carried out with a ProteoMiner Protein Enrichment Kit (Cat. # 163-3007; Bio-Rad laboratories, Hercules, CA, USA) according to the manufacturer's instructions. The proteins were dissolved in lysis buffer consisting of 8 M urea for denaturation afterwards. For cysteine alkylation, protein lysis was further subjected to 10 mM dithiothreitol (DTT, Cat. #10197777001, Sigma-Aldrich, Burlington, MA, USA) with incubation at 57 °C for 45 min, followed by 10 mM iodoacetamide (IAM, Cat. #I1149-5G, Sigma-Aldrich, Burlington, MA, USA) and incubation at room temperature in the dark for 1 h. A Bradford assay was used to determine the total protein concentration, for which 50 μg of protein of each sample was diluted four times with 100 mM triethylammonium bicarbonate (TEAB, Cat. #90114, Thermo Fisher Scientific, Waltham, MA, USA). Then, the protein solution was subjected to protein digestion with Trypsin Gold (Cat. #V5117; Promega, Madison, WI, USA). Trypsin Gold was added at a 1:40 (w/w) enzyme/protein ratio for further incubation at 37 °C for 18 h. HCl was added to a final concentration of 50 mM to stop the tryptic digestion. After trypsin digestion, the peptides were desalted with a Strata X C18 column (Phenomenex, Torrance, CA, USA) according to the manufacturer's protocol, and then vacuum-dried.

The digested peptides from 50 μg of protein were dissolved in 30 μL of 0.5 M TEAB and subjected to peptide labeling with an iTRAQ Reagent 8-plex Kit (SCIEX, Framingham, MA, USA) according to the manufacturer's instructions [25]: 113 and 114 for the CTRL group, 116 and 117 for the NP group, and 119 and 121 for the P group. The labeled peptides were combined and desalted with a Strata X C18 column followed by vacuum-drying. The peptides were subjected to a Shimadzu LC-20AB high-performance liquid chromatography (HPLC) pump system (Shimadzu, Kyoto, Japan) coupled with a high pH reversed-phase (RP) column to separate into 20 fractions. The following gradient was used for fractionation. The peptides were reconstituted with buffer A (5% acetonitrile (Cat. #900667-4 × 4L, Sigma-Aldrich, Burlington, MA, USA), 95% H$_2$O, pH 9.8) to 2 mL and loaded onto a column containing 5 μm of particles (Phenomenex, Torrance, CA, USA). The peptides were separated at a flow rate of 1 mL/min with a gradient of 5% buffer B (5% H$_2$O, 95% acetonitrile, pH 9.8) for 10 min, 5~35% buffer B for 40 min, and 35~95% buffer B for 1 min. The system was then maintained in 95% buffer B for 3 min and decreased to 5% within 1 min, before equilibrating with 5% buffer B for 10 min. Elution was monitored by measuring the absorbance at 214 nm, and fractions were collected every 1 min. The eluted peptides were pooled as 20 fractions and vacuum-dried. Each fraction was resuspended in 2% acetonitrile and 0.1% formic acid (Cat. #33015-500ML, Sigma-Aldrich, Burlington, MA, USA), and centrifuged at 20,000× g for 10 min. The supernatant was subjected to the following HPLC–MS analysis.

2.3. HPLC–MS and Bioinformatic Analysis

Each fraction was loaded onto a C18 trap column using a LC-20AD nano-HPLC instrument (Shimadzu, Kyoto, Japan) by an autosampler. Then, the peptides were eluted from the trap column and separated by an analytical C18 column (inner diameter of 75 μm) packed in-house, and then subjected to MS analysis with a TripleTOF 5600 System (SCIEX, Framingham, MA, USA) equipped with a Nanospray III source (SCIEX, Framingham, MA, USA). The following gradient was used for elution of the peptides for MS analysis: buffers A and B for elution were 2% acetonitrile with 0.1% formic acid, and 98% acetonitrile with 0.1% formic acid, respectively. The gradient was run at 300 nL/min, starting from 8~35% of buffer B for 35 min, then up to 60% for 5 min, maintained at 80% B for 5 min, and finally returned to 5% for 0.1 min and equilibrated for 10 min.

For the MS setting, the high-sensitivity mode was used for the whole data acquisition. The accumulation time for MS1 was 250 ms, and the mass ranges were from 350 to 1500 Da. Based on the intensity in the MS1 survey, as many as 30 product ion scans were collected if exceeding a threshold of 120 counts/s and with charge-state 2 + to 5 +, dynamic exclusion was set for 1/2 of the peak width (12 s). For iTRAQ data acquisition, the collision energy was adjusted to all precursor ions for collision-induced dissociation, and the Q2 transmission window for 100 Da was 100%. The raw MS/MS data were converted into MGF format by the ProteoWizard tool msConvert, and the exported files were searched using Mascot version 2.3.02 against the selected database Swissprot (Homo_sapiens, 201704). The fragment and peptide mass tolerance were set at 0.1 and 0.05 Da, respectively. The variable modifications were Oxidation (M) and iTRAQ8plex (Y), while the fixed modifications were Carbamidomethyl (C), iTRAQ8plex (N-term), and iTRAQ8plex (K). One missed cleavage was allowed. The false discovery rate (FDR) at 1%, which was based on the picked protein FDR strategy [26], was used for cut-off. Automated software IQuant Protein Quantification [27] was used to analyze the labeled peptides with isobaric tags. In this project, we set NP_1/CTRL_1, NP_2/CTRL_1, NP_1/CTRL_2, NP_2/CTRL_2, P_1/CTRL_1, P_1/CTRL_2, P_2/CTRL_1, P_2/CTRL_2, P_1/NP_1, P_1/NP_2, P_2/NP_1, and P_2/NP_2 as the comparison groups. The mean ratio of the protein expression in the pairwise comparison groups was calculated. For example, the mean ratio of NP vs. CTRL = (NP_1/CTRL_1 + NP_1/CTRL_2 + NP_2/CTRL_1 + NP_2/CTRL_2)/4. A protein with a mean ratio ≤0.83 or ≥1.2, a p-value < 0.05 by an independent t-test was considered as differentially expressed protein (DEP).

A Venn diagram for overlapping analysis was performed using Venny v2.1 [28]. The functions of the DEPs were analyzed using Protein Analysis Through Evolutionary Relationships (PANTHER) v15.0 [29] to demonstrate their Gene Ontology (GO) profiles. Detailed GO term descriptions at the level of DIRECT were obtained using the Database for Annotation, Visualization, and Integrated Discovery (DAVID) v6.8 [30]. A protein–protein interaction (PPI) network of the DEPs was constructed using the online Search Tool for the Retrieval of Interacting Genes (STRING) database [31]. The minimum required interaction score was set to medium confidence (0.4). The PPI results were exported and subjected to

Cytoscape v3.7.2 for visualization. The other results were visualized using PRISM v7.03. The mass spectrometry proteomics data have been deposited to the ProteomeXchange Consortium via the PRIDE [32] partner repository with the dataset identifier PXD023915.

2.4. Statistical Analysis

All results are presented as mean ± SD. Independent t-test, Kruskal–Wallis tests, or Mann–Whitney U tests were used for comparison studies. Statistical analysis was performed with SPSS 22. A p-value of <0.05 was considered statistically significant.

3. Results

3.1. Subject Characteristics

Among the 110 subjects in the dataset, a total of eight age-matched AIS subjects with a maximal Cobb angle of <30° at the first visit (baseline) without any prior treatment and who were skeletally immature (years since menarche of <two years; Risser sign of ≤four) were included in this study. The selection criteria for the AIS NP and AIS P subgroups and the clinical parameters are described in Table 2. None of the NP subjects received bracing or any treatment during the follow-up period, while all of the P group subjects received bracing treatment but still progressed and reached the surgical threshold. As shown in Tables 1 and 2, AIS subjects in the P group had a significantly later onset of menarche, lower tanner staging, and were skeletally less mature compared to the NP group, despite having a similar chronological age. The lean mass of the right and left arms and the trunk was statistically lower in the P group compared to the NP group. On the contrary, skeletal muscle mass, body fat mass, fat-free mass, right and left leg lean mass, and handgrip strength did not show a significant difference between the two AIS subgroups. Body weight, body height, arm span, and body mass index (BMI, calculated as body weight/arm span^2 [7]) showed no significant differences between the NP and P groups, although body weight, body height, and BMI were found to be significantly lower in the P group than in the CTRL group. The Cobb angle of the major curve in the two AIS groups showed no significant difference at their first visit.

Table 2. Selection criteria for the AIS subgroups and the subjects' information.

AIS Subgroups	Non-Progressive (NP)		Progressive (P)		p [1]
	Mean	SD	Mean	SD	
Selection criteria of the subgroups					
Cobb at first visit (°)	23.5	2.4	26.5	3	0.189
	(Individual: 21, 22, 25, 26)		(Individual: 23, 25, 29, 29)		
Change of Cobb angle at latest follow-up	Less than 6°		Final Cobb larger than 45°		/
	(Individual: 24, 21, 20, 28)		(Individual: 57, 59, 49, 50)		
With bracing	No (0/4)		Yes (4/4)		/
Sexual and skeletal maturity					
Time since onset of menarche (years)	1.6	0.8	−0.9	0.4	0.021
	(range: 0.62~2.57)		(range: −1.38~−0.34)		
Breast stage	3.3	0.5	2.0	0.8	0.044
	(range: 3~4)		(range: 1~3)		
Pubic hair	3.0	0.0	1.8	0.5	0.011
	(range: 3~3)		(range: 1~2)		
Risser sign	3.5	0.6	0.8	1.0	0.019
	(range: 3~4)		(range: 0~2)		
Body composition					
Skeletal muscle mass (kg)	16.8	2.7	14.1	1.2	0.149
Body fat mass (kg)	9.9	2.1	7.1	2.0	0.149
Fat-free mass (kg)	32.0	4.7	27.5	2.2	0.149

Table 2. Cont.

AIS Subgroups	Non-Progressive (NP)		Progressive (P)		p^1
	Mean	SD	Mean	SD	
Right arm lean mass (kg)	1.2	0.2	0.9	0.1	0.029
Left arm lean mass (kg)	1.2	0.2	0.9	0.1	0.043
Trunk lean mass (kg)	13.4	1.4	10.9	0.8	0.043
Right leg lean mass (kg)	4.9	1.2	3.8	0.3	0.083
Left leg lean mass (kg)	4.8	1.1	3.7	0.3	0.083
Handgrip strength					
Dominant hand (kg)	17.8	3.9	14.4	3.4	0.146
Non-dominant hand (kg)	18.4	5.3	13.8	3.6	0.149

[1] Mann–Whitney U-test was used. p in bold indicated a value of <0.05.

3.2. Up- and Downregulated DEPs in Pairwise Comparison Analysis

In total, 34,915 spectra were matched to 4749 peptides, and 1058 proteins were identified in all three groups of plasma samples (Table S1). Compared to the healthy control group, the non-progressive group had 127 upregulated and 185 downregulated DEPs, while the progressive group had 285 upregulated and 173 downregulated DEPs (Figure 2a). Compared to the non-progressive group, there were 375 proteins upregulated and 120 downregulated in the progressive group.

3.3. Gradually Changing DEPs Accompanying a Higher Risk of Scoliosis Progression

In order to discover those circulating DEPs that had gradually higher or lower levels accompanying a higher risk of scoliosis progression, the overlap of up and downregulated DEPs in all three comparison groups was determined. Only four proteins, namely, AIM1L (absent in melanoma 1-like), SOX2 (SRY-box 2), WDR7 (WD repeat domain 7), and DNM3 (dynamin 3), showed decreasing levels when comparing NP vs. CTRL, P vs. CTRL, and P vs. NP (Figure 2b). AIM1L, known as CRYBB2 (beta/gamma crystallin domain-containing protein 2), is biased in terms of expression in the esophagus and has functions in carbohydrate binding. WDR7 is a component in synaptic vesicles and is functionally involved in hematopoietic progenitor cell differentiation. DNM3 is a microtube-associated force-producing protein involved in producing microtubule bundles. SOX2 is a critical transcription factor regulating early embryogenesis.

On the contrary, 71 proteins showed upregulation when comparing NP vs. CTRL, P vs. CTRL, and P vs. NP (Figure 2c). GO analysis with PANTHER showed the distribution of these DEPs' annotation to be in three functional aspects (Figure 2d). For the molecular function (MF), the term "binding"—which includes protein–protein, protein–nucleic acid, and protein–lipid binding—was the most annotated term (59.06%). Catalytic activity was the second most annotated term (21.32%), which could indicate that some of the DEPs were enzymes. "Cellular process" (24.54%) was the most annotated biological process (BP) aspect, representing any process carried out at the cellular level, such as processes in a single cell, or cell–cell communication occurring at the cellular level. This term was followed by "cellular component organization or biogenesis" (15.10%) and "biological regulation" (11.90%). For the cellular component (CC), "cell" and "cell part" (both 19.24%) were the most annotated, followed by "organelle" and "organelle part" (12.83% and 11.32%, respectively).

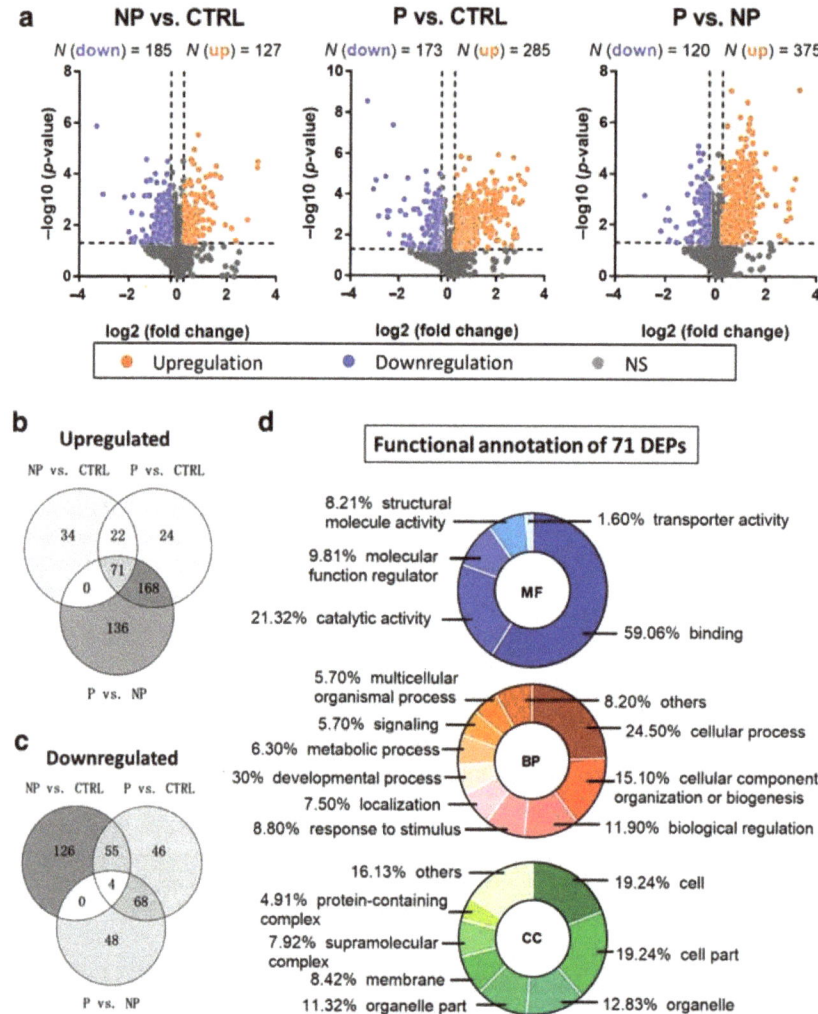

Figure 2. Analysis of differentially expressed proteins (DEPs). (**a**) Volcano plot of the relative quantitation results. A *t*-test was used between groups. Proteins with a ratio of ≤0.83 or ≥1.2 and a *p*-value < 0.05 were considered as DEPs. Blue and orange plots indicate down and upregulated DEPs, respectively. Gray plots represent non-significant (NS) proteins. (**b,c**) Venn diagrams show the overlap among all down and upregulated DEPs in the three comparison groups: NP vs. CTRL, P vs. CTRL, and P vs. NP. (**d**) PANTHER Gene Ontology (GO) functional categorization of upregulated DEPs presented in all of the comparison groups in (**b**). MF, BP, and CC represent the GO aspects molecular function, biological process, and cellular component, respectively. The percentage of each term was calculated as a protein hit the term/total function hits. The BP and CC terms less than 4% were combined as "others".

3.4. Shortlist of Muscle-Related DEPs

The gradually changed DEPs accompanying a higher risk of curve progression were analyzed using DAVID to determine their detailed function. None of the four gradually downregulated DEPs in Figure 2b were directly relevant to muscles according to GO annotation. Meanwhile, among the 71 upregulated DEPs in Figure 2c, 19 of them could annotate BP terms directly related to muscle activities in terms of including the keyword "muscle" (Table S2), such as "muscle contraction" and "muscle filament sliding". Due to the structural and functional similarities of skeletal, cardiac, and smooth muscle, many of the proteins can be expressed in more than one type of muscle. Calmodulin 1 (CALM1), for example, is expressed in all kinds of muscle cells and could regulate their contraction. Therefore, the GO terms related to all three muscle types were retained in our analysis. One of the DEPs, named angiotensinogen, which can annotate the GO term "response to muscle activity involved in regulation of muscle adaptation", was excluded from our list, since it was known to be generated and secreted by the liver and thus its modulating effect on muscle function is endocrine in nature only. The remaining 18 DEPs (Figure 3) were considered to be directly involved in muscle activities, while their circulating levels were associated with the risk of scoliosis progression.

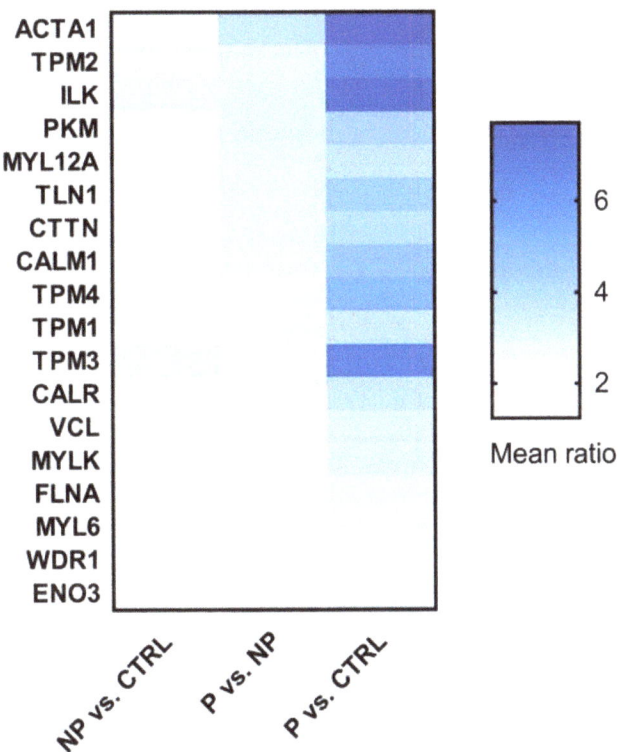

Figure 3. Heatmap of the upregulated DEPs that are functionally related to muscle. The DEPs are listed, sorted by the mean ratio of the P vs. NP groups. The mean ratio was calculated as the mean of four ratio values, e.g., the mean ratio of NP vs. CTRL = (NP_1/CTRL_1 + NP_1/CTRL_2 + NP_2/CTRL_1 + NP_2/CTRL_2)/4.

3.5. PPI Network of 18 Candidate DEPs

A PPI network of the 18 shortlisted DEPs was developed (Figure 4). The lines (interaction) thickness indicates the interaction score (range = 0.403~0.999) calculated by STRING, which represents the strength of data support. The size of the nodes (DEPs) indicates the mean ratio of the P vs. NP groups. ACTA1 (α-actin) had the largest expression ratio between the P vs. NP groups. The location of the DEPs was determined according to GO annotation and is represented by three colors. "Extracellular" represents all extracellular regions, including the extracellular matrix. "Membrane" includes both the membrane part and the cell junction. "Cell" indicates all parts inside the cell, such as the organelle part. The nodes were sorted by the degree of connectivity calculated by Cytoscape and listed in a circle. For example, VCL (vinculin), which is involved in cell matrix adhesion and cell–cell adhesion, had the highest connectivity, as it was shown to interact with 13 DEPs. The complex interactions among these DEPs indicate they are closely connected with one another and function as a network.

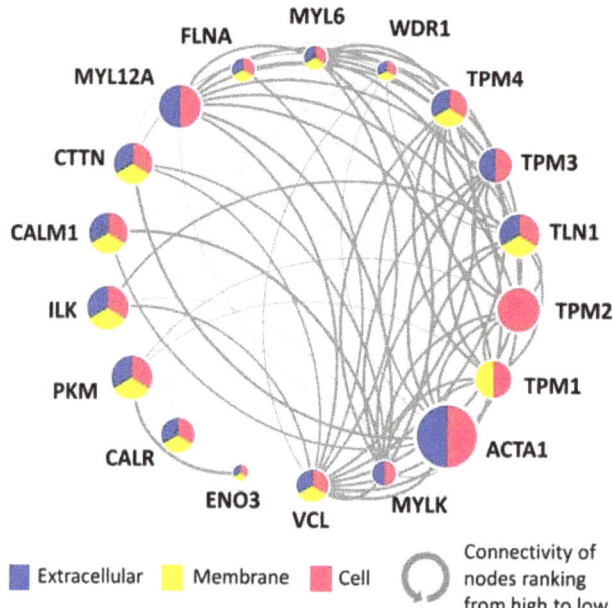

Figure 4. Protein–protein interaction (PPI) network among the upregulated muscle-related DEPs. The colors of each node (DEP) represent its location. The size of the node indicates its mean ratio of the P vs. NP groups. The nodes are sorted from VCL to ENO3 by the degree of connectivity calculated by Cytoscape and listed in a circle. The line (interaction) thickness indicates the interaction score calculated by STRING, which represents the strength of data support.

4. Discussion

As previous proteomic studies have only compared the profiles between the control and AIS groups [20,21], the current comparison analysis attempted to move a step further to compare the circulating protein profiles between healthy girls and girls with AIS, who were further divided into non-progressive and progressive AIS subgroups. This preliminary study demonstrated that the baseline muscle-related DEPs in the circulation of AIS subjects might represent a novel group of biomarkers for predicting curve progression to the surgical threshold.

A number of circulating proteins have been proposed as prognostic factors of AIS, such as melatonin and calmodulin [33–37]. Recently, our group proposed a composite model composed of plasma miR-145 and total procollagen type 1 N-terminal propeptide (P1NP) together with clinical parameters to predict the risk of curve progression in AIS, achieving a sensitivity of 72.2% and a specificity of 90% [38]. Despite there being a close interaction between bone and muscle, there are, as of yet, no muscle-related biomarkers for AIS. This proteomic study showed that among all of the upregulated DEPs in the progressive group, approximately 25% of DEPs (18 of 71) are found in muscles and play essential roles in muscle activities, such as muscle contraction and muscle regeneration. Among them, ACTA1 showed the highest fold change in the progressive vs. non-progressive AIS comparison, followed by another structural protein, TPM2 (tropomyosin beta chain). ACTA1 and TPM2 are only expressed in striated muscle. ACTA1 in the circulation is a well-reported candidate for muscle damage caused by physical damage or intensive exercise [39–42]. Injury could lead to an increase (up to 187 times) in ACTA1 levels in the serum [40]. Collectively, our preliminary results first suggest that there might be muscle structural damage to a certain extent in patients with AIS, which leads to the release of some cellular proteins into the bloodstream. Further in-depth investigation is warranted to determine whether these structural proteins originate from paraspinal muscles under asymmetric tension or a global phenomenon. In addition to ACTA1, some other DEPs are also associated with the etiopathogenesis of muscle-related diseases. ENO3 (beta-enolase) and its mutations can cause glycogen storage disorder XIII (GSD13, also known as Enolase-beta deficiency), which presents myalgia post exertion in adulthood and recurrent rhabdomyolysis [43]. Mutations of TPM2 and TPM3 (tropomyosin 3) have been reported to cause various congenital myopathies, such as CAP myopathy, Nemaline myopathy types 1 and 4, and congenital myopathies with fiber-type disproportion [44]. The close interactions among the 18 DEPs shown in the PPI network indicate that they function as a network; thus, the alternation of muscle fibers might not only be limited to structure, but also to affected muscle functions in patients with AIS. Most importantly, the upregulation of these DEPs in AIS in the progressive group was shown to have occurred prior to the Cobb angle progressing into a severe curvature, as the plasma were all collected at baseline, at which both the progressive and non-progressive AIS subjects had similar curve severities. Of note, the concurrent lower trunk and arm lean mass observed in the progressive group is in line with an abnormal muscle-related proteomic profile, further supporting the likelihood of impaired muscle functioning in the progressive group in the early stage.

The present study has its clinical implications. First, given the etiology of AIS remaining undetermined, the novel muscle-related DEP profiles observed in this study strongly indicate primary pathological changes in muscle tissues in AIS subjects, thus suggesting a new perspective for therapy to target the underlying etiology. Second, these proteomic markers from patients in the early stage of AIS provide potential predictors for curve progression. From the view that patients with AIS are recommended to visit the clinic regularly (e.g., every six months) until skeletal maturity to monitor curve progression, the predictors presented in this study could be helpful in risk stratification of AIS so that unnecessary clinical visits can be minimized, especially under conditions such as the COVID-19 pandemic. Third, screening muscle-related proteins in plasma samples has the potential to replace repeated X-ray measurements, which cause radiological toxicity, though further validation with larger sample sizes is warranted.

This study has some advantages compared to previous studies. (1) In order to perform a strict subgrouping of non-progressive AIS, the current study performed a six-year longitudinal follow-up until the patients reached skeletal maturity. (2) There have been studies reporting abnormal muscle morphology and functions in AIS, especially at paraspinal regions of the major curve. Nevertheless, these cross-sectional studies failed to answer whether the abnormal muscle phenotypes are primary or secondary to spinal curvature. Our study, conducted at baseline when the AIS subgroups had comparable severity, provides fresh evidence indicating the likelihood of abnormal muscle phenotypes at the protein level in AIS, which might contribute to curve progression. (3) iTRAQ-based proteomic analysis enables the simultaneous screening of thousands of proteins reflecting systemic changes of the whole body, and thus could provide enough candidates for further evaluation of biomarkers and for the establishment of a predication model of curve progression.

However, there are limitations in this study. (1) The findings of this pilot study, with a limited sample size in non-progressive and progressive AIS groups, requires further validation with larger and longitudinal cohorts. (2) Only female subjects were recruited in this study, which could have caused sampling bias. Despite there being higher AIS prevalence and risk of curve progression in girls, further investigations with cohorts including boys are necessary to validate our findings and to identify sex-specific DEPs in AIS. (3) Progressive and non-progressive subjects of similar ages and Cobb angles at the baseline were selected to minimize individual variation. However, differences in sexual and skeletal maturity between these two groups still exist and might be a cofounding factor partly contributing to the profile of DEPs. It should be noted that these unmatched factors might also contribute to the risk of progression, which should be taken into consideration in future similar studies. (4) Despite technological advancement, iTRAQ is still a costly approach when compared to well-established but less-sensitive methods such as 2D difference gel electrophoresis [45]. Therefore, the strategy of pooling plasma samples within one group was adopted, which is a common approach to reducing the variance of biological replicates in proteomics studies due to small sample sizes [46]. However, the pooling strategy has its own shortages, such as the effect of outlier samples. Therefore, verifying the levels of candidates in individual samples is desired in future validation studies.

In summary, this is the first study to hypothesize that there might be a higher level of circulating baseline muscle-related proteins in AIS, which might further link to the risk of curve progression. Herein, we proposed 18 proteins as potential candidates reflecting alternations of muscle phenotypes, which require further investigation to verify the circulating levels and biological functions of these biomarker candidates, and eventually a refined composite model for curve prediction.

Supplementary Materials: The following are available online at https://www.mdpi.com/article/10.3390/jcm10214927/s1. Table S1, All identified proteins with quantitative data; Table S2, Muscle activity-related GO terms in the aspect of biological function annotated by 19 upregulated DEPs.

Author Contributions: J.C. and W.L. conceived the study and its design; Y.W. performed the experiments and data analysis; Y.W. and W.L. drafted the manuscript; J.Z. assisted in the acquisition of the clinical parameters; H.C., A.H. and T.-p.L. collected the clinical samples and acquired the clinical data; J.C. performed critical revision of the manuscript; W.L. approved the submitted and final versions. All authors have read and agreed to the published version of the manuscript.

Funding: This work was partially supported by the Research Grants Council of the Hong Kong S.A.R., China (projects 14163517 and 14120818 to W.Y.W. Lee; project 14130216 to T.P. Lam), the Health and Medical Research Fund, the Food and Health Bureau, the Government of the Hong Kong Special Administrative Region (project 06170546 to W.Y.W. Lee), the NSFC/RGC Joint Research Scheme sponsored by the Research Grants Council of the Hong Kong Special Administrative Region, China and the National Natural Science Foundation of China (project numbers. N_CUHK416/16 and 8161101087 to T.P. Lam and Y. Qiu), the Hainan Provincial Natural Science Foundation of China (project 819QN365 to H. Chen) and the National Natural Science Foundation of China (project 81902270 to H. Chen).

Institutional Review Board Statement: This study was conducted according to the guidelines of the Declaration of Helsinki, and approved by the Institutional Review Board of The Chinese University of Hong Kong (CREC Ref. No. 2016.337, 1 August 2016).

Informed Consent Statement: Informed consent was obtained from all subjects and/or their guardians involved in the study.

Data Availability Statement: The mass spectrometry proteomics data were deposited to the ProteomeXchange Consortium via the PRIDE partner repository with the dataset identifier PXD023915.

Conflicts of Interest: The authors declare no conflict of interest.

References

1. Weinstein, S.L.; Dolan, L.A.; Cheng, J.C.; Danielsson, A.; Morcuende, J.A. Adolescent idiopathic scoliosis. *Nat. Rev. Dis. Primers* **2015**, *1*, 15030. [CrossRef]
2. Ueno, M.; Takaso, M.; Nakazawa, T.; Imura, T.; Saito, W.; Shintani, R.; Uchida, K.; Fukuda, M.; Takahashi, K.; Ohtori, S.; et al. A 5-year epidemiological study on the prevalence rate of idiopathic scoliosis in Tokyo: School screening of more than 250,000 children. *J. Orthop. Sci.* **2011**, *16*, 1–6. [CrossRef] [PubMed]

3. Luk, K.D.; Lee, C.F.; Cheung, K.M.; Cheng, J.C.; Ng, B.K.; Lam, T.P.; Mak, K.H.; Yip, P.S.; Fong, D.Y. Clinical Effectiveness of School Screening for Adolescent Idiopathic Scoliosis: A Large Population-Based Retrospective Cohort Study. *Spine* **2010**, *35*, 1607–1614. [CrossRef]
4. Weinstein, S.L.; Dolan, L.A.; Wright, J.G.; Dobbs, M.B. Effects of Bracing in Adolescents with Idiopathic Scoliosis. *N. Engl. J. Med.* **2013**, *369*, 1512–1521. [CrossRef]
5. Schiller, J.R.; Thakur, N.A.; Eberson, C.P. Brace Management in Adolescent Idiopathic Scoliosis. *Clin. Orthop. Relat. Res.* **2010**, *468*, 670–678. [CrossRef] [PubMed]
6. Martinez-Llorens, J.; Ramirez, M.; Colomina, M.J.; Bago, J.; Molina, A.; Caceres, E.; Gea, J. Muscle dysfunction and exercise limitation in adolescent idiopathic scoliosis. *Eur. Respir. J.* **2010**, *36*, 393–400. [CrossRef]
7. Yu, W.S.; Chan, K.Y.; Yu, F.W.P.; Yeung, H.Y.; Lee, K.M.; Ng, K.W.; Qiu, Y.; Lam, T.P.; Cheng, J.C.Y. Lower handgrip strength in girls with adolescent idiopathic scoliosis (AIS) a case-control study. *Stud. Health Technol. Inf.* **2012**, *176*, 175.
8. Lin, M.C.; Liaw, M.Y.; Chen, W.J.; Cheng, P.T.; Wong, A.M.; Chiou, W.K. Pulmonary function and spinal characteristics: Their relationships in persons with idiopathic and postpoliomyelitic scoliosis. *Arch. Phys. Med. Rehabil.* **2001**, *82*, 335–341. [CrossRef]
9. Bogduk NaM, J.E.; Pearcy, M.J. A universal model of the lumbar back muscles in the upright position. *Spine* **1992**, *17*, 897–913. [CrossRef]
10. Wong, C. Mechanism of right thoracic adolescent idiopathic scoliosis at risk for progression; a unifying pathway of development by normal growth and imbalance. *Scoliosis* **2015**, *10*, 2. [CrossRef]
11. Modi, H.N.; Suh, S.-W.; Yang, J.-H.; Hong, J.-Y.; Venkatesh, K.P.; Muzaffar, N. Spontaneous regression of curve in immature idiopathic scoliosis—Does spinal column play a role to balance? An observation with literature review. *J. Orthop. Surg. Res.* **2010**, *5*, 80. [CrossRef] [PubMed]
12. Zapata, K.A.; Wang-Price, S.S.; Sucato, D.J.; Dempsey-Robertson, M. Ultrasonographic Measurements of Paraspinal Muscle Thickness in Adolescent Idiopathic Scoliosis: A Comparison and Reliability Study. *Pediatr. Phys. Ther.* **2015**, *27*, 119–125. [CrossRef] [PubMed]
13. Mannion, A.F.; Meier, M.; Grob, D.; Müntener, M. Paraspinal muscle fibre type alterations associated with scoliosis: An old problem revisited with new evidence. *Eur. Spine J.* **1998**, *7*, 289–293. [CrossRef] [PubMed]
14. Stetkarova, I.; Zamecnik, J.; Bocek, V.; Vasko, P.; Brabec, K.; Krbec, M. Electrophysiological and histological changes of paraspinal muscles in adolescent idiopathic scoliosis. *Eur. Spine J.* **2016**, *25*, 3146–3153. [CrossRef] [PubMed]
15. Jiang, H.; Meng, Y.; Jin, X.; Zhang, C.; Zhao, J.; Wang, C.; Gao, R.; Zhou, X. Volumetric and Fatty Infiltration Imbalance of Deep Paravertebral Muscles in Adolescent Idiopathic Scoliosis. *Med. Sci. Monit.* **2017**, *23*, 2089–2095. [CrossRef]
16. Chan, Y.L.; Cheng, J.C.Y.; Guo, X.; King, A.D.; Griffith, J.F.; Metreweli, C. MRI evaluation of multifidus muscles in adolescent idiopathic scoliosis. *Pediatr. Radiol.* **1999**, *29*, 360–363. [CrossRef]
17. Jiang, H.; Meng, Y.; Jin, X.; Zhang, C.; Zhao, J.; Gao, R.; Zhou, X. Fiber Type-Specific Morphological and Cellular Changes of Paraspinal Muscles in Patients with Severe Adolescent Idiopathic Scoliosis. *Med. Sci. Monit.* **2020**, *26*, e924415.
18. Horgan, R.P.; Kenny, L.C. 'Omic' technologies: Genomics, transcriptomics, proteomics and metabolomics. *Obstet. Gynaecol.* **2011**, *13*, 189–195. [CrossRef]
19. Sun, Z.-J.; Jia, H.-M.; Qiu, G.-X.; Zhou, C.; Guo, S.; Zhang, J.-G.; Shen, J.-X.; Zhao, Y.; Zou, Z.-M. Identification of candidate diagnostic biomarkers for adolescent idiopathic scoliosis using UPLC/QTOF-MS analysis: A first report of lipid metabolism profiles. *Sci. Rep.* **2016**, *6*, 22274. [CrossRef]
20. Shen, N.; Chen, N.; Zhou, X.; Zhao, B.; Huang, R.; Liang, J.; Yang, X.; Chen, M.; Song, Y.; Du, Q. Alterations of the gut microbiome and plasma proteome in Chinese patients with adolescent idiopathic scoliosis. *Bone* **2019**, *120*, 364–370. [CrossRef]
21. Makino, H.; Seki, S.; Kitajima, I.; Motomura, H.; Nogami, M.; Yahara, Y.; Ejiri, N.; Kimura, T. Differential proteome analysis in adolescent idiopathic scoliosis patients with thoracolumbar/lumbar curvatures. *BMC Musculoskelet Disord.* **2019**, *20*, 247. [CrossRef]
22. Zhang, J.; Chen, H.; Leung, R.K.; Choy, K.W.; Lam, T.P.; Ng, B.K.; Qiu, Y.; Feng, J.Q.; Cheng, J.C.; Lee, W.Y. Aberrant miR-145-5p/β-catenin signal impairs osteocyte function in adolescent idiopathic scoliosis. *FASEB J.* **2018**, *32*, 6537–6549. [CrossRef] [PubMed]
23. Richards, B.S.; Bernstein, R.M.; D'Amato, C.R.; Thompson, G.H. Standardization of Criteria for Adolescent Idiopathic Scoliosis Brace Studies: SRS Committee on Bracing and Nonoperative Management. *Spine* **2005**, *30*, 2068–2075. [CrossRef] [PubMed]
24. Takagi, Y.; Yasuhara, T.; Gomi, K. Creatine kinase and its isozymes. *Rinsho Byori.* **2001**, *116*, 52–61. [PubMed]
25. iTRAQ Reagents—8plex Protocol. Available online: https://www.sciex.com/content/dam/SCIEX/pdf/brochures/mass-spectrometry-4375249C.pdf (accessed on 21 May 2021).
26. Savitski, M.M.; Wilhelm, M.; Hahne, H.; Kuster, B.; Bantscheff, M. A Scalable Approach for Protein False Discovery Rate Estimation in Large Proteomic Data Sets. *Mol. Cell Proteom.* **2015**, *14*, 2394–2404. [CrossRef]
27. Wen, B.; Zhou, R.; Feng, Q.; Wang, Q.; Wang, J.; Liu, S. IQuant: An automated pipeline for quantitative proteomics based upon isobaric tags. *Proteomics* **2014**, *14*, 2280–2285. [CrossRef]
28. Oliveros, J.C. VENNY. An Interactive Tool for Comparing Lists with Venn Diagrams. 2007. Available online: https://bioinfogp.cnb.csic.es/tools/venny/index.html (accessed on 17 September 2021).
29. Mi, H.; Muruganujan, A.; Ebert, D.; Huang, X.; Thomas, P.D. PANTHER version 14: More genomes, a new PANTHER GO-slim and improvements in enrichment analysis tools. *Nucleic Acids Res.* **2018**, *47*, D419–D426. [CrossRef]

30. Huang, D.W.; Sherman, B.T.; Lempicki, R.A. Systematic and integrative analysis of large gene lists using DAVID bioinformatics resources. *Nat. Protoc.* **2009**, *4*, 44–57. [CrossRef]
31. Szklarczyk, D.; Franceschini, A.; Wyder, S.; Forslund, K.; Heller, D.; Huerta-Cepas, J.; Simonovic, M.; Roth, A.; Santos, A.; Tsafou, K.P.; et al. STRING v10: Protein-protein interaction networks, integrated over the tree of life. *Nucleic Acids Res.* **2015**, *43*, D447–D452. [CrossRef]
32. Perez-Riverol, Y.; Csordas, A.; Bai, J.; Bernal-Llinares, M.; Hewapathirana, S.; Kundu, D.J.; Inuganti, A.; Griss, J.; Mayer, G.; Eisenacher, M.; et al. The PRIDE database and related tools and resources in 2019: Improving support for quantification data. *Nucleic Acids Res.* **2019**, *47*, D442–D450. [CrossRef]
33. Sadat-Ali, M.; Al-Habdan, I.; Al-Othman, A. Adolescent idiopathic scoliosis. Is low melatonin a cause? *Jt. Bone Spine* **2000**, *67*, 62–64.
34. Fagan, A.B.; Kennaway, D.J.; Sutherland, A.D. Total 24-Hour Melatonin Secretion in Adolescent Idiopathic Scoliosis: A Case-Control Study. *Spine* **1998**, *23*, 41–46. [CrossRef] [PubMed]
35. Kindsfater, K.; Lowe, T.; Lawellin, D.; Weinstein, D.; Akmakjian, J. Levels of platelet calmodulin for the prediction of progression and severity of adolescent idiopathic scoliosis. *JBJS* **1994**, *76*, 1186–1192. [CrossRef]
36. Lowe, T.G.; Burwell, R.G.; Dangerfield, P.H. Platelet calmodulin levels in adolescent idiopathic scoliosis (AIS): Can they predict curve progression and severity? Summary of an electronic focus group debate of the IBSE. *Eur. Spine J.* **2004**, *13*, 257–265. [CrossRef] [PubMed]
37. Noshchenko, A.; Hoffecker, L.; Lindley, E.M.; Burger, E.L.; Cain, C.M.; Patel, V.V.; Bradford, A.P. Predictors of spine deformity progression in adolescent idiopathic scoliosis: A systematic review with meta-analysis. *World J. Orthop.* **2015**, *6*, 537–558. [CrossRef]
38. Zhang, J.; Cheuk, K.Y.; Xu, L.; Wang, Y.; Feng, Z.; Sit, T.; Cheng, K.-L.; Nepotchatykh, E.; Lam, T.-P.; Liu, Z.; et al. A validated composite model to predict risk of curve progression in adolescent idiopathic scoliosis. *Eclinicalmedicine* **2020**, *18*, 100236. [CrossRef] [PubMed]
39. Martinez-Amat, A.; Boulaiz, H.; Prados, J.; Marchal, J.A.; Puche, P.P.; Caba, O.; Rodríguez-Serrano, F.; Aránega, A. Release of alpha-actin into serum after skeletal muscle damage. *Br. J. Sports Med.* **2005**, *39*, 830–834. [CrossRef]
40. Amat, A.M.; Corrales, J.A.M.; Serrano, F.R.; Boulaiz, H.; Salazar, J.C.P.; Contreras, F.H.; Perez, O.C.; Delgado, E.C.; Martín, I.; Jimenez, A.A. Role of alpha-actin in muscle damage of injured athletes in comparison with traditional markers. *Br. J. Sports Med.* **2007**, *41*, 442–446. [CrossRef]
41. Tekus, E.; Vaczi, M.; Horvath-Szalai, Z.; Ludany, A.; Koszegi, T.; Wilhelm, M. Plasma Actin, Gelsolin and Orosomucoid Levels after Eccentric Exercise. *J. Hum. Kinet.* **2017**, *56*, 99–108. [CrossRef]
42. Martínez-Amat, A.; Marchal, J.; Prados, J.; Hita, F.; Rodriguez-Serrano, F.; Boulaiz, H.; Martin, I.; Melguizo, C.; Caba, O.; Velez, C.; et al. Release of muscle α-actin into serum after intensive exercise. *Biol. Sport* **2010**, *27*, 263–268. [CrossRef]
43. Kanungo, S.; Wells, K.; Tribett, T.; El-Gharbawy, A. Glycogen metabolism and glycogen storage disorders. *Ann. Transl. Med.* **2018**, *6*, 474. [CrossRef] [PubMed]
44. Marttila, M.; Lehtokari, V.-L.; Marston, S.; Nyman, T.; Barnerias, C.; Beggs, A.; Bertini, E.; Ceyhan-Birsoy, Ö.; Cintas, P.; Gerard, M.; et al. Mutation update and genotype-phenotype correlations of novel and previously described mutations in TPM2 and TPM3 causing congenital myopathies. *Hum. Mutat.* **2014**, *35*, 779–790. [CrossRef] [PubMed]
45. Wu, W.W.; Wang, G.; Baek, S.J.; Shen, R.-F. Comparative Study of Three Proteomic Quantitative Methods, DIGE, cICAT, and iTRAQ, Using 2D Gel- or LC−MALDI TOF/TOF. *J. Proteome Res.* **2006**, *5*, 651–658. [CrossRef] [PubMed]
46. Diz, A.P.; Truebano, M.; Skibinski, D.O.F. The consequences of sample pooling in proteomics: An empirical study. *Electrophoresis* **2009**, *30*, 2967–2975. [CrossRef] [PubMed]

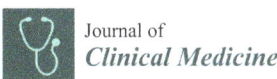

Article

Six-Month Results on Treatment Adherence, Physical Activity, Spinal Appearance, Spinal Deformity, and Quality of Life in an Ongoing Randomised Trial on Conservative Treatment for Adolescent Idiopathic Scoliosis (CONTRAIS)

Marlene Dufvenberg [1,*], Elias Diarbakerli [2,3], Anastasios Charalampidis [2,3], Birgitta Öberg [1], Hans Tropp [4,5,6], Anna Aspberg Ahl [7], Hans Möller [2,8], Paul Gerdhem [2,3] and Allan Abbott [1,6]

1 Department of Health, Medicine and Caring Sciences, Unit of Physiotherapy, Linköping University, SE 581 83 Linköping, Sweden; birgitta.oberg@liu.se (B.Ö.); allan.abbott@liu.se (A.A.)
2 Department of Clinical Science, Intervention and Technology (CLINTEC), Division of Orthopaedics and Biotechnology, Karolinska Institutet, SE 141 86 Stockholm, Sweden; elias.diarbakerli@sll.se (E.D.); anastasios.charalampidis@sll.se (A.C.); hans.moller@rkc.se (H.M.); paul.gerdhem@sll.se (P.G.)
3 Department of Reconstructive Orthopaedics, Karolinska University Hospital Huddinge, SE 141 86 Stockholm, Sweden
4 Department of Biomedical and Clinical Sciences, Linköping University, SE 581 83 Linköping, Sweden; hans.tropp@regionostergotland.se
5 Center for Medical Image Science and Visualization, Linköping University, SE 581 83 Linköping, Sweden
6 Department of Orthopaedics, Linköping University Hospital, SE 581 83 Linköping, Sweden
7 Department of Orthopaedics, Ryhov County Hospital, SE 551 85 Jönköping, Sweden; anna.aspberg.ahl@rjl.se
8 Stockholm Center for Spine Surgery, SE 171 64 Stockholm, Sweden
* Correspondence: marlene.dufvenberg@liu.se; Tel.: +46-7008-50750

Abstract: Adolescents with idiopathic scoliosis (AIS) often receive conservative treatments aiming to prevent progression of the spinal deformity during puberty. This study aimed to explore patient adherence and secondary outcomes during the first 6 months in an ongoing randomised controlled trial of three treatment interventions. Interventions consisted of physical activity combined with either hypercorrective Boston brace night shift (NB), scoliosis-specific exercise (SSE), or physical activity alone (PA). Measures at baseline and 6 months included angle of trunk rotation (ATR), Cobb angle, International Physical Activity Questionnaire short form (IPAQ-SF), pictorial Spinal Appearance Questionnaire (pSAQ), Scoliosis Research Society (SRS-22r), EuroQol 5-Dimensions Youth (EQ-5D-Y) and Visual Analogue Scale (EQ-VAS). Patient adherence, motivation, and capability in performing the intervention were reported at 6 months. The study included 135 patients (111 females) with AIS and >1-year estimated remaining growth, mean age 12.7 (1.4) years, and mean Cobb angle 31 (±5.3). At 6 months, the proportion of patients in the groups reporting high to very high adherence ranged between 72 and 95%, while motivation ranged between 65 and 92%, with the highest proportion seen in the NB group ($p = 0.014$, $p = 0.002$). IPAQ-SF displayed significant between group main effects regarding moderate activity ($F = 5.7$; $p = 0.004$; $\eta_{p^2} = 0.10$), with a medium-sized increase favouring the SSE group compared to NB. Walking showed significant between group main effects, as did metabolic equivalent (MET-min/week), with medium ($F = 6.8$, $p = 0.002$; $\eta_{p^2} = 0.11$, and large ($F = 8.3$, $p = < 0.001$, $\eta_{p^2} = 0.14$) increases, respectively, for the SSE and PA groups compared to NB. From baseline to 6 months, ATR showed significant between group medium-sized main effects ($F = 1.2$, $p = 0.019$, $\eta_{p^2} = 0.007$) favouring the NB group compared to PA, but not reaching a clinically relevant level. In conclusion, patients reported high adherence and motivation to treatment, especially in the NB group. Patients in the SSE and PA groups increased their physical activity levels without other clinically relevant differences between groups in other clinical measures or patient-reported outcomes. The results suggest that the prescribed treatments are viable first-step options during the first 6 months.

Citation: Dufvenberg, M.; Diarbakerli, E.; Charalampidis, A.; Öberg, B.; Tropp, H.; Aspberg Ahl, A.; Möller, H.; Gerdhem, P.; Abbott, A. Six-Month Results on Treatment Adherence, Physical Activity, Spinal Appearance, Spinal Deformity, and Quality of Life in an Ongoing Randomised Trial on Conservative Treatment for Adolescent Idiopathic Scoliosis (CONTRAIS). *J. Clin. Med.* **2021**, *10*, 4967. https://doi.org/10.3390/jcm10214967

Academic Editor: Theodoros B. Grivas

Received: 15 September 2021
Accepted: 23 October 2021
Published: 26 October 2021

Publisher's Note: MDPI stays neutral with regard to jurisdictional claims in published maps and institutional affiliations.

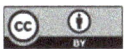

Copyright: © 2021 by the authors. Licensee MDPI, Basel, Switzerland. This article is an open access article distributed under the terms and conditions of the Creative Commons Attribution (CC BY) license (https://creativecommons.org/licenses/by/4.0/).

Keywords: idiopathic scoliosis; bracing; physiotherapeutic scoliosis-specific exercise; physical activity; adherence; spinal appearance; health-related quality of life

1. Introduction

Idiopathic scoliosis is a deformity of the spine, with most cases developing during puberty [1,2]. Spinal deformity can negatively affect health-related quality of life (HRQoL), including psychological distress, perception of spinal appearance, back pain, and pulmonary function in large curves [3–7]. Conservative treatments including a combination of bracing, scoliosis-specific exercise, and more general physical activity interventions are commonly used for patients with moderate-grade AIS, in order to prevent progression and to avoid surgical treatment [8].

Thoracolumbosacral braces are designed to provide three-dimensional correctional counterforces to the scoliosis curvature. Full-time bracing has been the usual care intervention for moderate-grade AIS [8]. A systematic review provides low-quality strength of evidence suggesting that full-time bracing is effective in approximately 75% of cases in preventing excessive progression of the spinal deformity during puberty [9]. More hours of brace wear have been associated with higher success rates [10]. However, full-time bracing can negatively affect patients' perceptions of body appearance, reduce quality of life, and cause back pain [11,12]. Hypercorrective night-time bracing aims to provide curve correction in supine position with reduced mechanical loading [13], and has shown comparable outcomes to full-time bracing in halting the progress of spine deformity [14,15]. Night-time bracing may also minimise potential limitation of daytime activities compared to full-time bracing, and may facilitate better treatment acceptability and adherence for a larger proportion of patients. This warrants investigating the viability of night-time bracing as a first-step approach before considering full-time bracing. This may potentially mitigate negative side effects and overtreatment of bracing [10,16,17].

Current international guidelines recommend scoliosis-specific exercise (SSE) to treat mild AIS (Cobb angle 11–24°), or adjunct to bracing for moderate-grade AIS [8]. However, it is unknown whether SSE is a viable first-step treatment for moderate-grade AIS. Standard features of SSE include three-dimensional spinal self-correction strategies and their integration in activities of daily living, stabilizing the corrected posture, and patient education [8,18]. This potentially influences neuromuscular and sensory integration effect mechanisms, aiming to prevent progression of AIS [19]. A recent systematic review comparing SSE with other conservative interventions for AIS displayed low-quality evidence for SSE causing greater improvements in function, HRQoL, self-image, mental health, and patient satisfaction. However, bracing displayed more effectiveness on measures of spinal deformity than SSE [20].

Physical activity is associated with health benefits for children, including improved muscle strength, motor development, aerobic fitness, and higher bone mineral density [21]. Children are recommended to perform a daily minimum of 60 min of physical activity of at least moderate intensity [21,22]. Current AIS guidelines also recommend sporting activities [8]. According to studies proposing low bone mineral density as a possible mechanism behind AIS [23,24], physical activity might be a possible alternative intervention [25]. However, research is needed in order to evaluate whether physical-activity-related intervention alone is also viable in preventing the progression of moderate-grade AIS [8].

Adherence can be defined as to what extent a person's behaviour corresponds to treatment recommendations [26]. Poor adherence is a reason for suboptimal clinical effect [26], and is therefore important to monitor in clinical trials where the treatment is self-managed and requires long-term maintenance.

An ongoing randomised controlled trial (RCT)—Conservative Treatment for Adolescent Idiopathic Scoliosis (CONTRAIS)—aims to investigate the effectiveness of conservative treatments of moderate-grade AIS in preventing progression and the need for surgical intervention [27]. The treatments consist of adequate self-mediated physical activity levels combined with either hypercorrective Boston brace night shift (NB), scoliosis-specific exercise (SSE), or active control with adequate self-mediated physical activity alone (PA).

Beyond assessment of Cobb angle and trunk rotation, it is of importance in the short-term to explore patients' adherence to treatments, physical activity levels, and potential effects on perception of spinal appearance and HRQoL, considering the long-term maintenance required for scoliosis treatments [28]. The aim of the present study was to explore patient adherence to treatment and secondary outcomes during the first 6 months in terms of physical activity, spinal appearance, spinal deformity, and quality of life within and between NB-, SSE-, and PA-based treatments for AIS in an ongoing RCT.

2. Materials and Methods

2.1. Study Design and Selection of Participants

The present study reports data at baseline and 6 months of an ongoing RCT. The study protocol has been previously published, and is available on clinicaltrials.gov (NCT0176130) [27]. Approval has been obtained by the Regional Ethical Board in Stockholm (Dnr 2012/172-31/4, 2015/1007-32, and 2017/609-32). Study centres were the orthopaedic departments at Karolinska University Hospital, Linköping University Hospital, Ryhov Hospital Jönköping, Eskilstuna Hospital, Västerås Hospital, and Sundsvall Hospital.

Inclusion criteria encompassed a diagnosis of idiopathic scoliosis in females and males; primary curve according to Cobb of 25–40° [29]; curve apex T7 or caudal; estimated remaining skeletal growth of at least one year; not more than one year after menarche; and age 9–17. Exclusion criteria were previous treatment for scoliosis or inability to understand Swedish. The enrolment of the patients took place consecutively between January 2013 and October 2018. Patients who declined participation were offered standard care, which consisted of full-time bracing. In total, 135 patients were randomised into one of three treatment groups: NB, SSE, or PA (Figure 1).

The present study concerns secondary outcomes based on clinical measurements and questionnaires at baseline and after 6 months of treatment. Questionnaires were completed without guidance of the health care provider (HCP), but guidance from the parents was allowed if requested by the patient. In the ongoing RCT, the primary outcome is failure of treatment, defined as an increase in Cobb angle of more than 6 degrees, as seen on two consecutive X-rays after 6 months in relation to the baseline X-ray. Our primary outcome will be reported in a future publication when all patients have reached the endpoint. The endpoint is defined as when the participant reaches skeletal maturity (less than 1.0 cm growth of body height in 6 months), or if the curve progresses by more than 6 degrees, as seen on two consecutive X-rays after 6 months in relation to the baseline X-ray.

A computer-generated concealed randomisation with varying block sizes, at a 1:1:1 ratio, was prepared a priori by an independent statistician. After informed consent, a central research coordinator was contacted for the randomisation process, after which the participants were assigned to the interventions. In this study, blinding of patients and therapists for treatment was not possible.

2.2. Interventions

To enhance desired behavioural outcomes—i.e., high adherence to the treatment plan and self-management—the capability, opportunity, motivation, and behaviour change model (COM-B) was applied for all allocated treatments [30]. The HCPs gave instructions and guidance to enable the patients' self-care ability, goal setting, progression, and follow-up of intervention prescription diary monitoring, as well as parents' participation in the treatment delivery. At an initial 60 min individual session with one out of four experienced physiotherapists, patients were instructed to increase physical activity for the entirety of the study. Instructions were given to perform adequate self-mediated physical activity of at least moderate intensity for $\geq$ 60 min daily in all groups [31]. A summary of the additional interventions is provided below, and in more detail in Figure S1. Abbreviations in Figure

S2. Every 6 months, reinforcement of the assigned intervention was performed Figure S1 at the clinic during an individual session of 60 min. Additional contact via telephone was used when needed.

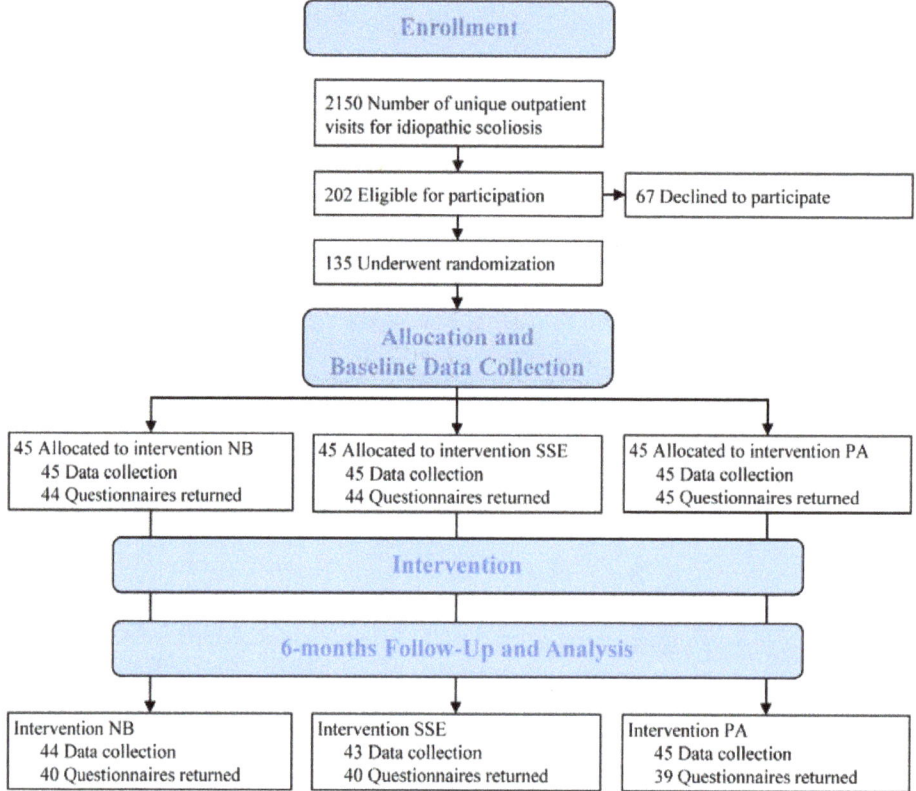

Figure 1. CONSORT flow diagram of the participants with AIS in the study.

2.2.1. Hypercorrective Boston Brace Night Shift

The NB group received a hypercorrective Boston brace night shift [32] tailored to the individual patients' scoliosis. and applying built-in correction in all three planes. The criterion for adequate brace correction was greater than or equal to 50% reduction in Cobb angle. Patients were advised to use the brace throughout every night for at least 8 h. The physiotherapist and orthotist educated the patient and parent when introducing the brace during the first session. The spine orthotist was available for outpatient brace adjustment when needed.

2.2.2. Scoliosis-Specific Exercise

The SSE group received supervised individual treatment by one out of four experienced physiotherapists, consisting of 3 × 60–90 min individual sessions with reiteration of skills learned and skill progression, once per month for the first 3 months. Additional single bolus sessions were given if required. Training goals were directed towards active self-correction in 3 dimensional planes, postural control, spinal stability, muscular stabilisation, and endurance in corrective postures, and were integrated into activities of daily living. Patients were initially asked to perform these specific exercises with 10 repetitions × 3 sets over 30 min, which was included in their prescription of 60 min self-mediated physical activity. When patients had mastered these exercises, they could additionally focus on transferring these skills to similar activities of daily living or individual sporting and recreational activities of interest. Patients were also instructed to use overcorrective side-shift postural strategies during activities of daily living involving relaxed sitting and standing positions. The SSE covered similar concepts and methods to those described in previous literature [33]. The physiotherapists were trained to ensure consistent treatment approach.

2.2.3. Active Control with Adequate Self-Mediated Physical Activity

The PA active control group were instructed to perform adequate self-mediated physical activity of at least moderate intensity for ≥ 60 min daily, for the entirety of the study, with no additional bracing or SSE intervention [31].

2.3. Measurements
Patient Characteristics and Clinical Measures

Patient data such as age, gender, weight, height, and angle of trunk rotation (ATR) assessed via scoliometer were assessed at baseline and at 6 months. Adverse events were reported at 6 months. The assessments took place at the orthopaedic departments, and were coordinated by a multiprofessional team consisting of physicians, nurses, and physiotherapists. Whole standing spine radiographs were performed at baseline and after 6 months. Two experienced spine surgeons not otherwise part of the research group performed blinded assessment of Cobb angle measurements of the largest curve on anonymised images without knowledge of age, sex, or treatment. The mean of the two blinded assessors' Cobb angle measurements of the largest curve was reported at baseline and 6 months.

2.4. Questionnaires, Self-Reported Data, and Health Care Provider Report

The questionnaires included self-report of maturity stages for breast/genitals and pubic hair (Tanner), treatment adherence, effects on HRQoL, perception of spinal appearance, and physical activity level.

2.4.1. Adherence, Motivation, and Capability

In line with the COM-B model [30], to gain knowledge of desired behavioural outcomes—i.e., adherence, motivation, and capability regarding the treatment plan—all study participants answered three additional questions "the grade to which you feel that you have completed the treatment (reported adherence)", "the grade to which you are motivated to carry out the treatment (reported motivation)" and, finally, "how confident are you in your own capability to perform the treatment? (reported capability)".

Additionally, the treating HCP team answered one question—"to what grade the patient has adhered to treatment plan" (reported patient adherence)—using the diary and after dialogue with the patients and families. The patients and HCPs were asked to rate each question on a scale from best "very sure" (1 point) to worst "not at all" (4 points). These questions were collected at the 6-month follow-up.

2.4.2. Physical Activity

Self-reported levels of physical activity during the prior 7 days were captured using the International Physical Activity Questionnaire short form (IPAQ-SF). The IPAQ-SF has acceptable measurement properties [34,35], and provides the achieved mean in minutes of daily activity at the levels of "walking", "moderate" and "vigorous" intensity activity, and "sitting". The volume of activity is computed by weighting each type of activity by its energy requirements as metabolic equivalents (MET). The mean total score of MET min/week is provided by summation of the duration (in min) and frequency (days) [35,36]. The total score ranges from 0 min/day to a maximum of 180 min/day.

2.4.3. Perception of Spinal Appearance

The pictorial part (pSAQ) [6] of the Spinal Appearance Questionnaire (SAQ) is based on the Walter Reed Visual Assessment Scale [37], and has shown good psychometric properties [38,39]. The patient's perception of spinal shape asymmetry is based on 7 categories: body curve, rib prominence, flank prominence, head–chest–hips relationship, head position over hips, shoulder level, and spine prominence. Each category is graded on a scale from "no" (1 point) to "most severe" spinal deformity (5 points). The total score ranges from "least" (7 points) to "most" (35 points) distorted appearance.

2.4.4. Health Related Quality of Life

The Scoliosis Research Society-22r (SRS-22r) is a valid and reliable scoliosis-specific patient-reported measure of HRQoL, and comprises 22 questions categorized into 5 domains (function, pain, self-image, mental health, and satisfaction) [40–42]. The domains, subscore (function, pain, self-image, mental health) and total score (all five domains) can range from "worst" (1 point) to "best" (5 points) [41]. The satisfaction domain and total score were included as measures after 6 months of treatment.

EuroQol 5-Dimensions Youth (EQ-5D-Y) is a valid and reliable generic questionnaire measuring HRQoL, where children from 8 years of age can report their own health [43–48]. The instrument comprises five dimensions: "mobility", "looking after myself", "doing usual activities", "having pain or discomfort" and "feeling worried, sad, or unhappy". Each dimension has three levels of severity: "no" (1 point), "some "(2 points) and "a lot of" (3 points) problems. A global assessment of current health state is measured with a visual analogue scale (EQ-VAS), from "worst" (0 points) to "best" (100 points) imaginable health state.

2.5. Statistical Methods and Analysis

This study's original sample size calculation was based on the primary outcome measure, with a failure of 15% in each of the NB and SSE groups, and 45% in the PA group [49]. With a significance level of 5%, a power of 80%, and consideration for dropout of up to 20%, 45 patients were required in each of the treatment groups [27].

Data was double-entered, and any discrepancies were checked and corrected. Inter-rater reliability of Cobb angle measurements performed by two blinded assessors was calculated via interclass correlation coefficient (ICC 2,1). Descriptive statistics at baseline were presented as mean and standard deviation (±), or as number and proportions (no, %). Patient–HCP agreement in reporting of adherence was estimated with linearly weighted kappa (K), and the relative strength of agreement according to poor <0.00, slight 0.00–0.20, fair 0.21–0.40, moderate 0.41–0.60, substantial 0.61–0.80, and almost perfect 0.81–1.00 [50]. Logistic regression was used to assess the association of two independent factors (motivation and capability) with adherence, applying dichotomised ratings "a very high grade and high grade" and "low grade and not at all". Statistics are presented as Nagelkerke pseudo R-squared (R^2) and odds ratio (OR).

To analyse differences within groups, paired-sample t-tests were performed. Effect size was estimated with Cohen's d as small 0.20, medium 0.50, and large 0.80 [51]. Between group analyses for continuous and categorical variables were performed using univariate analysis of variance (ANOVA) or chi-squared. For ANOVA, partial eta squared (η_p^2) was used as an estimated measure of effect size, where $\eta_p^2 = 0.01 \sim$ small effect, $\eta_p^2 = 0.06 \sim$ medium effect, and $\eta_p^2 = 0.14 \sim$ large effect [51]. Two-sided statistical significance was considered if $p < 0.05$. Paretian analysis presents a classification of health change in EQ-5D-Y from baseline to 6 months towards worse, unchanged, better, or indeterminable [52]. To avoid overestimation for IPAQ physical activity levels, outliers were excluded by truncating to 180 max min/day and a maximum of 21 h of activity/week [35]. All analyses were performed per protocol using statistical analysis performed using the Statistical Package for the Social Sciences (SPSS) statistical software for Windows (SPSS V26, IBM Corporation, New York, NY, USA).

3. Results

3.1. Participant Flow and Baseline Characteristics

Participant flow throughout the study is displayed in Figure 1. In total, 2150 patients were seen as outpatients during the inclusion period, and 135 patients were included and randomly allocated to 45 patients per group. The mean age was 12.7 ($\pm$1.4), and 111 were females (82%). There were two female questionnaire non-responders at baseline—one allocated to the NB group and one to the SSE group. Treatment groups did not differ at baseline regarding patient characteristics, clinical measures, or patient-reported outcomes (Tables 1–6).

Table 1. Baseline characteristics of the included patients.

	Overall Sample n = 135	NB n = 45	SSE n = 45	PA n = 45	p-Value
Age * (years)	12.7 (1.4)	12.7 (1.4)	12.6 (1.4)	12.6 (1.5)	0.892
Females (no.%)	111 (82)	39 (87)	33 (73)	39 (87)	0.161
Height * (cm)	158.1 (9.5)	157.2 (9.5)	158.1 (9.6)	159.0 (9.6)	0.678
Weight * (kg)	46.0 (9.2)	44.8 (9.3)	45.7 (9.0)	47.3 (9.4)	0.434
Body mass index *	18.3 (2.6)	18.0 (2.7)	18.2 (2.4)	18.6 (2.7)	0.504
Angle of trunk rotation * (degrees)	11.3 (3.1)	11.8 (2.7)	10.8 (3.3)	11.3 (3.1)	0.287
Tanner breast/genital N (%)					
I	8 (6)	2 (5)	5 (12)	1 (2)	
II	23 (18)	8 (19)	5 (12)	10 (24)	
III	65 (52)	22 (52)	20 (49)	23 (55)	0.521
IV	26 (21)	10 (24)	9 (22)	7 (17)	
V	3 (2)	-	2 (5)	1 (2)	
Tanner pubic hair N (%)					
I	16 (13)	5 (12)	6 (15)	5 (12)	
II	19 (15)	6 (15)	6 (15)	7 (17)	
III	33 (27)	14 (34)	9 (22)	10 (24)	0.595
IV	49 (40)	14 (34)	15 (38)	20 (48)	
V	6 (5)	2 (5)	4 (10)		
Cobb angle * (degrees)	31 (5.3)	32 (5.6)	31 (4.6)	31 (5.6)	0.433
Location of largest curve N (%)					
Thoracic	99 (73)	32 (73)	33 (73)	33 (73)	
Thoracolumbar	21 (16)	7 (16)	6 (13)	8 (18)	0.970
Lumbar	15 (11)	5 (11)	6 (13)	4 (9)	

* Values are given as mean and standard deviation (SD). N: number of patients; NB: hypercorrective Boston brace night shift; SSE: scoliosis-specific exercise; PA: adequate self-mediated physical activity; Tanner scale: breast/genitals and pubic hair I–V maturity stages; Cobb angle: largest curve of scoliosis measured with X-ray.

A total of 135 patients received the allocated treatment plan. At 6 months, there were 16 questionnaire non-responders (Figure 1), of whom 11 gave no reasons, 4 opted for a full-time brace, and 1 due to anxiety. This resulted at 6 months in 119 patients who provided patient-reported outcomes: 40 patients each in the NB and SSE groups, and 39 in the PA group. HCPs provided data collection regarding 132 patients: 44 in the NB group, 43 in the PA group, and 45 in the SSE group. At 6 months, patients or HCPs reported five adverse events in the NB group: sleeping problems during habituation period, awkwardness of staying overnight with friends, pressure towards ribs, redness and itchiness, and one unspecified. In the SSE group, one patient reported pain during treatment sessions, and one other patient reported muscle strain. No adverse events were reported in the PA group.

3.2. Adherence, Motivation, and Capability Regarding the Treatment Plan

Table 2 describes the reporting of adherence, motivation, and capability regarding the treatment plan at 6 months. In most cases a "high or very high grade" was reported by patients and practitioners. However, the NB group had a statistically significantly larger proportion of patients reporting a very high grade of adherence to the treatment plan compared to the PA group ($p = 0.014$). Furthermore, the NB group had a statistically significantly larger proportion of patients reporting a "very high grade" of motivation regarding the treatment plan compared to the PA group ($p = 0.002$). The NB group also had statistically significantly smaller proportion of patients reporting a lower grade of motivation regarding the treatment plan compared to the SSE and PA groups ($p = 0.002$). The strength of patient–HCP agreement in reported adherence to the treatment plan at 6 months was fair (K = 0.319). Patient–HCP proportional agreement on treatment adherence most frequently occurred within the "high grade–sure" ($n = 23/115$), and "very high grade–very sure" ($n = 22/115$) responses, but also had the largest mismatch between "high grade–very sure" ($n = 40/115$) responses.

Logistic regression highlighted that 37% of the variation in adherence at 6 months was explained by motivation and capability ($R^2 = 0.37$). Patients with high self-rated motivation had 3.6 times better odds of higher adherence to the treatment plan (OR 3.58, $p = 0.043$). Likewise, patients with high self-rated capability had 14.2 times better odds of higher adherence to the treatment plan (OR = 14.24, $p = 0.004$).

Table 2. Adherence, motivation, and capability regarding the treatment plan.

Patient and Practitioner Reporting Related to Performance of the Treatment Plan				
	NB N (%)	SSE N (%)	PA N (%)	p-Value
Patient-reported adherence to the treatment plan				0.014
Very high grade	**14 (37)** [a]	7 (18)	**4 (10)** [b]	
High grade	22 (58)	21 (54)	28 (74)	
Low grade	2 (5)	9 (23)	6 (16)	
Not at all	0 (0)	2 (5)	0 (0)	
Patient reported motivation regarding the treatment plan				0.002
Very high grade	**22 (56)** [a]	12 (30)	**6 (16)** [b]	
High grade	14 (36)	14 (35)	19 (50)	
Low grade	**2 (5)** [b]	**11 (27)** [a]	**11 (29)** [a]	
Not at all	1 (3)	3 (8)	2 (5)	
Patient-reported capability to adhere to the treatment plan				0.076
Very high grade	21 (54)	15 (38)	14 (37)	
High grade	17 (44)	22 (55)	18 (47)	
Low grade	1 (2)	1 (2)	6 (16)	
Not at all	0 (0)	2 (5)	0 (0)	
Practitioner-reported patient adherence to the treatment plan				0.129
Very sure	28 (67)	18 (44)	27 (64)	
Sure	11 (26)	10 (24)	10 (24)	
Unsure	2 (5)	8 (20)	3 (7)	
Not at all	1 (2)	5 (12)	2 (5)	

Patient–practitioner concordance in reporting of adherence to the treatment plan				
	Practitioner-reported patient adherence to the treatment plan			
	Very sure	Sure	Unsure	Not at all
Patient-reported adherence to the treatment plan				
Very high grade	22	2	1	0
High grade	40	23	8	0
Low grade	4	5	3	5
Not at all	0	0	0	2
Linear weighted Kappa = 0.319				

N: number of patients; NB: hypercorrective Boston brace night shift; SSE: scoliosis-specific exercise; PA: adequate self-mediated physical activity. Bold = statistical significance at $p < 0.05$, where row proportion [a] > [b].

3.3. Physical Activity Level

Results of the IPAQ-SF are displayed in Table 3. Regarding change from baseline to 6 months within groups, the NB group showed a small, statistically significant decrease in sitting time of 79 min/day ($p = 0.031$, $d = 0.45$). The SSE group had a statistically significant medium-sized increase in walking time of 20 min/day ($p = 0.002$, $d = 0.51$). The PA group had a small, statistically significant increase in moderate-intensity activity of 23 min/day ($p = 0.009$, $d = 0.49$), as well as an increase in walking of 15 min/day ($p = 0.033$, $d = 0.35$). Furthermore, the SSE and PA groups had statistically significant medium-sized increases of 1499 MET-min/week ($p = 0.001$, $d = 0.59$) and 1378 MET-min/week ($p = < 0.001$, $d = 0.73$), respectively.

Regarding between group differences in changes from baseline to 6 months, there was a statistically significant medium-sized main effect ($F = 5.7$, $p = 0.004$, $\eta_{p^2} = 0.10$) for moderate-intensity activity. This favoured the SSE group, with 37 min/day more than the NB group. Similarly, there was a statistically significant medium-sized main effect ($F = 6.8$; $p = 0.002$, $\eta_{p^2} = 0.11$) for walking, favouring the SSE and PA groups, with 27 min/day and 23 min/day more, respectively, compared to the NB group. The same pattern was displayed in MET-min/week, with a large, statistically significant main effect ($F = 8.3$, $p = < 0.001$, $\eta_{p^2} = 0.14$) favouring the SSE and PA groups, with 1880 and 1482 more MET-min/week, respectively, compared to the NB group.

Table 3. Physical activity levels for the IPAQ-SF in min/day and MET-min/week at baseline, within group change and between group differences in change between baseline to 6 months.

	Baseline	Within Group Changes from Baseline to 6 Months			Between Group Differences in Changes from Baseline to 6 Months	
IPAQ-SF min/day	Mean (SD)	Mean Change (SD)	p-Value	Cohen's d	Main Effects F; p-Value; η_{p^2}	Pairwise Comparison Mean difference (95% CI) p-Value
		Positive change = better outcome				Favoured group ↑
Vigorous					0.2; 0.844; 0.03	NA
NB	45 (54)	5 (49)	0.565			
SSE	47 (53)	9 (65)	0.392			
PA	40 (47)	9 (43)	0.228			
Moderate					5.7; **0.004**; 0.10	
NB	47 (60)	−10 (60)	0.318			NB-SSE ↑ = −37 (−64 to −10); **0.004**
SSE	65 (54)	11 (85)	0.417			SSE-PA= 10 (−17 to 38); >0.999
PA	39 (45)	23 (51)	**0.009**	0.49		NB-PA = −26 (−54 to 1); 0.066
Walking					6.8; **0.002**; 0.11	
NB	50 (46)	−14 (47)	0.073			NB-SSE ↑ = −27 (−46 to −8); **0.002**
SSE	38 (37)	20 (39)	**0.002**	0.51		SSE-PA= 4 (−15 to 23); >0.999
PA	39 (47)	15 (43)	**0.033**	0.35		NB-PA ↑ = −23 (−42 to −4); **0.014**
		Negative change = positive outcome				
Sitting					1.8; 0.167; 0.04	NA
NB	458 (199)	−79 (180)	**0.031**	0.45		
SSE	385 (184)	17 (134)	0.526			
PA	415 (153)	−9 (126)	0.693			
IPAQ-SF MET-min/week		Positive change = better outcome				Favoured group ↑
					8.3; **< 0.001**; 0.14	
NB	2751 (3522)	−411 (2508)	0.332			NB-SSE ↑ = −1880 (−3059 to −701); **0.001**
SSE	2693 (2098)	1499 (2525)	**0.001**	0.59		SSE-PA= 398 (−786 to 1582); >0.999
PA	2139 (1765)	1378 (2216)	**0.001**	0.73		NB-PA ↑= −1482 (−2667 to −297); **0.009**

IPAQ-SF: International Physical Activity Questionnaire short form; MET: metabolic equivalent; NB: hypercorrective Boston brace night shift; SSE: scoliosis-specific exercise; PA: adequate self-mediated physical activity. ↑ = Favoured group marked with an arrow, Bold = significant at $p < 0.05$; Cohen's d estimate = effect size; η_{p^2} = partial eta squared. NA = not applicable.

3.4. Perception of Spinal Appearance

There was a small, statistically significant mean decrease in pSAQ from baseline to 6 months for the SSE group (0.9 (±2.9), $p = 0.049$, $d = 0.34$). No between group differences in change from baseline to 6 months were displayed regarding pSAQ (Table 4).

3.5. Angle of Trunk Rotation and Cobb Angle

ATR showed a small, statistically significant within group mean change, increasing from baseline to 6 months for the SSE (1.2 (±2.4), $p = 0.004$) and PA groups (1.0 (±3.0), $p = 0.029$). A significant between group difference in change from baseline to 6 months was displayed favouring the NB group compared to the PA group (−1.5 (CI −3.0 to −0.1), $p = 0.037$), with a medium-sized main effect (F = 4.1, p-value = 0.019, $\eta_{p^2} = 0.07$) (Table 4).

Cobb angle showed a small, statistically significant within group mean change, increasing from baseline to 6 months for the NB group (2.3 (±4.3), $p = 0.001$). Likewise, there was a medium-sized within group mean change increasing for the SSE (3.7 (±7.0), $p = 0.001$) and PA groups (3.7 (±6.3), $p = < 0.001$). No between group differences in change from baseline to 6 months were displayed regarding Cobb angle (Table 4). The interrater reliability of Cobb angle measurements performed by two blinded assessors at baseline was ICC 2,1 = 0.817, and at 6 months ICC 2,1 = 0.888.

Table 4. Spinal appearance, angle of trunk rotation, and Cobb angles at baseline, within group changes from baseline to 6 months, and between group differences in changes from baseline to 6 months.

	Baseline	Within Group Changes from Baseline to 6 Months			Between Group Differences in Changes between Baseline and 6 Months	
	Mean (SD)	Mean Change (SD)	p-Value	Cohen's d	Main Effects F; p-Value; η_{p^2}	Pairwise Comparison Mean Difference (95% CI) p-Value
		Positive change = worse outcome				Favoured group ↑
pSAQ general (7–35)					0.7; 0.485; 0.01	NA
NB	11.7 (3.5)	0.1 (2.9)	0.784			
SSE	11.5 (3.1)	0.9 (2.9)	**0.049**	0.32		
PA	11.7 (2.8)	0.6 (3.2)	0.261			
Angle of trunk rotation (degrees)					4.1; **0.019**; 0.07	
NB	11.8 (2.7)	−0.6 (3.0)	0.172			NB-SSE= −1.5 (−3.1 to <0.1); 0.051
SSE	10.5 (3.0)	1.2 (2.4)	**0.004**	0.34		SSE-PA= −0.2 (−1.5 to 1.5); >0.999
PA	11.1 (2.8)	1.0 (3.0)	**0.029**	0.34		NB↑-PA= −1.5 (−3.0 to −0.1); **0.037**
Cobb angle					1.1; 0.332; 0.02	NA
NB	32 (5.6)	2.3 (4.3)	**0.001**	0.34		
SSE	31 (4.7)	3.7 (7.0)	**0.001**	0.50		
PA	31 (5.6)	3.7 (6.3)	**<0.001**	0.50		

pSAQ: pictorial Spinal Appearance Questionnaire; NB: hypercorrective Boston brace night shift; SSE: scoliosis-specific exercise; PA: adequate self-mediated physical activity. ↑ = Favoured group marked with an arrow, Bold = significant at $p < 0.05$; Cohen's d estimate = effect size; η_{p^2} = partial eta squared.

3.6. Health-Related Quality of Life

Results for the SRS-22r are displayed in Table 5. Regarding changes from baseline to 6 months within groups, the NB group had a small decrease in the function domain (−0.1 (±0.3), $p = 0.018$, $d = 0.36$), the PA group had a small decrease in the mental health domain (−0.2 (±0.5), $p = 0.009$, $d = 0.33$), and the SSE group had a small decrease in the SRS-22r subscore (−0.1 (±0.3), $p = 0.039$, $d = 0.22$). No between group differences in change from baseline to 6 months were displayed regarding SRS−22r domains or subscores. At 6 months, the SRS-22r satisfaction domain and total score displayed no significant differences between groups.

For EQ-VAS global health state, there were no statistically significant within group changes or between group differences in changes between baseline and 6 months (Table 5). The EQ-5D-Y dimensions and Paretian Classification of Health Change showed no statistically significant differences between groups at 6 months (Table 6).

Table 5. Health-related quality of life according to the SRS-22r and EQ-VAS global health scores at baseline, within group changes from baseline to 6 months, and between group differences in changes from baseline to 6 months.

	Baseline	Within Group Changes from Baseline to 6 Months			Between Group Differences in Changes between Baseline and 6 Months	
	Mean (SD)	Mean Change (SD)	p-Value	Cohen's d	Main Effects F; p-Value; η_p^2	Pairwise Comparison Mean Difference (95% CI) p-Value
		Negative Change = Worse Outcome				
SRS-22r Function (1–5)					1.2; 0.298; 0.02	NA
NB	4.8 (0.2)	−0.1 (0.3)	**0.018**	0.36		
SSE	4.7 (0.3)	−0.1 (0.4)	0.066			
PA	4.7 (0.3)	<−0.1 (0.3)	0.925			
SRS-22r Pain (1–5)					0.4; 0.658; 0.01	NA
NB	4.7 (0.6)	<−0.1 (0.4)	0.731			
SSE	4.6 (0.6)	<−0.1 (0.4)	0.486			
PA	4.7 (0.6)	<−0.1 (0.4)	0.943			
SRS-22r Self-image (1–5)					1.8; 0.170; 0.03	NA
NB	4.1 (0.7)	0.1 (0.5)	0.367			
SSE	4.2 (0.6)	−0.1 (0.5)	0.101			
PA	4.3 (0.5)	−0.1 (0.5)	0.200			
SRS-22r Mental health (1–5)					0.8; 0.437; 0.02	NA
NB	4.3 (0.6)	−0.1 (0.4)	0.325			
SSE	4.3 (0.6)	−0.1 (0.6)	0.152			
PA	4.3 (0.6)	−0.2 (0.5)	**0.009**	0.33		
SRS-22r Subscore (1–5)					0.9; 0.394; 0.02	NA
NB	4.5 (0.5)	<−0.1 (0.2)	0.493			
SSE	4.5 (0.4)	−0.1 (0.3)	**0.039**	0.22		
PA	4.5 (0.3)	−0.1 (0.3)	0.057			
SRS-22r Satisfaction (1–5)	At 6 months only				2.7; 0.074; 0.05	NA
NB	3.9 (0.8)					
SSE	3.5 (0.9)					
PA	3.4 (1.1)					
SRS-22r Total Score (1–5)	At 6 months only				0.8; 0.460; 0.01	NA
NB	4.4 (0.5)					
SSE	4.3 (0.5)					
PA	4.3 (0.4)					
EQ-VAS Global health (0–100)					0.2; 0.763; 0.01	NA
NB	88.2 (11.5)	−2.6 (10.4)	0.133			
SSE	88.0 (10.0)	−3.2 (15.0)	0.197			
PA	87.6 (10.6)	−1.0 (12.2)	0.620			

SRS-22r: The Scoliosis Research Society-22r; EQ-VAS: EuroQol Visual Analogue Scale; NB: hypercorrective Boston brace night shift; SSE: scoliosis-specific exercise; PA: adequate self-mediated physical activity. Bold = significant at $p < 0.05$; Cohen's d estimate = effect size; η_p^2 = partial eta squared. NA = not applicable.

Table 6. Health-related quality of life for the EQ-5D-Y dimensions, at baseline and 6 months, and changes in health state according to Paretian Classification of Health Change from baseline to 6 months.

EQ-5D-Y Dimensions	Mobility		Self-Care		Usual Activities		Pain/Discomfort		Anxiety/Depression	
	Baseline	6 Months	Baseline	6 Months	Baseline	6 Months	Baseline	6 Months	Baseline	6 Months
No problems										
NB-number (%)	44 (100)	39 (100)	44 (100)	38 (100)	42 (96)	38 (97)	34 (77)	30 (77)	28 (65)	25 (66)
SSE	43 (98)	39 (98)	44 (100)	40 (100)	41 (93)	37 (92)	33 (75)	26 (65)	31 (74)	29 (74)
PA	45 (100)	38 (100)	45 (100)	38 (100)	43 (96)	37 (97)	34 (76)	28 (74)	32 (71)	29 (76)
Moderate problems										
NB-number (%)	0 (0)	0 (0)	0 (0)	0 (0)	2 (4)	1 (3)	9 (20)	8 (20)	14 (33)	12 (32)
SSE	1 (2)	1 (2)	0 (0)	0 (0)	3 (7)	3 (8)	9 (20)	13 (32)	11 (26)	9 (23)
PA	0 (0)	0 (0)	0 (0)	0 (0)	2 (4)	1 (2)	10 (22)	9 (24)	12 (27)	8 (21)
Severe problems										
NB-number (%)	0 (0)	0 (0)	0 (0)	0 (0)	0 (0)	0 (0)	1 (2)	1 (3)	1 (2)	1 (3)
SSE	0 (0)	0 (0)	0 (0)	0 (0)	0 (0)	0 (0)	2 (4)	1 (2)	0 (0)	1 (3)
PA	0 (0)	0 (0)	0 (0)	0 (0)	0 (0)	0 (0)	1 (2)	1 (3)	1 (2)	1 (3)
Chi^2 p-Value	0.662	> 0.999	NA	NA	0.898	0.617	>0.999	0.869	0.852	0.906

Paretian Classification of Health Change, baseline to 6 months	Worse [1]	Unchanged [2]	Better [3]	Indeterminable [4]	Chi^2 p-Value
NB n = 38-number (%)					0.448
SSE n = 37-number (%)	8 (22)	22 (60)	6 (16)	1 (3)	
PA n = 38-number (%)	10 (26)	18 (47)	9 (24)	1 (3)	

EQ-5D-Y: EuroQol 5-Dimensions Youth; NB: hypercorrective Boston brace night shift; SSE: scoliosis-specific exercise; PA: adequate self-mediated physical activity; NA: not applicable—the distribution is a constant in self-care. Paretian Classification of Health Change: [1] The health state is worse in at least one dimension, and is no better in any other dimension; [2] the health state is exactly the same; [3] the health state is better in at least one dimension and is no worse in any other dimension; [4] the changes in health are "mixed"—better in one dimension, but worse in another.

4. Discussion

The present study's results highlight that differences exist in adherence and patient-reported outcomes after a 6-month period of either NB, SSE, or PA treatments for AIS. Overall, self-reported and HCP-reported assessments of patient adherence, motivation, and capability regarding the treatments were high, especially for the NB group (92–98%), while adherence and motivation for the PA and SSE treatments were statistically significantly lower by approximately 10–20%, respectively. Importantly, patient-reported capability to carry out the treatment plan over 6 months displayed no differences between groups. In contrast, a report from the World Health Organization showed lower proportions of adherence (50%) in long-term therapies, which further reduced if treatments were complex and self-managed [26]. This implies that the HCPs in this study successfully facilitated patient and parent understanding and physical ability to perform and self-manage the treatment plans over 6 months.

In line with the COM-B model [30] and other studies [26,53], high patient adherence had a significant positive association with patient capability and motivation. This suggests the importance of the HCP strategies in the delivery of the treatment plans. This not only serves to facilitate and maintain patient capabilities, but also to improve motivation, which may be important for long-term adherence to interventions. The COM-B model highlights the importance of providing sufficient opportunity to maintain a target behaviour. For example, the provision of extra HCP guidance if requested, the use of a training diary, and the promotion of the parent's role in guiding and motivating the patient can be important strategies that may help to influence motivation and treatment adherence.

Within the NB group, according to the IPAQ-SF, there was a decrease in time spent sitting, but no change in other physical activity levels during the 6-month period. In contrast, both the PA and SSE groups had a significant increase in walking, while moderate-intensity physical activity levels significantly increased in the PA group. This contributed to a significantly higher improvement in MET-min/week of physical activity in the PA and SSE groups compared to the NB group. Group means at baseline for IPAQ-SF levels, however, were already in line with recommendations for physical activity from the Public Health Ministry of Sweden [54], which are in line with the WHO´s recommendations [31]. Instead of increasing physical activity levels, one can speculate that the NB group was above all motivated to adhere to night-time bracing. This could be a potential factor influencing the higher patient ratings of adherence and motivation with the NB treatment plan [55]. George et al. [53] pointed out that adherence is rarely, if ever, an all-or-nothing phenomenon; more likely, some recommendations in a treatment plan are followed, while others receive less focus from the patient.

The patients in our sample had mean Cobb angle curves of 31 (±5.3) degrees at baseline, but perceived minimal spinal shape asymmetry according to the pSAQ [6]. The SAQ has been shown to be more sensitive and responsive to change than textual scales such as the SRS-22r self-image domain [28]. The SSE and PA groups had a small increase in ATR and a medium increase in Cobb angle, while small increases in pSAQ for the SSE group and Cobb angle for the NB group were seen at 6 months. However, the SRS-22r self-image domain displayed no differences during the study period. ATR displayed a medium-sized between group difference in changes from baseline to 6 months, favouring the NB group compared to the PA group. The observed changes in ATR and Cobb angle measurements in this study, however, were well below what can be considered clinically relevant, since both the scoliometer and digital Cobb angle measures have up to approximately 6 degrees standard error of measurement [56–59]. Schreiber et al. [60] found better general SAQ scores in AIS patients after 6 months of full-time bracing in combination with SSE compared to controls, in contrast to a previous study that showed more distorted perceived appearance in braced patients compared to non-braced patients [11]. It is possible that more intensive bracing [10] is required for patients to perceive changes in spinal appearance. However, when considering the risk of overtreatment, one may consider NB as a viable first step requiring lower dosage.

The SRS-22r satisfaction domain showed no between group differences despite the NB group reporting a significant decrease in the SRS-22r function domain over time. A previous study suggested that full-time brace wear can negatively impact different aspects of quality of life in 72% of the study population [12]. Conversely, another study found no decline in health in braced individuals compared to observation only [61]. The minimal important change for the SRS-22r function domain in moderate AIS has been reported to be 0.60 [62], which implies that the negative change in our study does not affect the patient in everyday activities.

The PA group showed a small, statistically significant decrease in the SRSr-22r mental health domain over the 6-month period. However, there were no statistically significant between group differences, and the PA group change was less than the minimal important change for the SRS-22r mental health domain in moderate AIS, which has been reported to be 0.55 [62]. The SSE group showed a small, statistically significant decrease in the SRSr-22r subscore over the 6-month period; this is in contrast to the findings of Monticone et al. [63], who evaluated the effect of SSE vs. traditional exercises in mild AIS, and found increased HRQoL favouring the SSE group. The SRS-22r subscores for patients in the present study, however, were slightly below normative values of 4.7 at baseline [64], but higher than previously reported values for braced, surgically treated, or untreated adults with AIS [7,65].

The EQ-VAS global health score in the present study population was high, and similar to normative data [46]. According to the EQ-5D-Y domain scores in the present study, patients very rarely reported problems with mobility, self-care, or usual activities, and none that were severe. When considering the anxiety/depression and pain/discomfort domains, severe problems were very rare, but 20–33% of the patients reported moderate problems at either baseline or 6 months, with no statistically significant between group differences in change over the 6 months. These proportions were similar to literature reporting Swedish general population normative EQ-5D-Y data for 12 and 16 year olds [46], but a little higher than normative EQ-5D scores for ages ≤ 19 [64]. Similar occurrence of pain has been reported with SRS-22r in a study of patients with AIS [4], but as high as 46% in full-time brace-treated populations evaluated with the Brace Questionnaire [12]. Anxiety and depression can be considered to be risk factors for chronic back pain [4]. This suggests the importance of helping patients showing signs of anxiety/depression and pain/discomfort to manage such problems throughout the treatment plan.

This RCT data collection was successfully carried out within the context of the Swedish public health care system. The study is therefore representative of the Swedish context, and generalizable to similar health care systems. The study's rigorous design, adequate sample size, patient adherence to treatment plan, and good retention in prospectively collected data provide lower risk of bias to findings compared to previous studies in the field. Another strength was the use of patient-reported outcome and experience measurements to capture the patient perspective regarding the three prescribed treatments. SSE in the current study covers similar concepts and methods to those described in previous literature on scoliosis-specific treatments [8,33]. However, the current study focused on patient self-management, with three supervised sessions as a first-step intervention during the first three months, and additional sessions if needed before the 6-month follow-up.

Key limitations of this study are that the evaluations of adherence, motivation, and capability are based on the entire treatment plan as a whole, and do not distinguish between the included parts of the treatment. Lower adherence toward one of the components in the treatment plan cannot be ruled out. This study only comprises subjective means of measuring adherence, including patient-administered questionnaires and HCP reports. Measuring adherence is complex, and overestimation [66] or underestimation among patients and HCPs is possible. Review of diaries at follow-up every 6 months was an initial strategy to maintain and report adherence as accurately as possible, but patient compliance with the use of a diary varied, with some patients filling their diaries in as an afterthought in conjunction with revisit. The current study was planned in 2011–2012, when the availability of objective and patient-friendly monitoring of adherence was in progress, as well as with telehealth to enhance adherence. Advances in new technologies and measurement methods enable objective measures of time spent in brace [10], along with pedometers and accelerometer-based devices to register physical activity, inactivity, and sleep [67]. However, objective measurements can be costly and technically demanding [26]. The current study had missing values ranging from 1.5 to 31%, where the IPAQ-SF sitting score had the highest number of missing values—possibly due to difficulty in reporting, because sitting occurs continually throughout the day. A mix of self-reported and reasonable objective measures could be the best way to capture adherence behaviour to a treatment plan [26], and to get a broad picture of health aspects in AIS [68].

5. Conclusions

After a 6-month intervention period, self-reported and HCP-reported patient adherence were high in all groups. Patients also reported motivation and capability to carry out and perform the treatment as high, especially in the NB group. Patients in exclusively active intervention groups increased their physical activity without other clinically relevant differences between groups on other clinical measures or patient-reported outcomes. The results suggest that prescribed interventions are viable first-step options during the first 6 months.

Supplementary Materials: The following are available online https://www.mdpi.com/article/10.3390/jcm10214967/s1: Figure S1: Detailed description of interventions within CONTRAIS; Figure S2: Abbreviations.

Author Contributions: Conceptualisation, P.G., A.A. and H.M.; methodology, M.D., B.Ö. and A.A.; software, A.A.; validation, A.A.; formal analysis, M.D., B.Ö. and A.A.; investigation, E.D., A.C., H.T., A.A.A., H.M., P.G. and A.A.; resources, P.G. and A.A.; data curation, M.D., A.C. and A.A.; writing—original draft preparation, M.D., B.Ö. and A.A.; writing—review and editing, M.D. and A.A.; visualization, M.D. and A.A.; supervision, B.Ö., H.T., P.G. and A.A.; project administration, A.A.; funding acquisition, P.G. and A.A. All authors have read and agreed to the published version of the manuscript.

Funding: This research was financially supported by The Swedish Research Council (Dnr 521-2012-1771); the regional agreement on medical training and clinical research (ALF) between Stockholm County Council, Karolinska Institutet, and Linköpings University; and the Swedish Society of Spinal Surgeons. Paul Gerdhem was supported by Region Stockholm (clinical research appointment).

Institutional Review Board Statement: This study was conducted in accordance with the guidelines of the Declaration of Helsinki and approved by the Regional Ethical Board in Stockholm (Dnr 2012/172-31/4, 2015/1007-32, and 2017/609-32).

Informed Consent Statement: Informed consent was obtained from all subjects involved in the study.

Data Availability Statement: The data that support the findings of this study are available from the CONTRAIS research group, and are thus not publicly available. The data are, however, available from the authors upon reasonable request.

Acknowledgments: The authors give thanks to Luigi Belcastro (research nurse and study coordinator) and Maria Wikzén (research nurse and study coordinator), as well as to Peter Endler, Kourosh Jalalpour, Panayiotis Savvides, Tomas Reigo, Anna Grauers, Björn Dahlman, Ylva Boden and, Ingrid Ekenman for patient recruitment. We also give thanks to Henrik Hedevik for statistical analysis, and the physiotherapists Sofia Berto and Suzanne Thorén. Acke Ohlin from Lund University and Kourosh Jalalpour from Karolinska University Hospital carried out all of the Cobb angle measurements.

Conflicts of Interest: The authors declare no conflict of interest.

Preregistration: Trial registration: NCT01761305 4 January 2013. Abbott, A.; Moller, H.; Gerdhem, P. CONTRAIS: Conservative Treatment for Adolescent Idiopathic Scoliosis: a randomised controlled trial protocol. BMC musculoskeletal disorders 2013, 14, 261, doi:10.1186/1471-2474-14-261. https://rdcu.be/cjWz2 (accessed on 4 January 2013).

References

1. Ekinci, S.; Ersen, O. Adolescent Idiopathic Scoliosis. *ACES* **2014**, *3*, 174–182. [CrossRef]
2. Weinstein, S.L.; Dolan, L.A. The Evidence Base for the Prognosis and Treatment of Adolescent Idiopathic Scoliosis: The 2015 Orthopaedic Research and Education Foundation Clinical Research Award. *J. Bone Jt. Surg. Am.* **2015**, *97*, 1899–1903. [CrossRef]
3. Weinstein, S.L.; Dolan, L.A.; Spratt, K.F.; Peterson, K.K.; Spoonamore, M.J.; Ponseti, I.V. Health and function of patients with untreated idiopathic scoliosis: A 50-year natural history study. *JAMA* **2003**, *289*, 559–567. [CrossRef]
4. Makino, T.; Kaito, T.; Sakai, Y.; Takenaka, S.; Yoshikawa, H. Health-related Quality of Life and Postural Changes of Spinal Alignment in Female Adolescents Associated With Back Pain in Adolescent Idiopathic Scoliosis: A Prospective Cross-sectional Study. *Spine* **2019**, *44*, E833–E840. [CrossRef]
5. Ramirez, N.; Johnston, C.E.; Browne, R.H. The prevalence of back pain in children who have idiopathic scoliosis. *J. Bone Jt. Surg. Am.* **1997**, *79*, 364–368. [CrossRef]
6. Savvides, P.; Gerdhem, P.; Grauers, A.; Danielsson, A.; Diarbakerli, E. Self-Experienced Trunk Appearance in Individuals With and Without Idiopathic Scoliosis. *Spine* **2020**, *45*, 522–527. [CrossRef]
7. Diarbakerli, E.; Grauers, A.; Danielsson, A.; Abbott, A.; Gerdhem, P. Quality of Life in Males and Females With Idiopathic Scoliosis. *Spine* **2019**, *44*, 404–410. [CrossRef]
8. Negrini, S.; Donzelli, S.; Aulisa, A.G.; Czaprowski, D.; Schreiber, S.; de Mauroy, J.C.; Diers, H.; Grivas, T.B.; Knott, P.; Kotwicki, T.; et al. 2016 SOSORT guidelines: Orthopaedic and rehabilitation treatment of idiopathic scoliosis during growth. *Scoliosis Spinal Disord.* **2018**, *13*, 3–51. [CrossRef]
9. Negrini, S.; Minozzi, S.; Bettany-Saltikov, J.; Chockalingam, N.; Grivas, T.B.; Kotwicki, T.; Maruyama, T.; Romano, M.; Zaina, F. Braces for idiopathic scoliosis in adolescents. *Cochrane Database Syst. Rev.* **2015**, *6*, CD006850. [CrossRef]
10. Dolan, L.A.; Donzelli, S.; Zaina, F.; Weinstein, S.L.; Negrini, S. Adolescent Idiopathic Scoliosis Bracing Success Is Influenced by Time in Brace: Comparative Effectiveness Analysis of BrAIST and ISICO Cohorts. *Spine* **2020**, *45*, 1193–1199. [CrossRef]
11. Danielsson, A.J.; Hasserius, R.; Ohlin, A.; Nachemson, A.L. Body appearance and quality of life in adult patients with adolescent idiopathic scoliosis treated with a brace or under observation alone during adolescence. *Spine* **2012**, *37*, 755–762. [CrossRef]
12. Piantoni, L.; Tello, C.A.; Remondino, R.G.; Bersusky, E.S.; Menendez, C.; Ponce, C.; Quintana, S.; Hekier, F.; Francheri Wilson, I.A.; Galaretto, E.; et al. Quality of life and patient satisfaction in bracing treatment of adolescent idiopathic scoliosis. *Scoliosis Spinal Disord.* **2018**, *13*, 26–37. [CrossRef] [PubMed]
13. Sattout, A.; Clin, J.; Cobetto, N.; Labelle, H.; Aubin, C.E. Biomechanical Assessment of Providence Nighttime Brace for the Treatment of Adolescent Idiopathic Scoliosis. *Spine Deform.* **2016**, *4*, 253–260. [CrossRef] [PubMed]
14. Ruffilli, A.; Fiore, M.; Barile, F.; Pasini, S.; Faldini, C. Evaluation of night-time bracing efficacy in the treatment of adolescent idiopathic scoliosis: A systematic review. *Spine Deform.* **2021**, *9*, 671–678. [CrossRef]
15. Costa, L.; Schlosser, T.P.C.; Jimale, H.; Homans, J.F.; Kruyt, M.C.; Castelein, R.M. The Effectiveness of Different Concepts of Bracing in Adolescent Idiopathic Scoliosis (AIS): A Systematic Review and Meta-Analysis. *J. Clin. Med.* **2021**, *10*, 2145. [CrossRef] [PubMed]
16. Simony, A.; Beuschau, I.; Quisth, L.; Jespersen, S.M.; Carreon, L.Y.; Andersen, M.O. Providence nighttime bracing is effective in treatment for adolescent idiopathic scoliosis even in curves larger than 35 degrees. *Eur. Spine J.* **2019**, *28*, 2020–2024. [CrossRef] [PubMed]
17. Janicki, J.A.; Poe-Kochert, C.; Armstrong, D.G.; Thompson, G.H. A comparison of the thoracolumbosacral orthoses and providence orthosis in the treatment of adolescent idiopathic scoliosis: Results using the new SRS inclusion and assessment criteria for bracing studies. *J. Pediatr. Orthop.* **2007**, *27*, 369–374. [CrossRef] [PubMed]
18. Weiss, H.R.; Klein, R. Improving excellence in scoliosis rehabilitation: A controlled study of matched pairs. *Pediatric Rehabil.* **2006**, *9*, 190–200. [CrossRef]
19. Berdishevsky, H.; Lebel, V.A.; Bettany-Saltikov, J.; Rigo, M.; Lebel, A.; Hennes, A.; Romano, M.; Bialek, M.; M'Hango, A.; Betts, T.; et al. Physiotherapy scoliosis-specific exercises—A comprehensive review of seven major schools. *Scoliosis Spinal Disord.* **2016**, *11*, 20. [CrossRef] [PubMed]
20. Thompson, J.Y.; Williamson, E.M.; Williams, M.A.; Heine, P.J.; Lamb, S.E. Effectiveness of scoliosis-specific exercises for adolescent idiopathic scoliosis compared with other non-surgical interventions: A systematic review and meta-analysis. *Physiotherapy* **2019**, *105*, 214–234. [CrossRef]
21. Janssen, I.; Leblanc, A.G. Systematic review of the health benefits of physical activity and fitness in school-aged children and youth. *Int. J. Behav. Nutr. Phys. Act.* **2010**, *7*, 40. [CrossRef]
22. World Health Organization. WHO Guidelines on Physical Activity and Sedentary Behaviour. Available online: https://apps.who.int/iris/bitstream/handle/10665/336657/9789240015111-eng.pdf (accessed on 16 February 2021).
23. Diarbakerli, E.; Savvides, P.; Wihlborg, A.; Abbott, A.; Bergstrom, I.; Gerdhem, P. Bone health in adolescents with idiopathic scoliosis. *Bone Jt. J.* **2020**, *102-B*, 268–272. [CrossRef] [PubMed]
24. Yip, B.H.; Yu, F.W.; Wang, Z.; Hung, V.W.; Lam, T.P.; Ng, B.K.; Zhu, F.; Cheng, J.C. Prognostic Value of Bone Mineral Density on Curve Progression: A Longitudinal Cohort Study of 513 Girls with Adolescent Idiopathic Scoliosis. *Sci. Rep.* **2016**, *6*, 39220. [CrossRef]

25. McKay, H.A.; Petit, M.A.; Schutz, R.W.; Prior, J.C.; Barr, S.I.; Khan, K.M. Augmented trochanteric bone mineral density after modified physical education classes: A randomized school-based exercise intervention study in prepubescent and early pubescent children. *J. Pediatr.* **2000**, *136*, 156–162. [CrossRef]
26. World Health Organization. Adherence to Long-Term Therapies: Evidence for Action/[Edited by Eduardo Sabateé]. 2003. Available online: https://apps.who.int/iris/handle/10665/42682 (accessed on 16 February 2021).
27. Abbott, A.; Moller, H.; Gerdhem, P. CONTRAIS: CONservative TReatment for Adolescent Idiopathic Scoliosis: A randomised controlled trial protocol. *BMC Musculoskelet. Disord.* **2013**, *14*, 261. [CrossRef] [PubMed]
28. Carreon, L.Y.; Sanders, J.O.; Diab, M.; Polly, D.W.; Diamond, B.E.; Sucato, D.J. Discriminative Properties of the Spinal Appearance Questionnaire Compared With the Scoliosis Research Society–22 Revised. *Spine Deform.* **2013**, *1*, 328–338. [CrossRef]
29. Negrini, S.; Aulisa, A.G.; Aulisa, L.; Circo, A.B.; de Mauroy, J.C.; Durmala, J.; Grivas, T.B.; Knott, P.; Kotwicki, T.; Maruyama, T.; et al. 2011 SOSORT guidelines: Orthopaedic and Rehabilitation treatment of idiopathic scoliosis during growth. *Scoliosis* **2012**, *7*, 3. [CrossRef] [PubMed]
30. Michie, S.; van Stralen, M.M.; West, R. The behaviour change wheel: A new method for characterising and designing behaviour change interventions. *Implement. Sci.* **2011**, *6*, 42. [CrossRef]
31. World Health Organization. WHO Guidelines Approved by the Guidelines Review Committee. Global Recommendations on Physical Activity for Health. Recommended Population Levels of Physical Activity for Health. Available online: https://www.ncbi.nlm.nih.gov/pubmed/26180873 (accessed on 4 September 2020).
32. Boston Orthotics and Prosthetics. Boston Brace Night Shift Scoliosis Brace. Available online: https://www.bostonoandp.com/products/scoliosis-and-spine/boston-night-shift/ (accessed on 4 September 2020).
33. Weiss, H.-R.; Maier-Hennes, A.; Romano, M.; Negrini, A.; Parzini, S.; Negrini, S.; Rigo, M.; Quera-Salva, G.; Villagrasa, M.; Ferrer, M.; et al. Various methods of Physiotherapy. In *Conservative Scoliosis Treatment: 1st SOSORT Instructional Course Lectures Book*; Grivas, T.B., Ed.; IOS Press, Incorporated: Amsterdam, The Netherlands, 2008; Volume 135, pp. 173–261.
34. Craig, C.L.; Marshall, A.L.; Sjostrom, M.; Bauman, A.E.; Booth, M.L.; Ainsworth, B.E.; Pratt, M.; Ekelund, U.; Yngve, A.; Sallis, J.F.; et al. International physical activity questionnaire: 12-country reliability and validity. *Med. Sci. Sports Exerc.* **2003**, *35*, 1381–1395. [CrossRef] [PubMed]
35. International Physical Activity Questionnaire. IPAQ Research Committee. Guidelines for Data Processing and Analysis of the International Physical Activity Questionnaire (IPAQ)—Short and Long Forms 2005. Available online: https://sites.google.com/site/theipaq/scoring-protocol (accessed on 17 January 2020).
36. The International Physical Activity Questionnaire (IPAQ). Available online: http://www.ipaq.ki.se/ (accessed on 17 January 2020).
37. Sanders, J.O.; Polly, D.W., Jr.; Cats-Baril, W.; Jones, J.; Lenke, L.G.; O'Brien, M.F.; Stephens Richards, B.; Sucato, D.J. Analysis of patient and parent assessment of deformity in idiopathic scoliosis using the Walter Reed Visual Assessment Scale. *Spine* **2003**, *28*, 2158–2163. [CrossRef] [PubMed]
38. Sanders, J.O.; Harrast, J.J.; Kuklo, T.R.; Bridwell, K.H.; Lenke, L.G.; Polly, D.W.; Diab, M.; Dormans, J.P.; Drummond, D.S.; Emans, J.B.; et al. The Spinal Appearance Questionnaire: Results of reliability, validity, and responsiveness testing in patients with idiopathic scoliosis. *Spine* **2007**, *32*, 2719–2722. [CrossRef] [PubMed]
39. Carreon, L.Y.; Sanders, J.O.; Polly, D.W.; Sucato, D.J.; Parent, S.; Roy-Beaudry, M.; Hopkins, J.; McClung, A.; Bratcher, K.R.; Diamond, B.E. Spinal appearance questionnaire: Factor analysis, scoring, reliability, and validity testing. *Spine* **2011**, *36*, E1240–E1244. [CrossRef]
40. Danielsson, A.J.; Romberg, K. Reliability and validity of the Swedish version of the Scoliosis Research Society-22 (SRS-22r) patient questionnaire for idiopathic scoliosis. *Spine* **2013**, *38*, 1875–1884. [CrossRef]
41. Asher, M.; Min Lai, S.; Burton, D.; Manna, B. Discrimination validity of the scoliosis research society-22 patient questionnaire: Relationship to idiopathic scoliosis curve pattern and curve size. *Spine* **2003**, *28*, 74–78. [CrossRef]
42. Asher, M.A.; Lai, S.M.; Glattes, R.C.; Burton, D.C.; Alanay, A.; Bago, J. Refinement of the SRS-22 Health-Related Quality of Life questionnaire Function domain. *Spine* **2006**, *31*, 593–597. [CrossRef] [PubMed]
43. Wille, N.; Badia, X.; Bonsel, G.; Burstrom, K.; Cavrini, G.; Devlin, N.; Egmar, A.C.; Greiner, W.; Gusi, N.; Herdman, M.; et al. Development of the EQ-5D-Y: A child-friendly version of the EQ-5D. *Qual. Life Res.* **2010**, *19*, 875–886. [CrossRef]
44. Burstrom, K.; Egmar, A.C.; Lugner, A.; Eriksson, M.; Svartengren, M. A Swedish child-friendly pilot version of the EQ-5D instrument–the development process. *Eur. J. Public Health* **2011**, *21*, 171–177. [CrossRef]
45. Bergfors, S.; Astrom, M.; Burstrom, K.; Egmar, A.C. Measuring health-related quality of life with the EQ-5D-Y instrument in children and adolescents with asthma. *Acta Paediatr.* **2015**, *104*, 167–173. [CrossRef]
46. Burström, K.; Bartonek, Å.; Broström, E.W.; Sun, S.; Egmar, A.C. EQ-5D-Y as a health-related quality of life measure in children and adolescents with functional disability in Sweden: Testing feasibility and validity. *Acta Paediatr.* **2014**, *103*, 426–435. [CrossRef] [PubMed]
47. Ravens-Sieberer, U.; Wille, N.; Badia, X.; Bonsel, G.; Burström, K.; Cavrini, G.; Devlin, N.; Egmar, A.C.; Gusi, N.; Olivares, P.R.; et al. Feasibility, reliability, and validity of the EQ-5D-Y: Results from a multinational study. *Qual. Life Res.* **2010**, *19*, 887–897. [CrossRef]
48. Cheung, P.W.H.; Wong, C.K.H.; Lau, S.T.; Cheung, J.P.Y. Responsiveness of the EuroQoL 5-dimension (EQ-5D) in adolescent idiopathic scoliosis. *Eur. Spine J.* **2018**, *27*, 278–285. [CrossRef] [PubMed]

49. Nachemson, A.L.; Peterson, L.E. Effectiveness of treatment with a brace in girls who have adolescent idiopathic scoliosis. A prospective, controlled study based on data from the Brace Study of the Scoliosis Research Society. *J. Bone Jt. Surg. Am.* **1995**, *77*, 815–822. [CrossRef] [PubMed]
50. Landis, J.R.; Koch, G.G. The measurement of observer agreement for categorical data. *Biometrics* **1977**, *33*, 159–174. [CrossRef] [PubMed]
51. Cohen, J. *Statistical Power Analysis for the Behavioral Sciences*, 2nd ed.; L. Erlbaum: Hillsdale, NJ, USA, 1988.
52. Devlin, N.; Parkin, D.; Browne, J. Using the EQ-5D as a Performance Measurement Tool in the NHS. Available online: http://openaccess.city.ac.uk/id/eprint/1502/1/Using_the_EQ-5D_as_a_performance_measurement_tool_in_the_NHS.pdf (accessed on 16 February 2021).
53. George, M. Adherence in Asthma and COPD: New Strategies for an Old Problem. *Respir. Care* **2018**, *63*, 818–831. [CrossRef]
54. Public Health Agency of Sweden. Living Conditions and Lifestyle, Physical Activity. Available online: https://www.folkhalsomyndigheten.se/the-public-health-agency-of-sweden/living-conditions-and-lifestyle/physical-activity/ (accessed on 16 February 2021).
55. Kazdin, A.E. Mediators and mechanisms of change in psychotherapy research. *Annu. Rev. Clin. Psychol.* **2007**, *3*, 1–27. [CrossRef] [PubMed]
56. Prowse, A.; Pope, R.; Gerdhem, P.; Abbott, A. Reliability and validity of inexpensive and easily administered anthropometric clinical evaluation methods of postural asymmetry measurement in adolescent idiopathic scoliosis: A systematic review. *Eur. Spine J.* **2016**, *25*, 450–466. [CrossRef]
57. Prowse, A.; Aslaksen, B.; Kierkegaard, M.; Furness, J.; Gerdhem, P.; Abbott, A. Reliability and concurrent validity of postural asymmetry measurement in adolescent idiopathic scoliosis. *World J. Orthop.* **2017**, *8*, 68–76. [CrossRef] [PubMed]
58. Bonagamba, G.H.; Coelho, D.M.; Oliveira, A.S. Inter and intra-rater reliability of the scoliometer. *Rev. Bras. Fisioter* **2010**, *14*, 432–438. [CrossRef] [PubMed]
59. Langensiepen, S.; Semler, O.; Sobottke, R.; Fricke, O.; Franklin, J.; Schonau, E.; Eysel, P. Measuring procedures to determine the Cobb angle in idiopathic scoliosis: A systematic review. *Eur. Spine J.* **2013**, *22*, 2360–2371. [CrossRef]
60. Schreiber, S.; Parent, E.C.; Moez, E.K.; Hedden, D.M.; Hill, D.; Moreau, M.J.; Lou, E.; Watkins, E.M.; Southon, S.C. The effect of Schroth exercises added to the standard of care on the quality of life and muscle endurance in adolescents with idiopathic scoliosis-an assessor and statistician blinded randomized controlled trial: "SOSORT 2015 Award Winner". *Scoliosis* **2015**, *10*, 24. [CrossRef]
61. Schwieger, T.; Campo, S.; Weinstein, S.L.; Dolan, L.A.; Ashida, S.; Steuber, K.R. Body Image and Quality-of-Life in Untreated Versus Brace-Treated Females With Adolescent Idiopathic Scoliosis. *Spine* **2016**, *41*, 311–319. [CrossRef] [PubMed]
62. Monticone, M.; Ambrosini, E.; Rocca, B.; Foti, C.; Ferrante, S. Responsiveness and Minimal Important Changes of the Scoliosis Research Society-22 Patient Questionnaire in Subjects With Mild Adolescent and Moderate Adult Idiopathic Scoliosis Undergoing Multidisciplinary Rehabilitation. *Spine* **2017**, *42*, E672–E679. [CrossRef] [PubMed]
63. Monticone, M.; Ambrosini, E.; Cazzaniga, D.; Rocca, B.; Ferrante, S. Active self-correction and task-oriented exercises reduce spinal deformity and improve quality of life in subjects with mild adolescent idiopathic scoliosis. Results of a randomised controlled trial. *Eur. Spine J.* **2014**, *23*, 1204–1214. [CrossRef]
64. Diarbakerli, E.; Grauers, A.; Gerdhem, P. Population-based normative data for the Scoliosis Research Society 22r questionnaire in adolescents and adults, including a comparison with EQ-5D. *Eur. Spine J.* **2017**, *26*, 1631–1637. [CrossRef]
65. Diarbakerli, E.; Grauers, A.; Danielsson, A.; Gerdhem, P. Health-Related Quality of Life in Adulthood in Untreated and Treated Individuals with Adolescent or Juvenile Idiopathic Scoliosis. *J. Bone Jt. Surg. Am.* **2018**, *100*, 811–817. [CrossRef]
66. Ekelund, U.; Sepp, H.; Brage, S.; Becker, W.; Jakes, R.; Hennings, M.; Wareham, N.J. Criterion-related validity of the last 7-day, short form of the International Physical Activity Questionnaire in Swedish adults. *Public Health Nutr.* **2006**, *9*, 258–265. [CrossRef] [PubMed]
67. Tudor-Locke, C. Outputs Available from Objective Monitors, Protocols for Data Collection, Management & Treatment and Resources for Data Interpretation and Reporting. In *The Objective Monitoring of Physical Activity: Contributions of Accelerometry to Epidemiology, Exercise Science and Rehabilitation*; Shephard, R.J., Tudor-Locke, C., Eds.; Springer: Cham, Switzerland, 2016; pp. 85–158.
68. Williams, M.A.; Heine, P.J.; Williamson, E.M.; Toye, F.; Dritsaki, M.; Petrou, S.; Crossman, R.; Lall, R.; Barker, K.L.; Fairbank, J.; et al. Active treatment for idiopathic adolescent scoliosis (ACTIvATeS): A feasibility study [with consumer summary]. *Health Technol. Assess.* **2015**, *19*, 1–242. [PubMed]

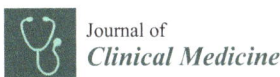

Article

A Pragmatic Benchmarking Study of an Evidence-Based Personalised Approach in 1938 Adolescents with High-Risk Idiopathic Scoliosis

Stefano Negrini [1,2], Sabrina Donzelli [3], Francesco Negrini [2,*], Chiara Arienti [4], Fabio Zaina [3] and Koen Peers [5,6]

1. Department of Biomedical, Surgical and Dental Sciences, University "La Statale", 20122 Milan, Italy; Stefano.negrini@unimi.it
2. IRCCS Istituto Ortopedico Galeazzi, 20161 Milan, Italy
3. ISICO (Italian Scientific Spine Institute), 20141 Milan, Italy; sabrina.donzelli@isico.it (S.D.); fabio.zaina@isico.it (F.Z.)
4. IRCCS Fondazione Don Gnocchi, 20148 Milan, Italy; carienti@dongnocchi.it
5. Department of Physical Medicine and Rehabilitation, University Hospital Leuven, 3000 Leuven, Belgium; koen.peers@uzleuven.be
6. Department of Development and Regeneration, University of Leuven, 3000 Leuven, Belgium
* Correspondence: Francesco.negrini@gmail.com; Tel.: +39-34-8598-8086

Citation: Negrini, S.; Donzelli, S.; Negrini, F.; Arienti, C.; Zaina, F.; Peers, K. A Pragmatic Benchmarking Study of an Evidence-Based Personalised Approach in 1938 Adolescents with High-Risk Idiopathic Scoliosis. *J. Clin. Med.* **2021**, *10*, 5020. https://doi.org/10.3390/jcm10215020

Academic Editor: Theodoros B. Grivas

Received: 21 September 2021
Accepted: 23 October 2021
Published: 28 October 2021

Publisher's Note: MDPI stays neutral with regard to jurisdictional claims in published maps and institutional affiliations.

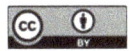

Copyright: © 2021 by the authors. Licensee MDPI, Basel, Switzerland. This article is an open access article distributed under the terms and conditions of the Creative Commons Attribution (CC BY) license (https://creativecommons.org/licenses/by/4.0/).

Abstract: Combining evidence-based medicine and shared decision making, current guidelines support an evidence-based personalised approach (EBPA) for idiopathic scoliosis in adolescents (AIS). EBPA is considered important for adolescents' compliance, which is particularly difficult in AIS. Benchmarking to existing Randomised Controlled Trials (RCTs) as paradigms of single treatments, we aimed to check the effectiveness and burden of care of an EBPA in high-risk AIS. This study's design features a retrospective observation of a prospective database including 25,361 spinal deformity patients < 18 years of age. Participants consisted of 1938 AIS, 11–45° Cobb, Risser stage 0–2, who were studied until the end of growth. EBPA included therapies classified for burdensomeness according to current guidelines. Using the same inclusion criteria of the RCTs on exercises, plastic, and elastic bracing, out of the 1938 included, we benchmarked 590, 687, and 884 participants, respectively. We checked clinically significant results and burden of care, calculating Relative Risk of success (RR) and Number Needed to Treat (NNT) for efficacy (EA) and intent-to-treat analyses. At the end of growth, 19% of EBPA participants progressed, while 33% improved. EBPA showed 2.0 (1.7–2.5) and 2.9 (1.7–4.9) RR of success versus Weinstein and Coillard's studies control groups, respectively. Benchmarked to plastic or elastic bracing, EBPA had 1.4 (1.2–1.5) and 1.7 (1.2–2.5) RR of success, respectively. The EBPA treatment burden was greater than RCTs in 48% of patients, and reduced for 24% and 42% versus plastic and elastic bracing, respectively. EBPA showed to be from 40% to 70% more effective than benchmarked individual treatments, with low NNT. The burden of treatment was frequently reduced, but it had to be increased even more frequently.

Keywords: adolescent idiopathic scoliosis; shared decision-making; personalised approach; bracing

1. Introduction

The practice of evidence-based medicine (EBM) combines evidence with physicians' expertise and patients' values [1]. As it comes mainly from the results of Randomised Controlled Trials (RCTs) focused on single treatments, a contradiction has been suggested between RCTs and personalised medicine/shared decision making [2,3], which has been shown to be important [4,5]. This contradiction also exists in clinical practice, where some practitioners prefer to follow strict protocols, and others propose highly personalised approaches. Extensive observational prospective studies can verify personalised approaches from a realistic everyday perspective [6] and verify the generalisability of RCTs [7]. In the case of conservative treatment of adolescent idiopathic scoliosis (AIS), RCTs [8–10] showed the efficacy of single treatments. Nevertheless, current clinical guidelines support an evidence-based approach, which clinicians can personalise within a range of different possible treatments for each clinical condition [11]: in this paper, we call this approach an evidence-based personalised approach (EBPA). EBPA is particularly advocated for adolescents because they are neither children doing what parents impose nor adults performing conscious choices. Still, they need to share decisions to adhere to treatments [11].

Scoliosis is a three-dimensional deformity of the spine and trunk with a prevalence of 2–3% in the general population [11]. The most common idiopathic type is classified according to the age at discovery, being most frequent in adolescence (AIS). AIS can have an aesthetic impact and cause in adulthood progressive deformities and back pain. Gold standard measures are Cobb degrees on a posteroanterior full-spine radiograph [11] where scoliosis is diagnosed as >10°, and health problems in adulthood are common at >50° and unusual at <30° [12–14]. A substantial percentage of adolescents rapidly progress during growth, with high risk between age ten and Risser bone maturity stage 2 [14,15].

The Bracing AIS Trial (BrAIST) RCT [8] confirmed the efficacy of plastic thoracolumbo-sacral orthosis (TLSO) for AIS of 20–40° consistently with a previous benchmarking controlled trial [16]. Results from cohort studies showed a various range of results from no efficacy to very high efficacy [17,18]. Population selection, research methodologies, patients' compliance, brace type, and construction, as well as expertise and management skills [11,19], can explain these differences. Minor side effects have been reported [8,20], with psychological impacts only occurring for braces extending to the cervical region [8,11,21]. Two RCTs have shown the efficacy of physiotherapeutic scoliosis-specific exercises (PSSE) [10] and elastic bracing (SpineCor) [9] in curves of 15–25° and 15–30°, respectively. The Cochrane Systematic Review on PSSE [22] is under revision to include other short-term RCTs that confirm the efficacy of PSSE, together with a pragmatic perspective [23] and one other design [24] study. Side effects have not been reported. There is no evidence for other conservative treatments [11].

Bracing and PSSE are demanding treatments proposed for asymptomatic adolescents to avoid curve progression to the reported risk thresholds [14]. These treatments last years until the end of growth. Consequently, compliance is one of the most significant issues [8,11,25]. Current clinical guidelines propose by consensus a range of possible treatments for each clinical condition, which experts must individually tailor through shared decision making. They also propose what we call here EBPA to achieve the best results to reduce the treatment burden and increase compliance through patients' adherence: this is achieved through a step-by-step path aimed to provide the most effective treatment with the lowest impact. Finally, they stress over- and under-treatment as well-known mistakes, since they cause unnecessary burden on patients or curve progression, respectively [11].

Nevertheless, we are not aware of any study on EBPA for AIS. We aimed to verify its results in a prospectively collected broad cohort of high-risk (Risser 0–2) AIS patients. We also wanted to compare two possible models of treatment diffused in the clinical world: EBPA versus per-protocol. This was done comparing existing RCTs (as a paradigm of per-protocol treatments) to subgroups of our EBPA cohort benchmarked (matched) for inclusion criteria. We expect these results to contribute to the debate about personalised decision making versus per-protocol approaches, particularly in adolescence when a personalised approach could be more appropriate than in adulthood. We also expect to verify the current evidence on AIS treatments generalising RCTs to everyday practice and determine the feasibility and importance of an EBPA.

2. Materials and Methods

2.1. Study Design and Participants

We designed a retrospective observational study nested in a prospective clinical database including all prospectively collected data of patients of a tertiary referral institute. The institute is specialised in the rehabilitation (conservative treatment) of spinal disorders at all ages, with specific attention to idiopathic scoliosis during growth. The prospective clinical data collection started in March 2003. At the time of data collection (31 December 2017), we included 29,859 individuals with spinal disorders, with 25,361 having had the first consultation before age 18.

We defined the following inclusion criteria: AIS diagnosis [11], curves 11–45° at the start, and a Risser stage between 0 and 2. Our institute receives many patients for a second opinion, so we only included those in charge, which we defined as adolescents who came at least three times to our facilities. The exclusion criteria were wearing a brace at first consultation and absence of X-rays in the three months before or after the start or end of treatment and observation. We found 1938 participants that fit the inclusion criteria (Figure 1). To compare the EBPA proposed in this study to standard treatments provided by RCTs, we selected three subgroups of participants paired to the existing end-of-growth RCTs using their inclusion criteria (Table 1). The Plastic Bracing (PB), Elastic Bracing (EB), and PSSE subgroups were compared to the BrAIST [8], SpineCor [9], and Monticone [10] papers, respectively. The 3 subgroups included 3 subsamples of the entire observed cohort of 1938 adolescents of 687, 884, and 590 participants, respectively,

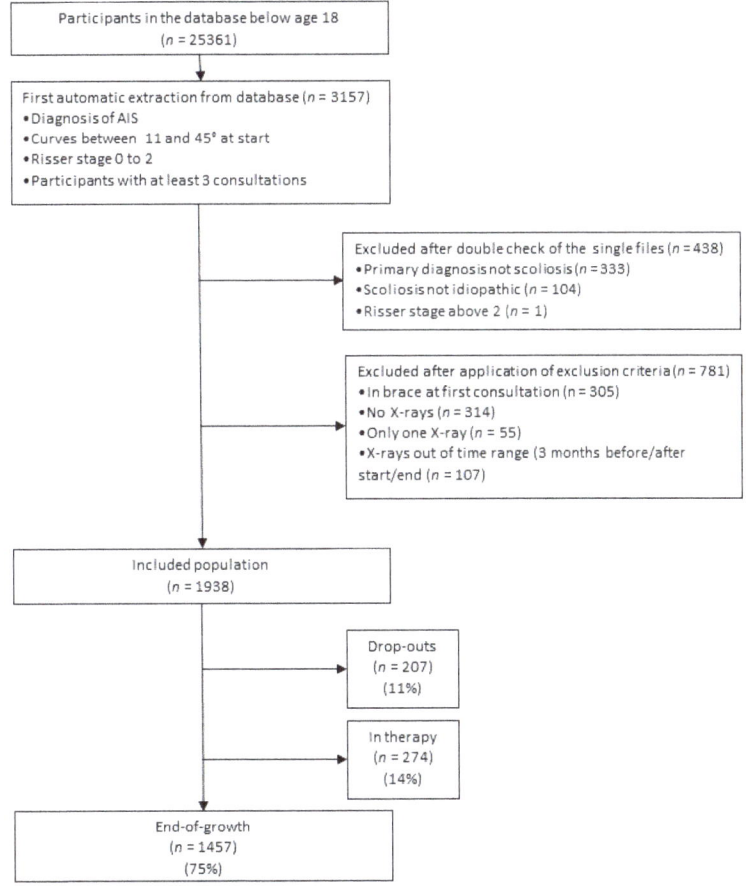

Figure 1. Selection of patients. Flow-chart of selection of participants from the clinical perspective. database. AIS, adolescent idiopathic scoliosis.

Table 1. Inclusion criteria of the existing end-of-growth Randomised Controlled Trials (RCTs) used for benchmarking in the current study.

Subgroup	Plastic Brace TLSO	Elastic Brace (SpineCor)	Physiotherapeutic Scoliosis-Specific Exercises
Acronym	BrAIST	EB	PSSE
Comparison RCT	Weinstein et al. [8]	Coillard et al. [9]	Monticone et al. [10]
Age (years)	10–15	8–15	10 or older
Risser (grade)	0–2	0–2	0–1
Menarche	pre-menarchal or 1-year post-menarchal	-	-
Cobb angle	20–40°	15–30°	11–25°
Curve	apex at, or caudal to T7	-	-
Previous treatments	not for AIS	-	-

Results of the patients treated with an evidence-based personalised approach (EBPA) in this study have been compared to the standard treatments received in the compared RCTs. BrAIST: Bracing Adolescent Idiopathic Scoliosis Trial; TLSO: Thoraco-Lumbo-Sacral Orthosis.

All parents provided written informed consent. The local Ethical Committee (Comitato Etico Milano Area B, Via F. Sforza 28, Milan, Italy-parere 801_2015bis, 15 December 2015) approved the study protocol, which is available at clinicaltrials.gov.

2.2. Procedures

Participants underwent a medical evaluation every 4–6 months, according to their growth rate. We prescribed a radiographic exam every two consultations, measuring Cobb degrees and recording the Risser stage.

Proposed treatments included observation, PSSE, and bracing. We proposed treatments according to the current situation and progression risk as determined by physician expertise by combining risk factors including Cobb degrees, growth, history, angle of trunk rotation (ATR), sagittal plane measures (radiographic measures of kyphosis and lordosis, pelvic parameters, and plumbline distances), aesthetics evaluated through the Trunk Aesthetic Clinical Evaluation (TRACE) scale, and others (e.g., family history) [11]. We proposed observation in low-degree, low-progression risk AIS to verify the effect of growth. PSSE followed mainly the SEAS (Scientific Exercises Approach to Scoliosis) approach [26], even if some participants autonomously chose other techniques; exercises were used in patients with a low degree and low to medium progression risk AIS to avoid bracing. An elastic brace (SpineCor 20 h/day) was used for 20–30° AIS not considered at high risk of progression. Plastic braces and included the rigid Sibilla, Lapadula [27], and PASB (Progressive-Action Short Brace) [28], and the very rigid [21] Sforzesco [27] braces. Plastic brace prescriptions ranged between 18 and 24 h/day according to progression risk. PSSE were always prescribed in combination with any brace prescription.

According to the SOSORT Guidelines [11], we defined the intensity of available treatments (Table 2) and a range of acceptable proposals for each clinical condition. These ranges fell within the range of possibilities proposed by the guidelines, so keeping an EBM approach. Each physician of our institute contributed to the definition of these protocols, which were gradually improved (as typical for EBM) with time, also with the introduction of new treatments (such as SpineCor since 2010). In front of single patients corresponding to each pre-defined clinical condition, physicians chose the treatment options remaining within the acceptable pre-defined range. The electronic patient record allowed checking the coherence between the protocols and the therapeutic proposals made by physicians, allowing to gradually improve the system. More information about the EBPA approach used in this study is reported in Appendix A.

Table 2. The intensity of treatment.

Intensity of Treatment	Treatment
0	Observation
1	Physiotherapeutic Scoliosis-Specific Exercises
2	Elastic brace (SpineCor)
3	Rigid plastic brace (Sibilla, Lapadula, PASB) brace 21 h/day or less
4	Rigid plastic brace (Sibilla, Lapadula, PASB) brace 22–24 h/day
5	Very rigid plastic brace (Sforzesco) brace 18–12 h/day
6	Very rigid plastic brace (Sforzesco) brace 22–24 h/day

In this table, treatments provided in the study have been ordered by intensity from the less to the most demanding. This corresponds also to the order from the least to the most effective. This order has been defined by expert consensus by the current SOSORT guidelines [11] and accepted by the SRS-SOSORT Consensus for research studies [14]. The ordinal scale used here has been adapted as follows: (1) night-time rigid bracing and scoliosis intensive rehabilitation were not present in our cohort and have been excluded; (2) according to the last Cochrane Review on bracing [21] we have differentiated between rigid and very-rigid braces; (3) half-time and part-time rigid bracing have been combined (categories 3 and 5) as well as full and total time (categories 4 and 6); (4) all observation categories with different time intervals between check-ups have been collapsed into the 0 category. PASB, Progressive-Action Short Brace. Note: the Sforzesco brace was developed between 2004 and 2005. Till then, the Lyon brace was the very rigid brace used.

To achieve an informed, shared decision, participants systematically received information from the treating physician about their clinical and aesthetic condition, progression risk, the importance of the 30°/50° thresholds [14], and how they could influence their health and possible results. We discussed alternatives to either reduce the burden of treatment or increase the probability of success. We finally proposed the prescription according to a risk/benefit ratio agreed upon with the patient and family. Hence, we can precisely describe the treatment provided only post hoc, since clinical decisions were always personalised. Appendix A provides examples of clinical decisions and the pathway followed by clinicians with patients to achieve the final individualised prescription. EBPA differs from a per-protocol approach in the quantity of information provided, full range of treatment alternatives proposed as effective, and the greater interaction with patient and family, with a final decision taken together on these bases.

After consultation, a trained scoliosis expert provided a cognitive–behavioural intervention (20–45 min) to answer questions and give information. An email question-and-answer service was also provided. In cases of bracing, in case of stability or improvement, a reward strategy was adopted with a gradual decrease every six months of 2 h/day. We kept an 18 h/day minimum dosage until Risser stage 3. Participants completed the study at bone maturity, defined as Risser stage 4, or at complete brace gradual weaning, if achieved after bone maturity.

2.3. Data Analysis

We analysed all data by sex, but it was not by race due to the uniformity of the Italian population. We defined the treatment intensity using an ordinal scale adapted from the current guidelines. We listed therapies in seven classes from the least (observation) to the most effective and burdening for participants (very rigid brace, 22–24 h/day) (Table 2). We used this scale to study the final results. We checked the scale application in our sample dividing all patients per treatment applied and verifying the Cobb degrees differences among groups.

Outcomes included the number of patients that achieved the primary outcomes of <30° and <50° [14]. Secondary outcomes included improvement or progression of >5° [14]. We also included achieving the current guidelines' [11] primary (optimal) and secondary (minimum desired achievement) treatment aims. Finally, we faced the concepts of under- and over-treatment. They are classically described as mistakes in AIS management since they mismatch between finally achieved results and applied treatments. These concepts start from the premise that increasing treatment intensity (as defined above) means higher efficacy and more patient demands. Consequently, under-treatment describes a therapy not effective enough to achieve desired targets, and over-treatment describes the opposite: therapies demand could have been lowered, since the results achieved were above the needs of the patients. We considered under- and over-treatment compared to the most relevant target, achieving adulthood with a curve below 30° [12–14]. We defined under-treatment as (1) when patients started treatment below 30° if the deformity progressed above 30°, and (2) when patients started treatment above 30° if they progressed at all. There is not a generally accepted definition of over-treatment (too demanding therapies), which is a concept stated in the guidelines [11] but not operationalised. For this paper, we needed such an operationalisation. Consequently, we defined over-treatment as any unnecessary improvement identified through a specific formula based on the 5° Cobb radiographic measurement error (Table 3). Improvements could be considered unnecessary when not changing the future of patients according to the known threshold of 30° for future problems in adulthood [14].

Table 3. Aims of treatments, over-, and under-treatment according to the different clinical situations.

Clinical Situation at the Start		Aims of Treatment According to Current Guidelines [11]		Thresholds of Over- and Under-Treatment	
Degree of scoliosis	°Cobb	Primary aim	Minimal aim	Over-treatment	Under-treatment
Low	11–20	End of growth < 20°	End of growth < 45°	Improvement > 5°	End of growth > 30°
Moderate	21–25			Improvement > 5° + $\left(\frac{°\text{Cobb start}-20°}{2}\right)$	
	26–30	End of growth < 30°			
	31–40				Progression > 5° #
Severe	41–45	End of growth < 45°	End of growth < 60° *		

Current guidelines [11] define the primary aim as the optimal desired achievement, while the minimal aim corresponds to the minimum desired achievement, in cases where it is impossible to obtain the primary aim. Keeping in mind the threshold of 30° [12–14], under-treatment has been defined when the deformity progressed above this significant threshold or, if already above, if it progressed at all. Conversely, over-treatment has been defined when there have been successful (1) improvements, for starting points below 21°; (2) important improvements according to a specific formula, reaching scoliosis below 30°, for starting points above 20°. * For severe curves, the guidelines propose postponing surgery [11]. We arbitrarily decided that a 60° curve requires immediate surgery, while below it is still possible to achieve results with conservative treatment [21] and set this threshold. # Only if therapy intensity was below 6.

We compared the PB, EB, and PSSE subgroups with the corresponding paired RCTs [8–10] for benchmarking purposes. We compared the baseline data using t-tests calculated using averages, standard deviations, and the number of patients. We used chi-square tests for percentages of different categories and final results. The outcomes for the paired RCTs were (1) ending at >50° for PB [8], (2) progression >5° for EB [9], and (3) progression > 3° for PSSE [10]. We performed an efficacy analysis, considering all patients who reached the end of treatment, and an intent-to-treat analysis (ITT). In the ITT, we hypothesised a worst-case scenario, with the patients who dropped out interpreted as failures. For EBPA and the treated group of the compared RCTs, we computed Relative Risk (RR) of success, Number Needed to Treat (NNT), and 95% Confidence Interval (95CI). These parameters could be calculated because our sample and those of the RCTs had been collected prospectively. Moreover, the comparison groups of the RCTs could offer natural history data to be compared to our subgroups, providing a successful pairing with similar baseline parameters in our subgroups and RCTs participants.

We collected data through software developed by our institute, managed with Excel, and analysed statistically with STATA 13 Texas 77845 USA.

3. Results

Out of 1938 participants, 274 (14%) were still in treatment and excluded, and 207 (11%) dropped out (Figure 1). We could not determine the reasons for dropping out due to the observational design of the study. The EBPA applied in the full cohort is described in Figure 2: each treatment group is statistically different from the others, with the exclusion of the comparison "Very rigid bracing (Sforzesco) 18–21 h per day" versus "Rigid bracing 22–24 h/day". The EBPA applied in every single subgroup benchmarked to an RCT is reported in Table 4. We could not benchmark our PSSE subgroup, since it included less mature (Risser stage) and 10 cm smaller participants than the paired RCT. For EB and PB subgroups, we found a few statistically but not clinically significant differences with the intervention and observation arms of corresponding RCTs at the baseline (Table 4).

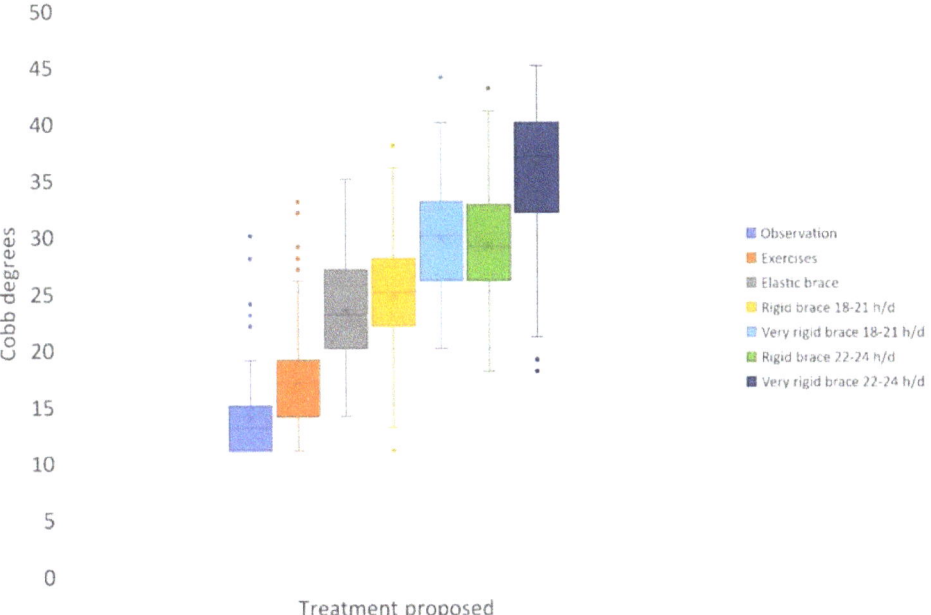

Figure 2. The intensity of treatments applied in the whole sample per Cobb degrees at the first consultation. All treatment groups were statistically different one from the other, with the only exception of "Very rigid bracing 18–21 h/day (h/d)" versus "Rigid bracing 22–24 h/d", where other determinants beyond Cobb degrees could play a role. Data of each single subgroup compared to RCTs are reported in Table 4.

Table 5 reports the individual choices made at the first patient–physician encounter (EBPA) throughout the 18 years of observation according to each clinical condition (determined according to the degree of scoliosis and Risser sign—see Appendix A). There is a percentage of patients who had a higher or lower treatment intensity. The same information about the subgroups and their benchmarked studies are reported in Table 4.

Due to the inclusion criteria, we had at baseline 69% of patients < 30°. At the end of treatment, this percentage increased to 78%, with 2% progressing above 50°. Improvement occurred in 33% and progression occurred in 19%. We reached the primary (optimal) guideline aims in 68% and the secondary (minimal) in 98%. Under- and over-treatment occurred in 13% and 10%, respectively.

Table 4. Comparison of baseline characteristics of subgroups BrAIST and EB in our study with paired RCTs [8,9]. Values are reported with ± Standard Deviation or 95% Confidence Intervals in parenthesis.

		BrAIST Subgroup vs. BrAIST RCT				EB Subgroup vs. Coillard RCT					PSSE Subgroup vs. Monticone RCT			
		BrAIST Subgroup of the Current Study	Comparison with BrAIST RCT Groups			Coillard Subgroup of the Current Study	Comparison with Coillard RCT Groups				PSSE Subgroup of the Current study	Comparison with Monticone RCT Groups		
			Observed	p	Treated		Observed	p	Treated	p		Observed	p	Treated	p
Number		687	96		146	884	36		21		590	55		55	
Age		12.7 ± 1.3	12.7 ± 1.2	NS	12.7 ± 1.0	NS	12.11 ± 1.5	12.2 ± 2	NS	12.2 ± 2	NS	12.6 ± 1.4	12.5 ± 1.1	NS	12.4 ± 1.1	NS
Female sex		83% (81–86)	90% (84–96)	0.13	92% (88–96)	0.01	82% (80–85)	86% (74–97)	0.68	85% (69–100)	0.88	82% (79–85)	71% (59-83)	0.07	75% (63–86)	0.23
Race	White	100%	76% (67–85)	<0.0001	79% (72–86)	<0.0001	100%	NA		NA		(100%)	NA		NA	
	Black	0	11% (11–11)		8% (8–8)		0	NA		NA		0	NA		NA	
	Other	0	9% (9–9)		5% (5–5)		0	NA		NA		0	NA		NA	
	Unknown	0	3% (3–3)		8% (8–8)		0	NA		NA						
Height		157.3 ± 9.1	153.6 ± 10.6	0.0002	156.5 ± 9.1	NS	158.7 ± 9.5					156.2 ± 9.1	146.3 ± 7.5	<0.0001	147.0 ± 5.7	<0.0001
Cobb angle of the largest curve		28.4 ± 5.8	30.3 ± 6.5	0.003	30.5 ± 5.8	<0.0001	22.3 ± 4.5	20.0 ± 4.1	0.002	22.0 ± 4.9	0.3	18.1 ± 4.1	19.3 ± 3.9	0.03	19.2 ± 2.5	0.05
Risser grade	0	56% (52–60)	64% (54–74)	NS	56% (48–64)	NS	48% (45–51)					69% (65–73)	45% (32–59)	0.0007	45% (32–59)	0.0007
	1	22% (19–25)	20% (12–28)		31% (23–39)		43% (40–46)					31% (27-35)	55% (41–68)		55% (41–68)	
	2	21% (18–24)	13% (6–20)		10% (5–15)		29% (26–32)									
Treatment intensity	0 Observation	1% (0–1)	100% (100–100)		0% (0–0)		1% (0–2)	100% (100–100)		0% (0–0)		6% (4–8)	100% (100–100)		0% (0–0)	
	1 PSSE (SEAS School)	14% (11–16)					41% (38–45)					60% (56–64)	0% (0–0)		100% (100–100)	
	2 Elastic brace (SpineCor)	9% (7–11)					10% (8–12)			100% (100–100)		8% (6–10)				

Table 4. Cont.

	BrAIST Subgroup vs. BrAIST RCT				EB Subgroup vs. Coillard RCT					PSSE Subgroup vs. Monticone RCT			
	BrAIST Subgroup of the Current Study	Comparison with BrAIST RCT Groups			Coillard Subgroup of the Current Study	Comparison with Coillard RCT Groups				PSSE Subgroup of the Current study	Comparison with Monticone RCT Groups		
		Observed	p	Treated	p		Observed	p	Treated	p		Observed	p	Treated	p
3 Rigid brace 18/21 h/d	29% (26–33)	0% (0–0)		100% (100–100)		31% (28–34)					20% (17–24)			
4 Rigid brace 22/24 h/d	11% (9–13)					5% (3–6)					2% (1–3)			
5 Very rigid brace (Sforzesco) 18–21 h/d	9% (7–11)					7% (5–9)					3% (2–4)			
6 Very rigid brace (Sforzesco) 22–24 h/d	28% (24–31)					5% (3–6)					1% (0–2)			

Table 5. Adherence of the entire population to the expected EBPA option.

Cobb Degrees	Risser Intensity of Treatment	0	1	2
10–20°	0	10%	6%	6%
	1	78%	80%	82%
	2	5%	4%	1%
	3	5%	10%	10%
	4	1%	0%	0%
	5	1%	1%	2%
	6	0%	0%	0%
21–30°	0	1%	1%	1%
	1	16%	18%	24%
	2	14%	9%	6%
	3	39%	45%	47%
	4	13%	7%	6%
	5	8%	11%	10%
	6	9%	8%	7%
31–40°	0	0%	0%	0%
	1	1%	0%	1%
	2	0%	1%	1%
	3	9%	7%	4%
	4	16%	15%	9%
	5	4%	17%	18%
	6	70%	59%	67%
Severe (41–45°)	0	0%	0%	0%
	1	0%	0%	0%
	2	0%	0%	0%
	3	0%	0%	0%
	4	2%	0%	0%
	5	0%	0%	7%
	6	98%	100%	93%

The treatment applied is listed for each clinical condition (defined according to the degree of scoliosis and Risser test—see Appendix A). The intensity of applied treatment follows this ordinal scale: 0. Observation, 1. PSSE (SEAS School), 2. Elastic brace (SpineCor), 3. Rigid brace 18/21 h/d, 4. Rigid brace 22/24 h/d, 5. Very rigid brace (Sforzesco) 18–21 h/d, 6. Very rigid brace (Sforzesco) 22–24 h/d. The yellow cells correspond to the expected EBPA. There are patients with treatment above or below the expected EBPA range. The choices performed for each subgroup are reported in Table 4 to compare with the benchmarked studies.

To check the efficacy of EBPA, we benchmarked our subgroups to RCTs controls (Figure 3). For the efficacy analysis, EBPA had 2.0 (1.7–2.5) and 2.9 (1.7–4.9) RR of success, with 2 (1.7–2.5) and 2.4 (1.6–4.8) NNT for BrAIST and SpineCor studies, respectively (Table 6). Failure rates of PB and EB were 2% and 19%, respectively, versus 52% and 75% in the observed arms of the BrAIST and SpineCor studies, respectively.

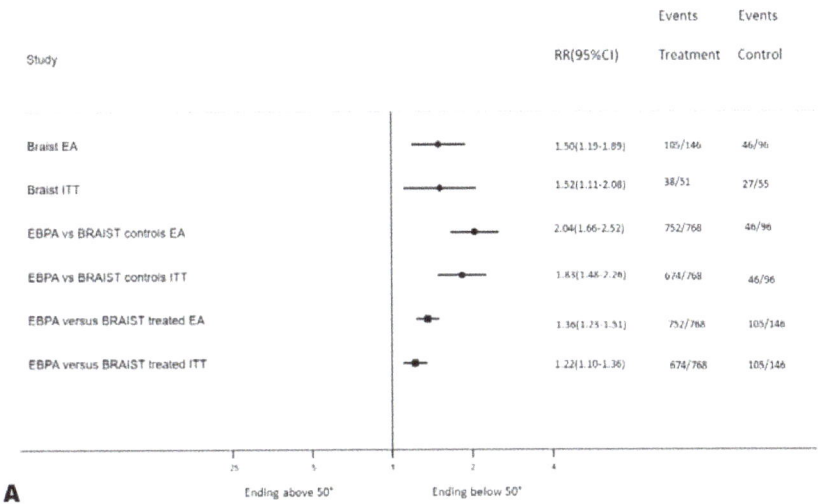
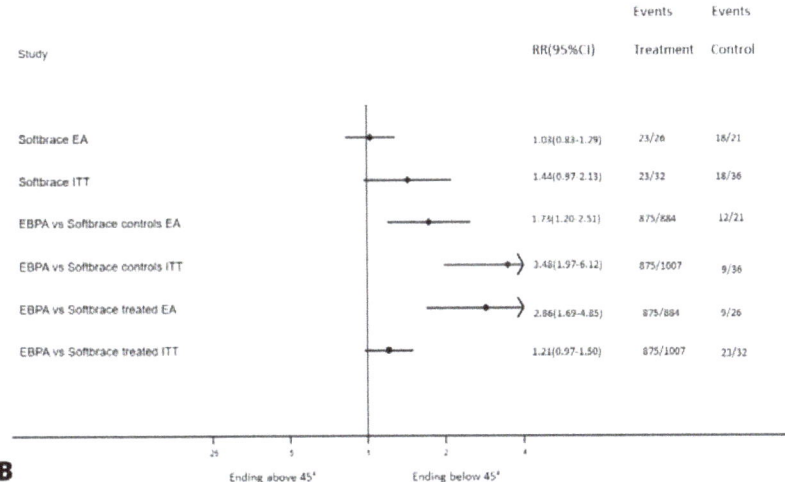

Figure 3. Relative Risk of success of the evidence-based personalised approach (EPBA) to paired RCTs [8,9]. Results in terms of Efficacy Analysis (EA) and Intention-to-Treat (ITT) are compared to the observational arms of each of the two studies. We used the Relative Risk (RR) of success since all data in RCTs and EBPA were collected prospectively. A higher RR shows the probability for a patient to achieve better results with one treatment vs. the other. The vertical line corresponds to the natural history data collected in every single RCT for the first four lines (for the original RCT, the first two lines, for the EBPA subgroups, the second two lines), while that in the last four corresponds to the comparison group coming from the RCTs (lines 3–4 to controls/natural history, lines 5–6 to the RCT treated group). The RCT on physiotherapeutic scoliosis-specific exercises (PSSE) [10] has not been compared since baseline populations were statistically significantly different. The same was true for the subgroups when we exclusively applied the treatment proposed in the RCTs.

Table 6. Comparison of evidence-based personalised approach (EBPA) with benchmarked Randomised Controlled Trials (RCTs): Plastic Brace (PB) and Elastic Brace (EB) subgroups with the BrAIST [8] and SpineCor [9] studies, respectively.

Analysis	Groups		Relative Risk (RR) of Success			Number Needed to Treat (NNT)	
	EBPA	RCT	RR	IC95	p	NNT	IC95
Comparison with BrAIST Study							
Efficacy	treated EBPA	controls BrAIST	2.0	1.7–2.5	$chi^2 = 307.4\ p < 0.001$	2.0	1.7–2.5
	treated EBPA	treated BrAIST	1.4	1.2–1.5	$chi^2 = 141.8\ p < 0.001$	3.8	2.9–5.3
Intent to Treat	treated EBPA	controls BrAIST	1.8	1.5–2.3	$chi^2 = 97.5\ p < 0.001$	2.5	2.0–3.3
	treated EBPA	treated BrAIST	1.2	1.1–1.4	$chi^2 = 24.46\ p < 0.001$	6.3	4.2–12.5
Comparison with SpineCor Study							
Efficacy	treated EBPA	controls SpineCor	1.7	1.2–2.5	$chi^2 = 184.2\ p < 0.001$	2.4	1.6–4.8
	treated EBPA	treated SpineCor	2.9	1.7–4.9	$chi^2 = 377.0\ p < 0.001$	1.6	1.2–2.2
Intent to Treat	treated EBPA	controls SpineCor	3.5	2.0–6.1	$chi^2 = 103.1\ p < 0.001$	1.6	1.3–2.1
	treated EBPA	treated SpineCor	1.2	0.97–1.5	$chi^2 = 5.96\ p = 0.05$ NS	6.7	3.2–100

RR: Relative Risk; NNT: Number Needed to Treat; IC95: Interval of Confidence 95%. In EBPA, we considered the subgroups comparable to the populations of RCTs. We used the Relative Risk (RR) of success since all data in RCTs and EBPA were collected prospectively. A higher RR shows the probability for a patient to achieve better results with one treatment vs. the other. It was in this way also possible to compare our subgroups to the control groups of RCTs, showing the superiority of EBPA on natural history. Note that the relative risk of success is different for the two comparisons: in BrAIST RCT, it was defined as remaining below 50° [8], while in SpineCor one, it was remaining below 45° [9].

To compare EBPA to single treatments, we benchmarked our subgroups to the RCTs treated groups (Figure 2). For the efficacy analysis, EBPA had 1.4 (1.2–1.5) and 1.7 (1.2–2.5) RR of success, with 3.8 (2.9–5.3) and 1.6 (1.2–2.2) NNT for plastic and elastic bracing, respectively. The above reported 2% and 19% failure rates of PB and EB compared to 28% and 34% in the treated arms of the BrAIST and SpineCor studies, respectively. EBPA treatment burden was more significant than RCTs in 48% of patients and reduced in 24% and 42% versus plastic and elastic bracing, respectively (Figure 4).

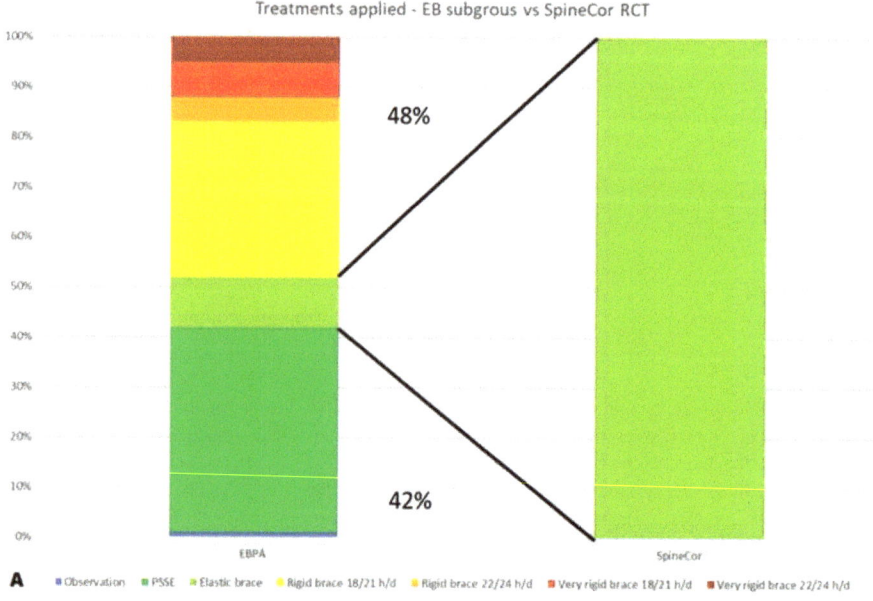

Figure 4. Cont.

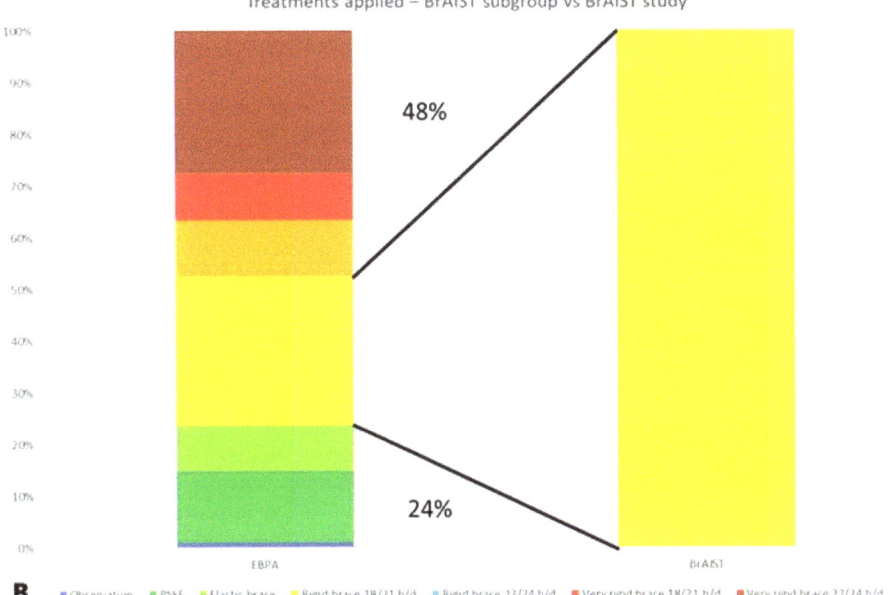

Figure 4. Comparison of the intensity of treatment for the evidence-based personalised approach (EPBA) versus paired RCTs [8,9]: (**A**) Thoraco-Lumbo-Sacral Orthosis (TLSO) [8] and (**B**) elastic braces [9]. The improvement in results of EBPA has been obtained using greater treatment intensity than paired RCTs in 48% of cases, but also a reduced treatment intensity in 24% of the BrAIST subgroup and 42% of the EB subgroup.

4. Discussion

This pragmatic observational study of a large prospective cohort benchmarked to published RCTs shows a higher efficacy of EBPA than standardised protocols. The probability of success of patients treated in EBPA is between 1.5 and 3.5 times that of natural history and between 1.2 and 2.9 when compared to per-protocol treated groups (RR in Table 6). This higher efficacy than what was reported in RCTs corresponds to a reduced burden of treatment for a high percentage of patients but also more demands on another important percentage of patients. The dropout, over-, and under-treatment rates are significant: 10%, 10%, and 13%, respectively.

The results of this study could be due to the real-world pragmatic approach of the EBPA we used vs. the artificial process of a research environment of a per-protocol RCT. It could very well be true that a real-world clinic that uses a strict protocol for all patients shows similar good results just because patients are motivated and not subject to an artificial randomisation and study process. Nevertheless, the study could also support the idea that a personalised approach based on shared decision making is superior to a standardised protocol. The latter is consistent with some papers based on different methodologies and other fields of medicine [5]; it is also coherent with the strong support given nowadays to patient-centred care. This is probably significant in AIS and adolescence [11] and could be specific to the field, but that is not necessarily the case. Shared decision making could improve compliance [2–5] and consequently final results, which could be particularly important in clinical areas where compliance is a problem, as in AIS [11,19,25,29]. We disagree with the contradiction suggested between EBM and shared decision making [2,3]. RCTs are one of the means to achieve EBM [1], but they do not coincide with it. The complete per-protocol application of RCT results is quite frequent among clinicians but not supported by EBM, and in the field of AIS, it can be one of the factors leading to the disparity of results reported in the literature [11,17].

As in previous studies [8,11,21], bracing has shown to be highly effective; personalisation increases its efficacy while reducing invasiveness whenever possible. Other elements can contribute to EBPA to explain the current results. Measured compliance was comparable to some studies [29] but much higher than others [8,30], which could explain our results and could be due to EBPA or the cognitive–behavioural approach [25]. The braces that we used are the most symmetric reported in the literature [18] with the precise aim of reducing visibility and increasing compliance [27]. Moreover, other brace-related technical and biomechanical factors could explain our results. Finally, we must consider that our braced patients always practised PSSE, too. This could influence final results as well as compliance [11].

This study confirms the possibility of stabilising AIS with PSSE [22,24] according to a pragmatic trial [23], but not a previous RCT [10] that reported improvements. This RCT population was different from all the other RCTs and our study, and the possible reduced progression risk due to higher bone maturity precluded any benchmarking.

The issue of under- and over-treatment is discussed in the AIS community [11], but we are not aware of any numerical definition. We proposed a specific approach internal to our EBPA population based on the most desired target of conservative treatment: an outcome below the 30° threshold [14] or, if not possible due to the starting deformity, approaching it as much as possible. Of note, we could also compare EBPA to per-protocol standard RCTs approach using the same concept. In this case, the higher percentage of bad results in RCTs could be considered under-treatment (i.e., not enough efforts are required for patients to achieve better results). Conversely, good results obtained with less invasive procedures with EBPA could be considered over-treatment by the RCTs (i.e., treatment invasive than what required by the clinical situation—as shown by EBPA being a less demanding treatment). Using this approach, under-treatment and over-treatment account for 48% and 25% for the standards TLSO 18 h/day in 20–40° AIS [8], and 48% and 42% for SpineCor in 15–30° AIS [9], respectively.

We had a 10% dropout rate, which may be due to the demands and length of treatment. On average, treatment lasted 3.7 ± 2.1 years, while dropouts stopped after 1.8 ± 0.8 years. Future studies should verify if these patients stopped treatment and their results at the end of growth. Nevertheless, at dropout, their results were not different from the other patients, and consequently, considering them total failures as we did in the ITT analysis is questionable.

The strengths of our study include the representation of everyday clinical reality, the possibility of checking many different factors and research hypotheses, a focus on the highest-risk population, and the large numbers achieved through a specific database. While this study reports real-world results, we also have to consider that the EBPA we used was developed in a tertiary referral institute. AIS is usually treated in tertiary referral institutes, particularly when it becomes important, but this is not always the case. Consequently, we cannot consider these results generalisable to everyday clinical life but only to tertiary referral institutes where high specific competencies are retrievable.

The limitations of our study include the non-randomised design that increases the rate of confounders. Nevertheless, RCTs for AIS are becoming difficult due to very high costs, large effect sizes that lead BrAIST to stop recruitment for ethical reasons [8], high failure rates, and recruitment difficulties [21]. Since the quality of evidence on AIS treatment is between low and very low [21,22], this study contributes to strengthening current evidence. This paper includes all patients who came to our institute according to specifically defined criteria, being representative of daily practice in a wide group of patients. Conversely, the subgroups compared to RCTs may not completely represent the everyday clinical reality, since they could share one possible problem of data from RCTs, which is the limited inclusion criteria leading to selection bias. However, the subgroups do demonstrate the success percentage in treatment per-protocol in an RCT compared to EBPA. The specialisation of our institute could reduce generalisability, but expertise is a prerequisite for EBPA. It is also theoretically possible that the rigor of data collection in clinical everyday life was reduced when compared to a research setting such as in RCTs. There are two main reasons why this should not happen: the electronic medical records of the institute provide a quality check of all individual patients and treating physicians need all data reported in this paper for their clinical follow-up. The only possibility would be not to report on the existence of a radiograph, but this does not happen. Future studies should verify the current definition of over- and under-treatment.

5. Conclusions

EBPA showed to be from 40% to 70% more effective than benchmarked individual treatments, with low NNT. The burden of treatment was frequently reduced, but it had to be increased even more frequently. These results contribute to the clinical and research debate about personalised medicine based on shared decision making versus standard protocols, particularly in adolescence. They impact practitioners because they confirm data on the efficacy of bracing and PSSE and stress their importance as components of a personalised approach. Guideline developers should continue to keep the concept of personalisation also in future recommendations [11]. Health policy managers should value an expert approach to scoliosis by tertiary referral practitioners. Finally, reducing patients requiring more invasive and costly procedures is highly relevant, particularly in low to middle-income countries where access to some treatments can be challenging.

Author Contributions: S.N.: conception and design of the work; acquisition, analysis, and interpretation of data; drafting of the work; final approval of the version to be published and agreement to be accountable for all aspects of the work. S.D.: acquisition, analysis, and interpretation of data; critical revision of the work; final approval of the version to be published and agreement to be accountable for all aspects of the work. F.N.: interpretation of data; critical revision of the work; final approval of the version to be published and agreement to be accountable for all aspects of the work. C.A.: analysis and interpretation of data; critical revision of the work; final approval of the version to be published and agreement to be accountable for all aspects of the work. F.Z.: acquisition, and interpretation of data; critical revision of the work; final approval of the version to be published and agreement to be accountable for all aspects of the work. K.P.: critical revision of the work. All authors have read and agreed to the published version of the manuscript.

Funding: This research received no external funding. Publication was funded through research grants of the Italian Ministry of Health (Ricerca Corrente).

Institutional Review Board Statement: The local Ethical Committee (Comitato Etico Milano Area B, Via F. Sforza 28, Milan, Italy-parere 801_2015bis, 15 December 2015) approved the study protocol available in clinicaltrials.gov (accessed on 21 September 2021).

Informed Consent Statement: Informed consent was obtained from all subjects involved in the study.

Data Availability Statement: The data presented in this study are openly available in Zenodo at https://doi.org/10.5281/zenodo.5517156 (accessed on 20 September 2021).

Acknowledgments: Alberto Negrini conceived with S.N., developed, and maintains with the ISICO software team the program for data collection and the database. Gianfranco Marchini developed with S.N. the SPoRT concept of bracing and the Sforzesco Brace. Antonio Negrini e Nevia Verzini developed the SEAS approach, which evolved to the current version thanks to the work mainly of Michele Romano and Alessandra Negrini. All physicians working in ISICO contributed daily to data acquisition and improvements of medical evaluation and treatment. All physiotherapists working in ISICO contributed daily to improvements of the PSSE approach. The orthotists of COL Centro Ortopedico Lombardo Milan, CPO Centro Presidi Ortopedici Parma, COV Centro Ortopedico Vigevanese Vigevano (PV), Officina Ortopedica Orthotecnica Gardolo (TN), Ortopedia IMAR Pescara, ITOP Palestrina (Rome), EL AR Barcellona Pozzo di Gotto (Me) work every day with ISICO to build and improve the braces studied here.

Conflicts of Interest: S.N. has a stock of ISICO (Italian Scientific Spine Institute). S.D., F.N., C.A., F.Z. and K.P. have no conflict of interests to declare.

Appendix A. Description of the Evidence-Based Personalised Approach (EBPA) Used in This Study

Current Clinical Guidelines developed by the Society on Scoliosis Orthopedic and Rehabilitation Treatment (SOSORT) have been developed following an evidence-based clinical approach; they also followed a step-by-step approach to current treatments, where for each clinical condition, a different range of possible treatment could be proposed (Table A1) [11].

Table A1. Possible range of treatments proposed by the SOSORT Guidelines [11].

		Low (up to 20°)		Moderate (21–40°)		Severe (>40°)	
		Min	Max	Min	Max	Min	Max
Infantile		Obs 3	Obs 3	Obs 3	TTRB	TTRB	Su
Juvenile			PPSE	PSSE		HTRB	
Adolescent	Risser 0	Obs 6	SSB	HTRB	FTRB	TTRB	Su
	Risser 1					FTRB	
	Risser 2			PSSE		FTRB	
	Risser 3					FTRB	
	Risser 4	Obs12	SIR				
Adult up to 25 y		Nothing	PSSE	Obs12	SIR	Obs6	HTRB
Adult	No Pain			PSSE		Obs12	
	Pain	PSSE	SSB	HTRB		PSSE	Su
Elderly	No Pain	Nothing	PSSE	Obs36	PSSE	Obs12	HTRB
	Pain	PSSE	SSB	PSSE	HTRB	PSSE	Su
	Trunk decompensation	Obs6			PTRB		

For each clinical condition, treatment is proposed from a minimum (Min) to a maximum (Max) intensity. In progressive order of intensity, treatments are Obs: observation (with number of months from a minimum intensity of follow-up every 12 months to a maximum every 3 months); PSSE: Physiotherapeutic Scoliosis-Specific Exercises; SIR: Scoliosis Inpatient Rehabilitation; SSB: scoliosis soft brace; PTRB: part-time (12–15 h per day) rigid bracing; HTRB: half-time (16–18 h per day) rigid bracing; FTRB: full-time (19–22 h per day) rigid bracing; TTRB: total-time (23–24 h per day) rigid bracing; Su: surgery.

In this paper, we followed what was proposed by the SOSORT Guidelines, and we called our treatment an Evidence-Based Personalised Approach (EBPA). Consequently, per each clinical condition, we proposed a range of possible treatments according to Table A2 that is within the range proposed by SOSORT. Each physician in our Institute followed this protocol, and compliance was checked through our clinical data recording system. Regular monthly team meetings were held to improve the system and check variances–obviously accepted in individual cases.

Figure A1 reports a graphical description of the three stages of an evidence-based approach according to the current clinical guidelines and the triad of evidence-based medicine [11].

The first step of the EBPA is the evaluation of the clinical situation according to the current evidence. At this moment in time, for adolescents with idiopathic scoliosis (AIS), Risser score between 0 and 2, we have the RCTs reported in the figure and described in the main text: Monticone 2014 showing the efficacy of Physiotherapeutic Scoliosis-Specific Exercises (PSSE) above "wait & see" for curves 15–25° Cobb; Coillard 2012 showing the efficacy of SpineCor above "wait & see" for curves 15–30° Cobb; Wong 2018 showing the efficacy of plastic braces above SpineCor for curves 20–30°; Weinstein 2014 showing the efficacy of plastic braces above "wait & see" for curves 20–40° Cobb; Lusini 2012 showing the efficacy of very rigid plastic braces above "wait & see" for curves 45–60° Cobb with a reduction of the need of surgery of 50%.

Table A2. Range of treatments proposed in this study (EBPA) (yellow lines) compared to SOSORT Clinical Guidelines (white lines).

Guidelines	EBPA		Risser 0	Risser 1	Risser 2
Low (10–20°)		Minimum	Observation (6 months)		
	10–20°	Minimum	0. Observation (3 months)	0. Observation (6 months)	
		Maximum	2. Soft Scoliosis Brace	1. Physiotherapeutic Scoliosis Specific Exercises	
		Maximum	Soft Scoliosis Brace		
Moderate (21–40°)		Minimum	Half-Time Rigid Bracing	Physiotherapeutic Scoliosis Specific Exercises	
	21–30°	Minimum	1. Physiotherapeutic Scoliosis-Specific Exercises		
		Maximum	5. Half-Time Very Rigid Bracing		
	31–40°	Minimum	3. Half-Time Rigid Bracing		
		Maximum	6. Full-Time Very Rigid Bracing		
		Maximum	Surgery		
Severe (>40°)		Minimum	6. Total-Time Rigid Bracing	6. Full-Time Rigid Bracing	
	41–45°	Minimum	6. Full-Time Very Rigid Bracing		
		Maximum	6. Total-Time Very Rigid Bracing		
		Maximum	Surgery		

The Moderate (21–40°) range of scoliosis of the Guidelines is split into two EBPA subgroups (21–30° and 31–40°). For each clinical condition, treatment is proposed by Guidelines and EBPA from a minimum (Min) to a maximum (Max) intensity. The SOSORT Guidelines propose the following intensity progression reported in this table: observation, Physiotherapeutic Scoliosis-Specific Exercises, Soft Scoliosis Brace, half-time (16–18 h per day) rigid bracing, full-time (19–22 h per day) rigid bracing, total-time (23–24 h per day) rigid bracing. In this study, the intensity follows the same progression but with a slight difference: 0 Observation, 1 PSSE (SEAS School), 2 Elastic brace (SpineCor), 3 Rigid brace 18/21 h/d, 4 Rigid brace 22/24 h/d, 5 Very rigid brace (Sforzesco) 18–21 h/d, 6 Very rigid brace (Sforzesco) 22–24 h/d.

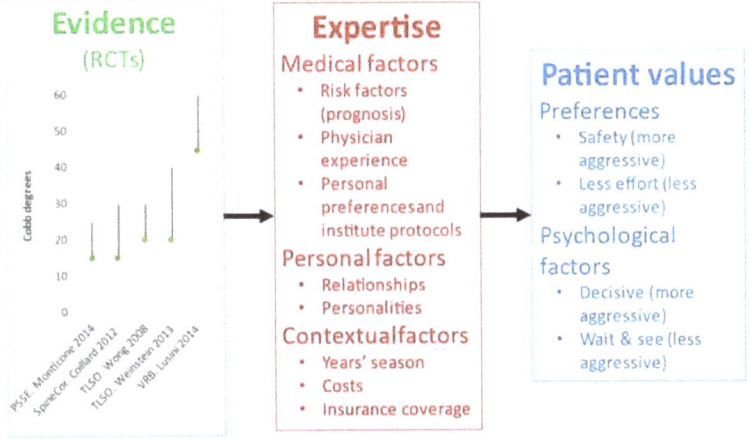

Figure A1. Graphical description of the three stages of an evidence-based approach according to the current clinical guidelines and the triad of evidence-based medicine used in the study. All details and explanations are reported in the Appendix A.

The second step of the EBPA is to apply the clinical expertise of the treating clinicians. This takes into account multiple factors, including:

- Medical factors: they include commonly described risk factors determining the prognosis, even if without a complete certainty; physician experience drives to a more or less conservative or aggressive attitude; physicians' preferences and institute protocols greatly influence the dosage (number of hours per day of treatment), since there are no strong scientific data on the topic.

- Personal factors: they include the relationships with patient and family, the evaluation of the personalities of patient and family, and how they could influence treatment.

Contextual factors: they include the years' season (e.g., in the summer, plastic braces are more demanding), treatment costs, and insurance coverage.

The third step of EBPA is patients' values. They include multiple factors, including the following:

- Preferences: the need for safety with as few risks as possible drives to a more aggressive attitude (more demanding treatments), while more significant attention to care and psychological well-being can lead to the opposite.
- Psychological factors: a more significant internal locus of control or an aggressive attitude will lead to more demanding treatments, while the opposite will become true on the other extreme of the psychological spectrum.

The physician will first evaluate the clinical situation and identify a range of possible treatments according to the current evidence and guidelines. Expertise will allow the clinician to "weigh" this range of possibilities according to the factors mentioned above. As a result, he/she will have a preferential proposal for the patient while providing all information to her/him and the family about the whole range of possibilities and the risk/demand ratio of each choice (a more demanding treatment decreases the risk of progression, and vice versa). According to the current knowledge, the pathology and progression probability are also described, including the current and future health risks. Finally, the clinician presents and discusses the prognosis and other "expertise-based" factors with their current strength of evidence. This process allows the patient and family to orientate the final decision, expressing their values in an interactive process, including open questions and answers sessions. Sometimes, the third step continues after the consultation, during the cognitive–behavioural session described in the text, and/or through other contacts in the subsequent days with clinicians. In addition, there could be an agreement for a time-buying strategy, i.e., a less demanding treatment with reduced follow-up time to closely check the outcomes and eventually change therapy as soon as possible.

In some cases, the situation is crystal clear, such as when there is no pathology (no need of treatment), or, at the other side of the spectrum, when there is a surgical case with the patient and family willing to try to avoid it (immediate most demanding treatment for the longest time). In these cases, there is no discussion; it is a black or white situation. On the contrary, in most cases, there are multiple possible options in terms of treatment or dosage. In these gray situations, there is plenty of space for discussion and shared decisions. The usual length of the first consultation, including this process and a proper history taking and clinical exam, lasts on average 30/40 min for an expert clinician, with a range between 50% and 200% of this time.

In Figures A2–A4, we exemplify the process described above. All three cases consider AIS of patients at age 11, Risser score 0, and triradiate cartilage open (i.e., maximum progression risk according to the current knowledge).

In case the scoliosis is of 15° Cobb (Figure A2), we have first to take into account the measurement error, which leads to a range between 10° and 20°. With these possibilities, we could consider a range of possible treatments from observation to SpineCor. Factors such as prominence, rigidity, sagittal plane, family history, and other prognostic elements will drive the clinician's preference and proposal. The decision will finally be achieved by discussing it with the patient and family.

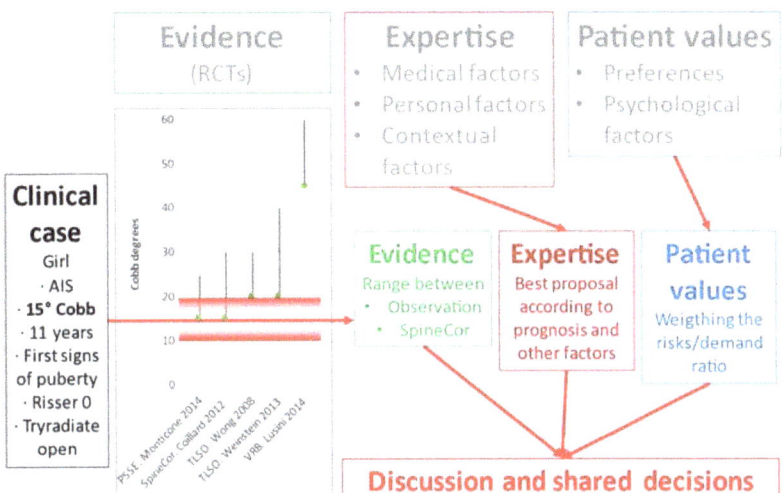

Figure A2. Application of an Evidence Based Clinical Approach to the theoretical Clinical case 1: age 11, Risser score 0, triradiate cartilage open, scoliosis of 15° Cobb.

In case the scoliosis is of 25° Cobb (Figure A3), the measurement error leads to a range between 20° and 30°; the possible treatments range between PSSEs and full-time plastic rigid brace. The last could be proposed for example in case of an important prominence or rigidity, while the first in case of an important postural component with no big signs of deformity and perhaps being in full summer for a patient living at the seaside: in this case, a closer follow-up would also be proposed. The final decision will always rely on the patient and family risk/demand ratio evaluation.

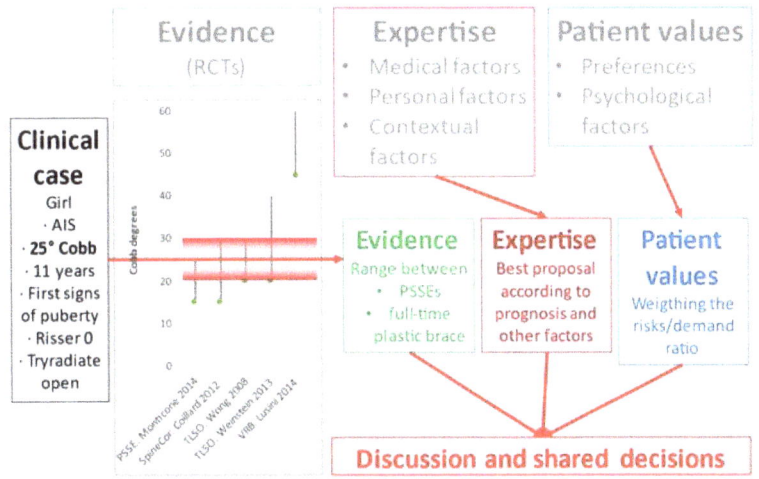

Figure A3. Application of an Evidence Based Clinical Approach to the theoretical Clinical case 2: age 11, Risser score 0, triradiate cartilage open, scoliosis of 25° Cobb.

Finally, in case of scoliosis at the top range of this study, with 40° Cobb (Figure A4) and a range between 35° and 45° to be considered, a brace is unavoidable according to the current evidence. The expertise will play a role in proposing a part-time (18 h per day) rigid plastic brace in case of good prognosis versus a full-time (23/24 h per day) very rigid brace in case of a patient considered at high risk of surgery due to other features (important prominence, high rigidity, big decompensation, flat back, etc). Contrarily to all the other cases, for the latter, very bad prognosis situation, very little space will be given to patient and family discussion.

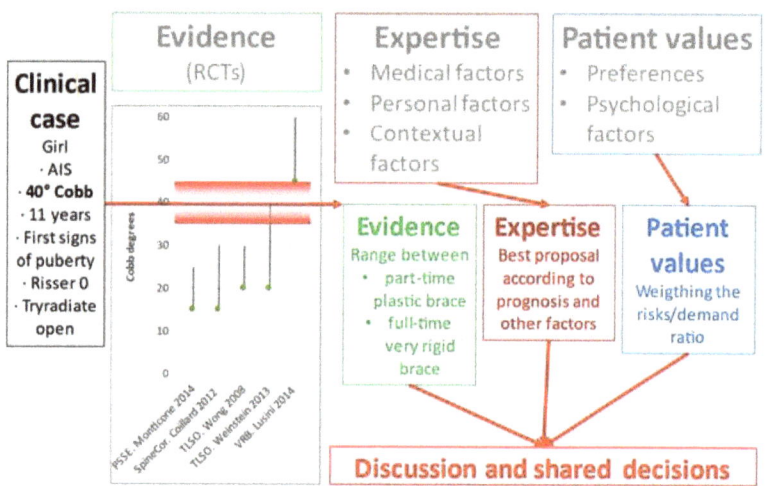

Figure A4. Application of an Evidence Based Clinical Approach to the theoretical Clinical case 3: age 11, Risser score 0, triradiate cartilage open, scoliosis of 40° Cobb.

References

1. Sackett, D.L.; Rosenberg, W.M.; Gray, J.A.; Haynes, R.B.; Richardson, W.S. Evidence Based Medicine: What It Is and What It Isn't. *BMJ* **1996**, *312*, 71–72. [CrossRef]
2. Ansmann, L.; Pfaff, H. Providers and Patients Caught Between Standardization and Individualization: Individualized Standardization as a Solution Comment on "(Re) Making the Procrustean Bed? *Standardization and Customization as Competing Logics in Healthcare."* *Int. J. Health Policy Manag.* **2017**, *7*, 349–352. [CrossRef]
3. Barratt, A. Evidence Based Medicine and Shared Decision Making: The Challenge of Getting Both Evidence and Preferences into Health Care. *Patient Educ. Couns.* **2008**, *73*, 407–412. [CrossRef]
4. McCormack, J.; Elwyn, G. Shared Decision Is the Only Outcome That Matters When It Comes to Evaluating Evidence-Based Practice. *BMJ Evid.-Based Med.* **2018**, *23*, 137–139. [CrossRef] [PubMed]
5. Jacke, C.O.; Albert, U.S.; Kalder, M. The Adherence Paradox: Guideline Deviations Contribute to the Increased 5-Year Survival of Breast Cancer Patients. *BMC Cancer* **2015**, *15*, 734. [CrossRef]
6. Garber, A.M.; Tunis, S.R. Does Comparative-Effectiveness Research Threaten Personalized Medicine? *N. Engl. J. Med.* **2009**, *360*, 1925–1927. [CrossRef] [PubMed]
7. Vandenbroucke, J.P. Why Do the Results of Randomised and Observational Studies Differ? *BMJ* **2011**, *343*, d7020. [CrossRef] [PubMed]
8. Weinstein, S.L.; Dolan, L.A.; Wright, J.G.; Dobbs, M.B. Effects of Bracing in Adolescents with Idiopathic Scoliosis. *New Engl. J. Med.* **2013**, *369*, 1512–1521. [CrossRef]
9. Coillard, C.; Circo, A.B.; Rivard, C.H. A Prospective Randomized Controlled Trial of the Natural History of Idiopathic Scoliosis versus Treatment with the Spinecor Brace. Sosort Award 2011 Winner. *Eur. J. Phys. Rehabil. Med.* **2014**, *50*, 479–487.
10. Monticone, M.; Ambrosini, E.; Cazzaniga, D.; Rocca, B.; Ferrante, S. Active Self-Correction and Task-Oriented Exercises Reduce Spinal Deformity and Improve Quality of Life in Subjects with Mild Adolescent Idiopathic Scoliosis. Results of a Randomised Controlled Trial. *Eur. Spine J.* **2014**, *23*, 1204–1214. [CrossRef]
11. Negrini, S.; Donzelli, S.; Aulisa, A.G.; Czaprowski, D.; Schreiber, S.; de Mauroy, J.C.; Diers, H.; Grivas, T.B.; Knott, P.; Kotwicki, T.; et al. 2016 SOSORT Guidelines: Orthopaedic and Rehabilitation Treatment of Idiopathic Scoliosis during Growth. *Scoliosis Spinal. Disord* **2018**, *13*, 3. [CrossRef]
12. Weinstein, S.L.; Dolan, L.A.; Spratt, K.F.; Peterson, K.K.; Spoonamore, M.J.; Ponseti, I.V. Health and Function of Patients with Untreated Idiopathic Scoliosis: A 50-Year Natural History Study. *JAMA* **2003**, *289*, 559–567. [CrossRef] [PubMed]
13. Mayo, N.E.; Goldberg, M.S.; Poitras, B.; Scott, S.; Hanley, J. The Ste-Justine Adolescent Idiopathic Scoliosis Cohort Study. Part III: Back Pain. *Spine* **1994**, *19*, 1573–1581. [CrossRef]

14. Negrini, S.; Hresko, T.M.; O'Brien, J.P.; Price, N.; SOSORT Boards; SRS Non-Operative Committee. Recommendations for Research Studies on Treatment of Idiopathic Scoliosis: Consensus 2014 between SOSORT and SRS Non-Operative Management Committee. *Scoliosis* **2015**, *10*, 8. [CrossRef] [PubMed]
15. Di Felice, F.; Zaina, F.; Donzelli, S.; Negrini, S. The Natural History of Idiopathic Scoliosis During Growth: A Meta-Analysis. *Am. J. Phys. Med. Rehabil.* **2018**, *97*, 346–356. [CrossRef] [PubMed]
16. Nachemson, A.L.; Peterson, L.E. Effectiveness of Treatment with a Brace in Girls Who Have Adolescent Idiopathic Scoliosis. A Prospective, Controlled Study Based on Data from the Brace Study of the Scoliosis Research Society. *J. Bone Jt. Surg. Am.* **1995**, *77*, 815–822. [CrossRef] [PubMed]
17. Dolan, L.A.; Weinstein, S.L. Surgical Rates after Observation and Bracing for Adolescent Idiopathic Scoliosis: An Evidence-Based Review. *Spine* **2007**, *32*, S91–S100. [CrossRef]
18. Zaina, F.; De Mauroy, J.C.; Grivas, T.; Hresko, M.T.; Kotwizki, T.; Maruyama, T.; Price, N.; Rigo, M.; Stikeleather, L.; Wynne, J.; et al. Bracing for Scoliosis in 2014: State of the Art. *Eur. J. Phys. Rehabil. Med.* **2014**, *50*, 93–110.
19. Negrini, S.; Grivas, T.B.; Kotwicki, T.; Rigo, M.; Zaina, F.; International Society on Scoliosis Orthopaedic and Rehabilitation Treatment (SOSORT). Guidelines on "Standards of Management of Idiopathic Scoliosis with Corrective Braces in Everyday Clinics and in Clinical Research": SOSORT Consensus 2008. *Scoliosis* **2009**, *4*, 2. [CrossRef] [PubMed]
20. Dunn, J.; Henrikson, N.B.; Morrison, C.C.; Blasi, P.R.; Nguyen, M.; Lin, J.S. Screening for Adolescent Idiopathic Scoliosis: Evidence Report and Systematic Review for the US Preventive Services Task Force. *JAMA* **2018**, *319*, 173–187. [CrossRef] [PubMed]
21. Negrini, S.; Minozzi, S.; Bettany-Saltikov, J.; Chockalingam, N.; Grivas, T.B.; Kotwicki, T.; Maruyama, T.; Romano, M.; Zaina, F. Braces for Idiopathic Scoliosis in Adolescents. *Cochrane Database Syst. Rev.* **2015**, *6*, CD006850. [CrossRef]
22. Romano, M.; Minozzi, S.; Bettany-Saltikov, J.; Zaina, F.; Chockalingam, N.; Kotwicki, T.; Maier-Hennes, A.; Negrini, S. Exercises for Adolescent Idiopathic Scoliosis. *Cochrane Database Syst. Rev.* **2012**, *8*, CD007837. [CrossRef]
23. Negrini, S.; Donzelli, S.; Negrini, A.; Parzini, S.; Romano, M.; Zaina, F. Specific Exercises Reduce the Need for Bracing in Adolescents with Idiopathic Scoliosis: A Practical Clinical Trial. *Ann. Phys. Rehabil. Med.* **2019**, *62*, 69–76. [CrossRef] [PubMed]
24. Fusco, C.; Zaina, F.; Atanasio, S.; Romano, M.; Negrini, A.; Negrini, S. Physical Exercises in the Treatment of Adolescent Idiopathic Scoliosis: An Updated Systematic Review. *Physiother. Theory Pract.* **2011**, *27*, 80–114. [CrossRef] [PubMed]
25. Karol, L.A.; Virostek, D.; Felton, K.; Wheeler, L. Effect of Compliance Counseling on Brace Use and Success in Patients with Adolescent Idiopathic Scoliosis. *J. Bone Jt. Surg. Am.* **2016**, *98*, 9–14. [CrossRef]
26. Romano, M.; Negrini, A.; Parzini, S.; Tavernaro, M.; Zaina, F.; Donzelli, S.; Negrini, S. SEAS (Scientific Exercises Approach to Scoliosis): A Modern and Effective Evidence Based Approach to Physiotherapic Specific Scoliosis Exercises. *Scoliosis* **2015**, *10*, 3. [CrossRef]
27. Negrini, S.; Marchini, G.; Tessadri, F. Brace Technology Thematic Series—The Sforzesco and Sibilla Braces, and the SPoRT (Symmetric, Patient Oriented, Rigid, Three-Dimensional, Active) Concept. *Scoliosis* **2011**, *6*, 8. [CrossRef] [PubMed]
28. Aulisa, A.G.; Mastantuoni, G.; Laineri, M.; Falciglia, F.; Giordano, M.; Marzetti, E.; Guzzanti, V. Brace Technology Thematic Series: The Progressive Action Short Brace (PASB). *Scoliosis* **2012**, *7*, 6. [CrossRef] [PubMed]
29. Donzelli, S.; Zaina, F.; Negrini, S. In Defense of Adolescents: They Really Do Use Braces for the Hours Prescribed, If Good Help Is Provided. Results from a Prospective Everyday Clinic Cohort Using Thermobrace. *Scoliosis* **2012**, *7*, 12. [CrossRef]
30. Katz, D.E.; Herring, J.A.; Browne, R.H.; Kelly, D.M.; Birch, J.G. Brace Wear Control of Curve Progression in Adolescent Idiopathic Scoliosis. *J. Bone Jt. Surg. Am.* **2010**, *92*, 1343–1352. [CrossRef]

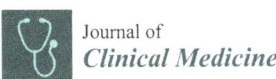

Review

Sclerostin and Its Involvement in the Pathogenesis of Idiopathic Scoliosis

Elias S. Vasiliadis [1,*], Dimitrios Stergios Evangelopoulos [1], Angelos Kaspiris [2], Christos Vlachos [1] and Spyros G. Pneumaticos [1]

[1] 3rd Department of Orthopaedics, School of Medicine, National and Kapodistrian University of Athens, KAT Hospital, 16541 Athens, Greece; ds.evangelopoulos@gmail.com (D.S.E.); christosorto@gmail.com (C.V.); spirospneumaticos@gmail.com (S.G.P.)
[2] Laboratory of Molecular Pharmacology, Division for Orthopaedic Research, School of Health Sciences, University of Patras, 26504 Rion, Greece; angkaspiris@hotmail.com
* Correspondence: eliasvasiliadis@yahoo.gr; Tel.: +30-2132-086-000

Abstract: Idiopathic scoliosis is a disorder of unknown etiology. Bone biopsies from idiopathic scoliosis patients revealed changes at cellular and molecular level. Osteocytic sclerostin is downregulated, and serum level of sclerostin is decreased. Osteocytes in idiopathic scoliosis appear to be less active with abnormal canaliculi network. Differentiation of osteoblasts to osteocytes is decelerated, while Wnt/β-catenin signaling pathway is overactivated and affects normal bone mineralization that leads to inferior mechanical properties of the bone, which becomes susceptible to asymmetrical forces and causes deformity of the spinal column. Targeting bone metabolism during growth by stimulating sclerostin secretion from osteocytes and restoring normal function of Wnt/β-catenin signaling pathway could, in theory, increase bone strength and prevent deterioration of the scoliotic deformity.

Keywords: idiopathic scoliosis; sclerostin; osteocytes; β-catenin; Wnt signaling pathway

1. Introduction

Idiopathic scoliosis is a disorder of unknown etiology. Numerous factors have been involved in its pathogenesis either by initiating or by contributing to the progression of the deformity [1]. Sclerostin has been recognized as a negative regulator of bone formation through inhibition of canonical Wnt signaling pathway in osteoblast lineage cells [2], and its role was first recognized in the study of two rare high bone mass disorders, namely sclerosteosis [3] and van Buchem's disease [4]. Systematic research into sclerostin's biology and mechanisms of action revealed that it is involved in the pathogenesis of many skeletal disorders.

Low bone mass is a common finding among idiopathic scoliosis patients, and osteopenia is considered a prognostic factor for curve progression [5,6]. In addition, structural changes of bone micro-structure have been reported, [7] suggesting that there are changes at the cellular and molecular level. Abnormal differentiation of osteoblasts and a reduction in the population of osteocytes were found in bone tissues from idiopathic scoliosis patients [8]. Osteocytes in idiopathic scoliosis appear to be less active with abnormal canaliculi network, which affects normal bone mineralization [9]. Furthermore, sclerostin expression was found decreased, while β-catenin was overexpressed in bone lining cells derived from patients with idiopathic scoliosis [9]. The present review article summarizes the current knowledge on sclerostin structure, expression, and regulation and also discusses its role in the pathogenesis of idiopathic scoliosis.

2. Sclerostin Structure, Expression, and Regulation

Sclerostin is a 190-amino-acid secreted glycoprotein that is encoded by SOST, a gene identified in sclerosteosis and van Buchem's disease patients [10]. SOST gene is localized

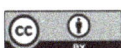

in chromosome 17q12–q21, [11] and encodes a 27 kDa–213 amino-acid pro-peptide, with the first 23 amino acids as part of a signal sequence for secretion. Sclerostin, the SOST gene product, is rarely detected as the expected 27 kDa protein, as it is secreted predominantly in a dimeric form [12]. It has two glucosylation sites and contains a cystin-knot motif that covers residues 80–167 [13], indicating that sclerostin is closely related to the DAN protein family although its amino-acid similarity to the members of the DAN family is rather limited [14]. A similar sequence of the cystin-knot is present in TGFb superfamily. DAN family proteins antagonize BMPs signaling [15]. Although the role of sclerostin as a direct BMPs antagonist is not clear [2], there is evidence that it downregulates BMPs action by preventing BMPs binding to its receptors [16]. Sclerostin is also considered as an inhibitor of the canonical Wnt signaling pathway that plays a central role in the regulation of bone growth and remodeling through its binding to the Wnt LRP 5/6 co-receptors.

Sclerostin is considered as an osteocyte specific protein [16]. The SOST gene has been detected in numerous other organs, such as the lung, kidney, aorta, heart, liver, and bone [13,15,17]. By using SOST promoter LacZ reporter, SOST gene expression was documented in the epididymis, pyloric sphincter, carotid arteries, and parts of the cerebellum [18]. The presence of congenital hand disorders in patients with sclerosteosis [3] suggests that SOST is expressed in the developing embryo. LacZ reporter was detected in the distal limb bud ectoderm and gradually is restricted to the digits as gestational age progresses [18].

SOST gene expression has also been detected in articular cartilage [16], mineralized hypertrophic chondrocytes [19], cementocytes [19], and osteoclasts [20], suggesting that sclerostin is expressed by terminally differentiated cells within mineralized matrices [19].

Although sclerostin is found in numerous tissues, it is predominately produced by osteocytes and is associated with high bone mass disorders in humans [3,4]. SOST knockout mice also appear with an increased bone mass phenotype due to enhanced osteogenesis [21]. These findings assign sclerostin as a key negative regulator of bone formation through inhibition of canonical Wnt signaling pathway and antagonizing BMPs.

Activation of canonical Wnt signaling pathway is initiated by ligands, such as Wnt proteins, which bind to Frizzled receptors, and its co-receptors of low-density lipoprotein-related receptor (LRP) proteins, LRP5 and LRP6. An inhibition of GSK-3β follows inside the cytoplasm, leading to accumulation of β-catenin, which then translocates into the nucleus and induces gene transcription [22]. Through this mechanism, differentiation of mesenchymal stem cells is controlled in favor of osteoblastic differentiation. Osteoblastic differentiation predominates, apoptosis of osteoblast precursor cells is suppressed, and chondrogenic, myogenic, and adipogenic differentiation is restrained, indicating that canonical Wnt signaling pathway is essential for MSCs differentiation to osteoblast lineage cells. Numerous LRP5 mutations were found to reduce sclerostin binding and result in high bone mass diseases, similar to sclerosteosis. These findings further support the role of sclerostin in regulating Wnt activity [23,24].

Furthermore, in osteoblast lineage cells, the activation of canonical Wnt signaling pathway enhances the secretion of osteoprotegerin (OPG), the decoy receptor for receptor activator of nuclear factor kappa-B ligand (RANKL), and suppresses osteoclast differentiation of osteoclast precursors [22]. SOST knock-out mice showed an anabolic effect with increased bone formation without elevation of bone resorption markers [21]. The increase in bone mass corresponds to improved microstructure with relative proteoglycan content, lower apatite crystal maturity, and lower matrix mineralization, which are related with increased resistance to maximum load, stiffness, and energy to failure [25].

Additionally, in osteocytes, sclerostin increases the expression of cathepsin K, tartrate-resistant acid phosphatase (TRAP), and carbonic anhydrase-2 in vitro, which are proteins involved in bone resorption and remodeling of extracellular matrix [26].

There are two regions that regulate SOST gene expression: the upstream promoter region and the downstream enhancer, evolutionary conserve region 5(ECR5). Interestingly, ECR5 is required for sclerostin production only in osteocytes and not in cells from other tissues [27]. These regulatory regions are sites where numerous transcription factors bind in response to cytokines and growth factors. In van Buchem's disease, there is a homozygous absence of ECR5 region, which has binding sites for the myocyte enhancer factor (Mef2c) transcription factor [28], suggesting that the binding of Mef2c to the ECR5 region of the SOST gene is important for SOST gene expression. The upstream promoter region has binding sequences for osteoblast transcription factor runt-related transcription factor 2 (Runx2) [29] and also contains a methylation site. Demethylation of this region during osteoblast-osteocyte transition results in increased SOST expression [30].

Reports regarding the role of vitamin D in regulation of SOST gene expression are not consistent. Vitamin D was found either to induce SOST expression [31] or to decrease the transcriptional activity of the SOST promoter [32].

Current data demonstrated that sclerostin was also implicated in bone fracture healing process and in the pathophysiology of osteoarthritis and spinal deformities or disc degeneration via its angiogenetic activities [33]. Micro-CT analysis for vasculogenesis demonstrated that application of sclerostin antibody was associated with neo-angiogenesis improvement during the second post-fractural week. On the contrary, there was not any difference regarding vascularization at the sixth or ninth week. Contrariwise, no significant improvement was detected in total vessel volume or diameter during the eighth week after the injury [34]. Recently, it was displayed that the application of sclerostin antibodies [35] were involved in the cartilage preservation and chondrocyte metabolism inhibiting the expression of catabolic angiogenetic molecules, like Vascular Endothelial Growth Factor (VEGF) [17]. In-vitro studies demonstrated that sclerostin significantly induces Primary Human Umbilical Vein Endothelial Cells (HUVEC) cell proliferation, an effect that is exerted by VEGF [36]. Moreover, sclerostin angiogenic activity in vivo was evaluated with chorioallantoic membrane (CAM) assay, and it was comparable to the VEGF-induced proangiogenic effects [36]. Similarly, the expression of anti-angiogenic Pigment Epithelium-Derived Factor (PEDF), whose down-regulation was closely associated with the progression of skeletal angiogenic deformities and was spatially expressed in areas of endochondral ossification and bone remodeling, was strongly inhibited by the expression of sclerostin [37]. These activities of sclerostin were also associated with increased recruitments of osteoclasts and their circulating monocyte progenitors and with reduced expression of osteoblastic genes and bone mineralization [36]. Based on these findings, it was suggested that sclerostin not only induced angiogenesis and can be classified with other Wnt antagonists already known for their angiogenic properties but can be considered as a critical growth factor for angiogenesis-osteogenesis coupling effect [36].

Sclerostin is expressed by osteocytes in mineralized bone and by mineralizing chondrocytes in articular cartilage and the growth plate in most primary bone tumors, such as osteoma, osteoid osteoma, osteoblastoma, and osteosarcoma [38]. Furthermore, sclerostin is expressed by tumor cells in most high-grade osteosarcomas and pariosteal osteosarcomas. In human osteosarcoma Saos2 cell line, Runx2 was found to increase SOST gene expression by binding to the proximal promoter [39]. The precise role of sclerostin is not clear, and evidence regarding the role of Wnt-signaling pathway in osteosarcoma is contradictory. Wnt-signaling pathway was reported either to facilitate osteosarcoma [40] or to suppress cellular proliferation and metastases [41].

Serum sclerostin levels were found to be age dependent [38,39]. Older women had 46% higher serum sclerostin levels than younger women [38]. Conversely, both young and aged women had similar bone SOST mRNA levels, implying that other tissues may be responsible for increased sclerostin secretion with age [38].

Furthermore, sclerostin was expressed by tumor cells in most high-grade osteosarcomas and pariosteal osteosarcomas. In human osteosarcoma Saos2 cell line, Runx2 was found to increase SOST gene expression by binding to the proximal promoter [39]. The precise role of sclerostin is not clear and evidence regarding the role of Wnt-signaling pathway in osteosarcoma is contradictory. Wnt-signaling pathway was reported either to facilitate osteosarcoma [40], or to suppress cellular proliferation and metastases [41].

Serum sclerostin levels were found to be age dependant [42,43]. Older women had 46% higher serum sclerostin levels than younger women [42]. Conversely, both young and aged women had similar bone SOST mRNA levels, implying that other tissues may be responsible for increased sclerostin secretion with age [42].

3. Osteocytes in Idiopathic Scoliosis

In bone tissues from patients with idiopathic scoliosis, the population of bone lining cells was found different than controls. Number of osteocytes was lower, osteoblasts were higher, and osteoclasts were found unaltered [9]. Osteocytes are key regulators of bone remodeling by transforming mechanical forces into structural changes of bone microenvironment through regulation of bone homeostasis. Osteocytes are considered as the main mechano-sensors of bone, and their impact of mechano-transduction is determined by numerous signaling networks, which are involved in skeletal growth and function [44].

Osteocytes are located in cavities in mineralized matrix called lacunae and form a well-organized network of small canals, the canaliculi. Canaliculi are occupied by osteocyte cellular extensions, the dendrites, which allow communication with other cells and are filled by canalicular fluid, which carries nutrients and biological factors and transmits mechanical signals [45]. Mechanical loading exerted on bone matrix is amplified through fluid flow inside lacunae and canaliculi [46] and stimulates osteocytes, which transduce the mechanical signal into biochemical reaction [47]. In idiopathic scoliosis, osteocytes' canaliculi were found disorganized and less in number, with shortening of their dendrites' length [9].

In response to mechanical loading, osteocytes produce numerous biological factors that regulate bone homeostasis and remodeling. Following mechanical loading, osteocytes secrete sclerostin, prostaglandins [48], and other inflammatory factors, such as TNF, leukemia inhibitory factor, and oncostatin M, which downregulate sclerostin expression [49].

Abnormal osteocyte function in idiopathic scoliosis results in impaired bone mineralization and inferior mechanical properties of the bone, which is susceptible to asymmetric forces that cause deformity of the spine [50].

4. Sclerostin and Idiopathic Scoliosis

Osteocytic sclerostin is downregulated by mechanical loading in wild-type mice, resulting in increase of new bone formation after canonical Wnt-signaling pathway activation, while in human SOST transgenic mice (DMP1-SOST), the anabolic response to loading was disrupted [51]. Suppression of sclerostin after mechanical loading is caused, among other mechanisms, by the increased periostin secretion, by periosteal osteoblasts [52], and the involvement of prostaglandin E2 and nitric oxide [47,52].

Osteocytes from bone biopsies of patients with idiopathic scoliosis had decreased SOST gene expression as well as lower sclerostin secretion. Osteocytes derived from CTNNB1 knocking down osteoblasts from patients with idiopathic scoliosis SOST gene expression and sclerostin secretion were found significantly elevated [9]. These findings provide evidence that sclerostin antagonizes Wnt/β-catenin signaling pathway.

In bone marrow mesenchymal stem cells derived from idiopathic scoliosis patients, miRNAs miR-17-5p, miR-106a-5p, miR-106b-5p, miR-16-5p, miR-93-5p, and miR-181b-5p were found up-regulated. Their role was identified as osteogenic differentiation and bone-formation suppressors. Additionally, up-regulation of miR-15a-5p was involved in regulation of cell apoptosis [53]. There are several studies in the literature that negatively corelate miRNAs with sclerostin. Higher serum levels of miRNA-21 were coupled with lower levels of sclerostin [54], while inhibition of miRNA-218-5p promoted SOST gene expression [55]. Serum level of SOST was negatively correlated with plasma miR-145, and serum level of SOST miR-145 knockdown in osteoblasts from idiopathic scoliosis patients improved osteocyte function possibly by maturation of osteocytes and dendrite formation and not by osteoblast differentiation [9]. Decreased levels of sclerostin may be explicated due to elevated levels of miRNAs in bone biopsies from idiopathic scoliosis patients.

Wnt signaling pathway was found overactivated in bone biopsies from scoliotic patients as active β-catenin was found significantly elevated [50]. Similar findings were reported in zebrafish scoliotic model, where β-catenin activity was related to the deformity of the spine through the enzyme tyrosine kinase 7 [56]. Although Wnt/β-catenin activation increases bone mass, overactivation of Wnt/β-catenin signaling pathway in idiopathic scoliosis halt osteoblasts from differentiation to osteocytes [57] and compromise matrix mineralization [58]. Additionally, Runx2, an early bone formation marker, was found decreased in idiopathic scoliosis bone tissues, meaning that bone formation was impaired due to Wnt/β-catenin signaling pathway overexpression [7]. Overactivation of Wnt/β-catenin signaling pathway may play a role in the progression of the deformity through abnormal function of muscles [59], the intervertebral disc [60], and the vertebral growth plate [61]. One possible explanation of asymmetrical muscle contraction between convex and concave side of a scoliotic curve is the role of cadmodulin and its relation to Wnt/β-catenin signaling pathway and sclerostin expression. Cadmodulin concentration in paraspinal muscles was found increased at the convex side and decreased at the concave side of patients with idiopathic scoliosis [62]. Calmodulin after binding with calcium activates myosin light chain and contributes in smooth muscle contraction [63]. Cadmodulin downregulation was found to affect calcitonin and consequently calcium blood levels and G proteins activation [64]. Calcitonin downregulation subsequently downregulates sclerostin expression [65] and activates Wnt/β-catenin signaling pathway in osteoblastic differentiation of bone marrow stem cells [66]. Similarly, G proteins induce Wnt/β-catenin signaling [51] and show higher expression in the vertebral bodies from the convex side of the scoliotic spine [67]. One possible explanation of sclerostin downregulation in patients with idiopathic scoliosis is through the cadmodulin/calcitonin interaction.

Asymmetric mechanical forces over a vulnerable spinal column during growth may cause deformity of the spine. The origin of asymmetric mechanical forces is unknown. There are numerous etiologic concepts in the literature that involve relative anterior spinal overgrowth [68]; rib cage asymmetry [69]; handedness [70]; central nervous system abnormalities [71,72]; deficits of the vestibular system, which may affect the tone of paraspinal muscles [73]; decreased leptin levels in the peripheral blood [74]; and the double neuroosseous theory, which results in the loss of co-ordination between autonomic and somatic nervous systems of the spine and trunk [75]. A direct association between mechanical loading and sclerostin expression is documented in the literature. Enhanced loading of the ulna in rodents reduced osteocyte expression of sclerostin, and parts of cortical bone sustaining greater strain demonstrated a more profound reduction of sclerostin staining osteocytes [76]. Numerous genes associated with activation of Wnt-signaling pathway in wild-type mice were upregulated after loading, but in DMP1-SOST mice, this response was not evidenced [77]. Mechanical loading was associated with inhibition of bone loss in response to unloading in SOST knock-out mice [78]. Stroke patients, who experience mechanical unloading due to long-term immobilization, were found with increased levels of serum sclerostin [79]. Anti-sclerostin antibodies prevented unloading induced bone loss in a hindlimb-immobilization rat model [80]. Mechanical loading was found to suppress TGFβ signaling in osteocytes, which is required for SOST gene expression, resulting in sclerostin suppression [81]. Although sclerostin-independent changes in bone formation after loading has been reported [82], sclerostin downregulation is critical for the osteogenic response to mechanical loading by relieving inhibition of Wnt-signaling pathway. Although increased mechanical forces decrease sclerostin expression from osteocytes, there is no evidence for how asymmetrical loading may affect sclerostin in idiopathic scoliosis. Further studies are required to investigate this association.

Wnt/β-catenin signaling pathway overexpression and sclerostin downregulation by osteocytes could be progressive factors for the development of idiopathic scoliosis. Although sclerostin is a negative regulator of bone formation, it could play a role in Wnt/β-catenin signaling pathway downregulation. In theory, by restoring bone metabolism during growth at a molecular level through Wnt/β-catenin signaling pathway downregulation and stimulating sclerostin secretion from osteocytes at a cellular level, bone vulnerability could be alleviated, and the scoliotic deformity could be improved. Further studies are needed in order to test this hypothesis, and care should be taken to minimize the possible side effects of Wnt/β-catenin signaling pathway and sclerostin action at sites other than the spinal column.

Author Contributions: E.S.V.; conceptualization, methodology, writing—original draft preparation, D.S.E.; writing—review and editing, A.K.; investigation, data curation, C.V.; writing—original draft preparation, S.G.P.; Supervision. All authors have read and agreed to the published version of the manuscript.

Funding: This research received no external funding.

Institutional Review Board Statement: Not applicable.

Informed Consent Statement: Not applicable.

Conflicts of Interest: The authors declare no conflict of interest.

References

1. Cheng, J.C.; Tang, N.L.; Yeung, H.Y.; Miller, N. Genetic association of complex traits: Using idiopathic scoliosis as an example. *Clin. Orthop. Relat. Res.* **2007**, *462*, 38–44. [CrossRef]
2. van Bezooijen, R.L.; Roelen, B.A.; Visser, A.; van der Wee-Pals, L.; de Wilt, E.; Karperien, M.; Hamersma, H.; Papapoulos, S.E.; ten Dijke, P.; Löwik, C.W. Sclerostin is an osteocyte-expressed negative regulator of bone formation, but not a classical BMP antagonist. *J. Exp. Med.* **2004**, *199*, 805–814. [CrossRef]
3. Hamersma, H.; Gardner, J.; Beighton, P. The natural history of sclerosteosis. *Clin. Genet.* **2003**, *63*, 192–197. [CrossRef] [PubMed]
4. Van Buchem, F.S.P.; Hadders, H.N.; Hansen, J.F.; Woldring, M.G. Hyperostosis Corticalis Generalisata: Report of Seven Cases. *Am. J. Med.* **1962**, *33*, 387–397. [CrossRef]
5. Cheng, J.C.; Guo, X.; Sher, A.H. Persistent osteopenia in adolescent idiopathic scoliosis. A longitudinal follow up study. *Spine* **1999**, *24*, 1218–1222. [CrossRef] [PubMed]
6. Hung, V.W.; Qin, L.; Cheung, C.S.; Lam, T.P.; Ng, B.K.; Tse, Y.K.; Guo, X.; Lee, K.M.; Cheng, J.C. Osteopenia: A new prognostic factor of curve progression in adolescent idiopathic scoliosis. *J. Bone Jt. Surg. Am.* **2005**, *87*, 2709–2716.
7. Wang, Z.; Chen, H.; Yu, Y.E.; Zhang, J.; Cheuk, K.; Ng, B.K.; Qiu, Y.; Guo, X.E.; Cheng, J.C.; Lee, W.Y. Unique local bone tissue characteristics in iliac crest bone biopsy from adolescent idiopathic scoliosis with severe spinal deformity. *Sci. Rep.* **2017**, *7*, 40265. [CrossRef]
8. Tanabe, H.; Aota, Y.; Nakamura, N.; Saito, T. A histomorphometric study of the cancellous spinal process bone in adolescent idiopathic scoliosis. *Eur. Spine J.* **2017**, *26*, 1600–1609. [CrossRef]
9. Zhang, J.; Chen, H.; Leung, R.K.K.; Choy, K.W.; Lam, T.P.; Ng, B.K.W.; Qiu, Y.; Feng, J.Q.; Cheng, J.C.Y.; Lee, W.Y.W. Aberrant miR-145-5p/b-catenin signal impairs osteocyte function in adolescent idiopathic scoliosis. *FASEB J.* **2018**, *32*, 6537–6549. [CrossRef]
10. Balemans, W.; Van Den Ende, J.; Paes-Alves, F.; Dikkers, F.G.; Willems, P.J.; Vanhoenacker, F.; de Almeida-Melo, N.; Alves, C.F.; Stratakis, C.A.; Hill, S.C.; et al. Localization of the gene for sclerosteosis to the van Buchem disease-gene region on chromosome 17q12-q21. *Am. J. Hum. Genet.* **1999**, *64*, 1661–1669. [CrossRef]
11. Van Hul, W.; Balemans, W.; Van Hul, E.; Dikkers, F.G.; Obee, H.; Stokroos, R.J.; Hildering, P.; Vanhoenacker, F.; Van Camp, G.; Willems, P.J. Van Buchem disease (hyperostosis corticalis generalisata) maps to chromosome 17q12-q21. *Am. J. Hum. Genet.* **1998**, *62*, 391–399. [CrossRef]
12. Hernandez, P.; Whitty, C.; Wardale, R.J.; Henson, F.M.D. New insights into the location and form of sclerostin. *Biochem. Biophys. Res. Commun.* **2014**, *446*, 1108–1113. [CrossRef]
13. Brunkow, M.E.; Gardner, J.C.; Van Ness, J.; Paeper, B.W.; Kovacevich, B.R.; Proll, S.; Skonier, J.E.; Zhao, L.; Sabo, P.J.; Fu, Y.; et al. Bone dysplasia sclerosteosis results from loss of the SOST gene product, a novel cystine knot-containing protein. *Am. J. Hum. Genet.* **2001**, *68*, 577–589. [CrossRef]
14. Weidauer, S.E.; Schmieder, P.; Beerbaum, M.; Schmitz, W.; Oschkina, H.; Mueller, T.D. NMR structure of the Wnt modulator protein Sclerostin. *Biochem. Biophys. Res. Commun.* **2009**, *380*, 160–165. [CrossRef] [PubMed]
15. Balemans, W.; Ebeling, M.; Patel, N.; Van Hul, E.; Olson, P.; Dioszegi, M.; Lacza, C.; Wuyts, W.; Van Den Ende, J.; Willems, P.; et al. Increased bone density in sclerosteosis is due to the deficiency of a novel secreted protein (SOST). *Hum. Mol. Genet.* **2001**, *10*, 537–543. [CrossRef] [PubMed]
16. Winkler, D.G.; Sutherland, M.K.; Geoghegan, J.C.; Yu, C.; Hayes, T.; Skonier, J.E.; Shpektor, D.; Jonas, M.; Kovacevich, B.R.; Staehling-Hampton, K.; et al. Osteocyte control of bone formation via sclerostin, a novel BMP antagonist. *EMBO J.* **2003**, *22*, 6267–6276. [CrossRef]

17. Weivoda, M.M.; Youssef, S.J.; Oursler, M.J. Sclerostin expression and functions beyond the osteocyte. *Bone* **2017**, *96*, 45–50. [CrossRef]
18. Collette, N.M.; Yee, C.S.; Muruquesh, D.; Sebastian, A.; Taher, L.; Gale, N.W.; Economides, A.N.; Harland, R.M.; Loots, G.G. Sost and its paralog Sostdc1 coordinate digit number in a Gli-3dependent manner. *Dev. Biol.* **2013**, *383*, 90–105. [CrossRef]
19. Van Bezooijen, R.L.; Bronckers, A.L.; Gortzak, R.A.; Hogendoorn, P.C.; Van der Wee-Pals, L.; Balemans, W.; Oostenbroek, H.J.; Van Hul, W.; Hamersma, H.; Dikkers, F.G.; et al. Sclerostin in mineralized matrices and van Buchem disease. *J. Dent. Res.* **2009**, *88*, 569–574. [CrossRef]
20. Kusu, N.; Laurikkala, J.; Imanishishi, M.; Usui, H.; Konischi, M.; Miyake, A.; Thesleftt, I.; Itoh, N. Sclerostin is a novel secreted osteoclast-derived bone morphogenetic protein antagonist wtih unique ligand specificity. *J. Biol. Chem.* **2003**, *278*, 24113–24117. [CrossRef] [PubMed]
21. Li, X.; Ominsky, M.S.; Niu, Q.T.; Sun, N.; Daughterty, B.; D'Agostin, D.; Kurahara, C.; Gao, Y.; Cao, J.; Gong, J.; et al. Targeted deletion of the sclerostin gene in mice results in increased bone formation and bone strength. *J. Bone Miner. Res.* **2008**, *23*, 860–869. [CrossRef]
22. Maeda, K.; Kobayashi, Y.; Koide, M.; Uehara, S.; Okamoto, M.; Ishihara, A.; Kayama, T.; Saito, M.; Marumo, K. The Regulation of Bone Metabolism and Disorders by Wnt Signaling. *Int. J. Mol. Sci.* **2019**, *20*, 5525. [CrossRef] [PubMed]
23. Semenov, M.V.; He, X. LRP5 mutations linked to high bone mass diseases cause reduced LRP5 binding and inhibition by SOST. *J. Biol. Chem.* **2006**, *281*, 38276–38284. [CrossRef]
24. Van Wesenbeeck, L.; Cleiren, E.; Gram, J.; Beals, R.K.; Benichou, O.; Scopelliti, D.; Key, L.; Renton, T.; Bartels, C.; Gong, Y.Q.; et al. Six novel missense mutations in the LDL receptor-related protein 5 (LRP5) gene in different conditions with an increased bone density. *Am. J. Hum. Genet.* **2003**, *72*, 763–771. [CrossRef] [PubMed]
25. Hassler, N.; Roschger, A.; Gamsjaeger, S.; Kramer, I.; Lueger, S.; van Lierop, A.; Roschger, P.; Klaushofer, K.; Paschalis, E.P.; Kneissel, M.; et al. Sclerostin Deficiency Is Linked to Altered Bone Composition. *J. Bone Miner. Res.* **2014**, *29*, 2144–2151. [CrossRef] [PubMed]
26. Wijenayaka, A.R.; Kogawa, M.; Lim, H.P.; Bonewald, L.F.; Findlay, D.M.; Atkins, G.J. Sclerostin stimulates osteocyte support of osteoclast activity by a RANKL-dependent pathway. *PLoS ONE* **2011**, *6*, e25900. [CrossRef] [PubMed]
27. Collette, N.M.; Genetos, D.C.; Economides, A.N.; Xie, L.; Shahnazari, M.; Yao, W.; Lane, N.E.; Harland, R.M.; Loots, G.G. Targeted deletion of Sost distal enhancer increases bone formation and bone mass. *Proc. Natl. Acad. Sci. USA* **2012**, *109*, 14092–14097. [CrossRef]
28. Koide, M.; Kobayashi, Y. Regulatory mechanisms of sclerostin expression during bone remodeling. *J. Bone Miner. Metab.* **2019**, *37*, 9–17. [CrossRef]
29. Komori, T. Regulation of Proliferation, Differentiation and Functions of Osteoblasts by Runx2. *Int. J. Mol. Sci.* **2019**, *20*, 1694. [CrossRef]
30. Delgado-Calle, J.; Sanudo, C.; Bolado, A.; Fernandez, A.F.; Arozamena, J.; Pascual-Carra, M.A.; Rodriguez-Rey, J.C.; Fraga, M.F.; Bonewald, L.; Riancho, J.A. DNA methylation contributes to the regulation of sclerostin expression in human osteocytes. *J. Bone Miner. Res.* **2012**, *27*, 926–937. [CrossRef]
31. Wijenayaka, A.R.; Prideaux, M.; Yang, D.; Morris, H.A.; Findlay, D.M.; Anderson, P.H.; Atkins, G.J. Early response of the human SOST gene to stimulation by 1α,25-dihydroxyvitamin D3. *J. Steroid Biochem. Mol. Biol.* **2016**, *164*, 369–373. [CrossRef] [PubMed]
32. St John, H.C.; Hansen, S.J.; Pike, J.W. Analysis of SOST expression using large minigenes reveals the MEF2C binding site in the evolutionarily conserved region (ECR5) enhancer mediates forskolin, but not 1,25-dihydroxyvitamin D or TGFbeta responsiveness. *J. Steroid Biochem. Mol. Biol.* **2016**, *164*, 277–280. [CrossRef]
33. Sakellariou, G.T.; Iliopoulos, A.; Konsta, M.; Kenanidis, E.; Potoupnis, M.; Tsiridis, E.; Gavana, E.; Sayegh, F.E. Serum levels of Dkk-1, sclerostin and VEGF in patients with ankylosing spondylitis and their association with smoking, and clinical, inflammatory and radiographic parameters. *Jt. Bone Spine* **2017**, *84*, 309–315. [CrossRef] [PubMed]
34. Suen, P.K.; Zhu, T.Y.; Chow, D.H.; Huang, L.; Zheng, L.Z.; Qin, L. Sclerostin Antibody Treatment Increases Bone Formation, Bone Mass, and Bone Strength of Intact Bones in Adult Male Rats. *Sci. Rep.* **2015**, *5*, 15632. [CrossRef] [PubMed]
35. Liu, Y.; Rui, Y.; Cheng, T.Y.; Huang, S.; Xu, L.; Meng, F.; Lee, W.Y.; Zhang, T.; Li, N.; Li, C.; et al. Effects of Sclerostin Antibody on the Healing of Femoral Fractures in Ovariectomised Rats. *Calcif. Tissue Int.* **2016**, *98*, 263–274. [CrossRef] [PubMed]
36. Oranger, A.; Brunetti, G.; Colaianni, G.; Tamma, R.; Carbone, C.; Lippo, L.; Mori, G.; Pignataro, P.; Cirulli, N.; Zerlotin, R.; et al. Sclerostin stimulates angiogenesis in human endothelial cells. *Bone* **2017**, *101*, 26–36. [CrossRef]
37. He, X.; Cheng, R.; Benyajati, S.; Ma, J.X. PEDF and its roles in physiological and pathological conditions: Implication in diabetic and hypoxia-induced angiogenic diseases. *Clin. Sci.* **2015**, *128*, 805–823. [CrossRef]
38. Inagaki, Y.; Hookway, E.S.; Kashima, T.G.; Munemoto, M.; Tanaka, Y.; Hassan, A.B.; Oppermann, U.; Athanasou, N.A. Sclerostin expression in bone tumours and tumour-like lesions. *Histopathology* **2016**, *69*, 470–478. [CrossRef]
39. Sevetson, B.; Taylor, S.; Pan, Y. Cbfa1/RUNX2 directs specific expression of the sclerosteosis gene (SOST). *J. Biol. Chem.* **2004**, *279*, 13849–13858. [CrossRef]
40. Techavichit, P.; Gao, Y.; Kurenbekova, L.; Shuck, R.; Donehower, L.A.; Yustein, J.T. Secreted Frizzled-Related Protein 2 (sFRP2) promotes osteosarcoma invasion and metastatic potential. *BMC Cancer* **2016**, *16*, 869. [CrossRef]

41. Baker, E.K.; Taylor, S.; Gupte, A.; Chalk, A.M.; Bhattacharya, S.; Green, A.C.; Martin, T.J.; Strbenac, D.; Robinson, M.D.; Purton, L.E.; et al. Wnt inhibitory factor 1 (WIF1) is a marker of osteoblastic di_erentiation stage and is not silenced by DNA methylation in osteosarcoma. *Bone* **2015**, *73*, 223–232. [CrossRef]
42. Roforth, M.M.; Fujita, K.; McGregor, U.I.; Kirmani, S.; McCready, L.K.; Peterson, J.M.; Drake, M.T.; Monroe, D.G.; Khosla, S. Effects of age on bone mRNA levels of sclerostin and other genes relevant to bone metabolism in humans. *Bone* **2014**, *59*, 1–6. [CrossRef] [PubMed]
43. Mödder, U.I.; Hoey, K.A.; Amin, S.; McCready, L.K.; Achenbach, S.J.; Riggs, B.L.; Melton, L.J.; Khosla, S. Relation of age, gender, and bone mass to circulating sclerostin levels in women and men. *J. Bone Miner. Res.* **2011**, *26*, 373–379. [CrossRef] [PubMed]
44. Papachristou, D.J.; Papachroni, K.K.; Basdra, E.K.; Papavassiliou, A.G. Signalimg networks and transcription factors regulating mechanotransduction in bone. *BioEssays* **2009**, *31*, 794–804. [CrossRef] [PubMed]
45. Palumbo, C.; Palazzini, S.; Marotti, G. Morphological study of intercellular junctions during osteocyte differentiation. *Bone* **1990**, *11*, 401–406. [CrossRef]
46. Zeng, Y.; Cowin, S.C.; Weinbaum, S. A fiber matrix model for fluid flow and streaming potentials in the canaliculi of an osteon. *Ann. Biomed. Eng.* **1994**, *22*, 280–292. [CrossRef]
47. Genetos, D.C.; Toupadakis, C.A.; Raheja, L.F.; Wong, A.; Papanicolaou, S.E.; Fyhrie, D.P.; Loots, G.G.; Yellowley, C.E. Hypoxia decreases sclerostin expression and increases Wnt signaling in osteoblasts. *J. Cell Biochem.* **2010**, *110*, 87–96. [CrossRef] [PubMed]
48. Klein-Nulend, J.; Bakker, A.D.; Bacabac, R.G.; Vatsa, A.; Weinbaum, S. Mechanosensation and transduction in osteocytes. *Bone* **2013**, *54*, 182–190. [CrossRef] [PubMed]
49. Walker, E.C.; McGregor, N.E.; Poulton, I.J.; Solano, M.; Pompolo, S.; Fernandes, T.J.; Constable, M.J.; Nicholson, G.C.; Zhang, J.G.; Nicola, N.A.; et al. Oncostatin M promotes bone formation independently of resorption when signaling through leukemia inhibitor factor in mice. *J. Clin. Investig.* **2010**, *120*, 582–592. [CrossRef]
50. Cheng, J.C.; Castelein, R.M.; Chu, W.C.; Danielsson, A.J.; Dobbs, M.B.; Grivas, T.B.; Gurnett, C.A.; Luk, K.D.; Moreau, A.; Newton, P.O.; et al. Adolescent idiopathic scoliosis. *Nat. Rev. Dis. Primers* **2015**, *1*, 15030. [CrossRef]
51. Tu, X.; Rhee, Y.; Condon, K.W.; Bivi, N.; Allen, M.R.; Dwyer, D.; Stollina, M.; Turner, C.H.; Robling, A.G.; Plotkin, L.I.; et al. Sost downregulation and local Wnt signaling are required for the osteogenic response to mechanical loading. *Bone* **2012**, *50*, 209–217. [CrossRef] [PubMed]
52. Bonnet, N.; Standley, K.N.; Bianchi, E.N.; Stadelmann, V.; Foti, M.; Conway, S.J.; Ferrari, S.L. The matricellular protein Periostin is required for Sclerostin inhibition and the anabolic response to mechanical loading and physical activity. *J. Biol. Chem.* **2009**, *284*, 35939–35950. [CrossRef] [PubMed]
53. Hui, S.; Yang, Y.; Li, J.; Li, N.; Xu, P.; Li, H.; Zhang, Y.; Wang, S.; Lin, G.; Li, S.; et al. Differential miRNAs profile and bioinformatics analyses in bone marrow mesenchymal stem cells from adolescent idiopathic scoliosis patients. *Spine J.* **2019**, *19*, 1584–1596. [CrossRef] [PubMed]
54. Suarjana, I.N.; Isbagio, H.; Soewondo, P.; Rachman, I.A.; Sadikin, M.; Prihartono, J.; Malik, S.G.; Soeroso, J. The Role of Serum Expression Levels of Microrna-21 on Bone Mineral Density in Hypostrogenic Postmenopausal Women with Osteoporosis: Study on Level of RANKL, OPG, TGFβ-1, Sclerostin, RANKL/OPG Ratio, and Physical Activity. *Acta Med. Indones* **2019**, *51*, 245–252. [PubMed]
55. Liao, H.; Zhang, Z.; Liu, Z.; Lin, W.; Huang, J.; Huang, Y. Inhibited microRNA-218-5p attenuates synovial inflammation and cartilage injury in rats with knee osteoarthritis by promoting sclerostin. *Life Sci.* **2021**, *267*, 118893. [CrossRef]
56. Hayes, M.; Gao, X.; Yu, L.X.; Paria, N.; Henkelman, R.M.; Wise, C.A.; Ciruna, B. ptk7 mutant zebrafish models of congenital and idiopathic scoliosis implicate dysregulated Wnt signalling in disease. *Nat. Commun.* **2014**, *5*, 4777. [CrossRef]
57. Rodda, S.J.; McMahon, A.P. Distinct roles for hedgehog and canonical Wnt signaling in specification, differentiation and maintenance of osteoblast progenitors. *Development* **2006**, *133*, 3231–3244. [CrossRef]
58. Regard, J.B.; Cherman, N.; Palmer, D.; Kuznetsov, S.A.; Celi, F.S.; Guettier, J.M.; Chen, M.; Bhattacharyya, N.; Wess, J.; Coughlin, S.R.; et al. Wnt/b-catenin signaling is differentially regulated by Ga proteins and contributes to fibrous dysplasia. *Proc. Natl. Acad. Sci. USA* **2011**, *108*, 20101–20106. [CrossRef]
59. Cisterna, P.; Henriquez, J.P.; Brandan, E.; Inestrosa, N.C. Wnt signaling in skeletal muscle dynamics: Myogenesis, neuromuscular synapse and fibrosis. *Mol. Neurobiol.* **2014**, *49*, 574–589. [CrossRef]
60. Kondo, N.; Yuasa, T.; Shimono, K.; Tung, W.; Okabe, T.; Yasuhara, R.; Pacifici, M.; Zhang, Y.; Iwamoto, M.; Enomoto-Iwamoto, M. Intervertebral disc development is regulated by Wnt/beta -catenin signaling. *Spine* **2011**, *36*, E513–E518. [CrossRef]
61. Tamamura, Y.; Otani, T.; Kanatani, N.; Koyama, E.; Kitagaki, J.; Komori, T.; Yamada, Y.; Costantini, F.; Wakisaka, S.; Pacifici, M.; et al. Developmental regulation of Wnt/beta-catenin signals is required for growth plate assembly, cartilage integrity, and endochondral ossification. *J. Biol. Chem.* **2005**, *280*, 19185–19195. [CrossRef]
62. Acaroglu, E.; Akel, I.; Alanay, A.; Yazici, M.; Marcucio, R. Comparison of the melatonin and calmodulin in paravertebral muscle and platelets of patients with or without adolescent idiopathic scoliosis. *Spine* **2009**, *34*, E659–E663. [CrossRef] [PubMed]
63. Tansey, M.G.; Luby-Phelps, K.; Kamm, K.E.; Stull, J.T. Ca(2+) dependent phosphorylation of myosin light chain kinase decreases the Ca2+ sensitivity of light chain phosphorylation within smooth muscle cells. *J. Biol. Chem.* **1994**, *269*, 9912–9920. [CrossRef]
64. Nishizawa, Y.; Okui, Y.; Inaba, M.; Okuno, S.; Yukioka, K.; Miki, T.; Watanabe, Y.; Morii, H. Calcium/Cadmodulin-mediated action of calcitonin on lipid metabolism in rats. *J. Clin. Investig.* **1988**, *82*, 1165–1172. [CrossRef] [PubMed]

65. Gooi, J.H.; Pompolo, S.; Karsdal, M.A.; Kulkarni, N.H.; Kalajzic, I.; McAhren, S.H.; Han, B.; Onyia, J.E.; Ho, P.W.; Gillespie, M.T.; et al. Calcitonin impairs the anabolic effect of PTH in young rats and stimulates expression of sclerostin by osteocytes. *Bone* **2010**, *46*, 1486–1497. [CrossRef]
66. Zhou, R.; Yuan, Z.; Liu, J.; Liu, J. Calcitonin gene-related peptide promotes the expression of osteoblastic genes and activates the WNT signal transduction pathway in bone marrow stromal stem cells. *Mol. Med. Rep.* **2016**, *13*, 4689–4696. [CrossRef] [PubMed]
67. Xu, E.; Lin, T.; Jiang, H.; Ji, Z.; Shao, W.; Meng, Y.; Gao, R.; Zhou, X. Asymmetric expression of GPR126 in the convex/concave side of the spine is associated with spinal skeletal malformation in adolescent idiopathic scoliosis population. *Eur. Spine J.* **2019**, *28*, 1977–1986. [CrossRef]
68. Murray, D.W.; Bulstrode, C.J. The development of adolescent idiopathic scoliosis. *Eur. Spine J.* **1996**, *5*, 251–257. [CrossRef] [PubMed]
69. Grivas, T.B.; Burwell, G.R.; Vasiliadis, E.S.; Webb, J.K. A segmental radiological study of the spine and rib–cage in children with progressive infantile idiopathic scoliosis. *Scoliosis* **2016**, *1*, 17. [CrossRef] [PubMed]
70. Grivas, T.B.; Vasiliadis, E.S.; Polyzois, V.D.; Mouzakis, V. Trunk asymmetry and handedness in 8245 school children. *Pediatr. Rehabil.* **2006**, *9*, 259–266. [CrossRef] [PubMed]
71. Shi, L.; Wang, D.; Chu, W.C.; Burwell, R.G.; Freeman, B.J.; Heng, P.A.; Cheng, J.C. Volume-based morphometry of brain MR images in adolescent idiopathic scoliosis and healthy control subjects. *Am. J. Neuroradiol.* **2009**, *30*, 1302–1307. [CrossRef]
72. Chau, W.W.; Chu, W.C.; Lam, T.P.; Ng, B.K.; Fu, L.L.; Cheng, J.C. Anatomical Origin of Abnormal Somatosensory-Evoked Potential (SEP) in Adolescent Idiopathic Scoliosis with Different Curve Severity and Correlation With Cerebellar Tonsillar Level Determined by MRI. *Spine* **2016**, *41*, E598–E604. [CrossRef]
73. Byl, N.N.; Holland, S.; Jurek, A.; Hu, S.S. Postural imbalance and vibratory sensitivity in patients with idiopathic scoliosis: Implications for treatment. *J. Orthop. Sports Phys. Ther.* **1997**, *26*, 60–68. [CrossRef]
74. Qiu, Y.; Sun, X.; Qiu, X.; Li, W.; Zhu, Z.; Zhu, F.; Wang, B.; Yu, Y.; Qian, B. Decreased circulating leptin level and its association with body and bone mass in girls with adolescent idiopathic scoliosis. *Spine* **2007**, *32*, 2703–2710. [CrossRef]
75. Burwell, R.G.; Aujla, R.K.; Grevitt, M.P.; Dangerfield, P.H.; Moulton, A.; Randell, T.L.; Anderson, S.I. Pathogenesis of adolescent idiopathic scoliosis in girls—A double neuro-osseous theory involving disharmony between two nervous systems, somatic and autonomic expressed in the spine and trunk: Possible dependency on sympathetic nervous system and hormones with implications for medical therapy. *Scoliosis* **2009**, *4*, 24.
76. Robling, A.G.; Niziolek, P.J.; Baldridge, L.A.; Condon, K.W.; Allen, M.R.; Alam, I.; Mantila, S.M.; Gluhak-Heinrich, J.; Bellido, T.M.; Harris, S.E.; et al. Mechanical stimulation of bone in vivo reduces osteocyte expression of Sost/sclerostin. *J. Biol. Chem.* **2008**, *283*, 5866–5875. [CrossRef]
77. Robinson, J.A.; Chatterjee-Kishore, M.; Yaworsky, P.J.; Cullen, D.M.; Zhao, W.; Li, C.; Kharode, Y.; Sauter, L.; Babij, P.; Brown, E.L.; et al. Wnt/beta-catenin signaling is a normal physiological response to mechanical loading in bone. *J. Biol. Chem.* **2006**, *281*, 31720–31728. [CrossRef]
78. Lin, C.; Jiang, X.; Dai, Z.; Guo, X.; Weng, T.; Wang, J.; Li, Y.; Feng, G.; Gao, X.; He, L. Sclerostin Mediates Bone Response to Mechanical Unloading Through Antagonizing Wnt/b-Catenin Signaling. *J. Bone Miner. Res.* **2009**, *24*, 1651–1661. [CrossRef] [PubMed]
79. Gaudio, A.; Pennisi, P.; Bratengeier, C.; Torrisi, V.; Lindner, B.; Mangiafico, R.A.; Pulvirenti, I.; Hawa, G.; Tringali, G.; Fiore, C.E. Increased sclerostin serum levels associated with bone formation and resorption markers in patients with immobilization-induced bone loss. *J. Clin. Endocrinol. Metab.* **2010**, *95*, 2248–2253. [CrossRef]
80. Tian, X.; Jee, W.S.S.; Li, X.; Paszty, C.; Ke, H.Z. Sclerostin antibody increases bone mass by stimulating bone formation and inhibiting bone resorption in a hindlimb-immobilization rat model. *Bone* **2011**, *48*, 197–201. [CrossRef] [PubMed]
81. Nguyen, J.; Tang, S.Y.; Nguyen, D.; Alliston, T. Load Regulates Bone Formation and SclerostinExpression through a TGFb-Dependent Mechanism. *PLoS ONE* **2013**, *8*, e53813. [CrossRef]
82. Morse, A.; McDonald, M.M.; Kelly, N.H.; Melville, K.M.; Schindeler, A.; Kramer, I.; Kneissel, M.; van der Meulen, M.C.H.; Little, D.G. Mechanical load increases in bone formation via a sclerostin-independent pathway. *J. Bone Miner. Res.* **2014**, *29*, 2456–2467. [CrossRef] [PubMed]

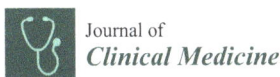

Article

Morphology, Development and Deformation of the Spine in Mild and Moderate Scoliosis: Are Changes in the Spine Primary or Secondary?

Theodoros B. Grivas [1,*], George Vynichakis [1], Michail Chandrinos [1], Christina Mazioti [2], Despina Papagianni [3], Aristea Mamzeri [4] and Constantinos Mihas [5]

1. Department of Orthopedics & Traumatology, "Tzaneio" General Hospital of Piraeus, 185 36 Piraeus, Greece; vini_gio@windowslive.com (G.V.); ChandrinosMichail@gmail.com (M.C.)
2. Health Visitor, "Tzaneio" General Hospital of Piraeus, 185 36 Piraeus, Greece; maziotix@gmail.com
3. School Nurse—Health Visitor, Special Primary School of Rafina, 190 09 Attica, Greece; papdes2009@hotmail.com
4. Health Visitor, TOMY Attica Square, 104 45 Athens, Greece; mamzeri_aristea@hotmail.com
5. Department of Internal Medicine, Kymi General Hospital—Health Centre, 340 03 Euboea (Evia), Greece; gas521@yahoo.co.uk
* Correspondence: tgri69@otenet.gr

Citation: Grivas, T.B.; Vynichakis, G.; Chandrinos, M.; Mazioti, C.; Papagianni, D.; Mamzeri, A.; Mihas, C. Morphology, Development and Deformation of the Spine in Mild and Moderate Scoliosis: Are Changes in the Spine Primary or Secondary? *J. Clin. Med.* **2021**, *10*, 5901. https://doi.org/10.3390/jcm10245901

Academic Editor: Hiroyuki Katoh

Received: 21 November 2021
Accepted: 14 December 2021
Published: 16 December 2021

Publisher's Note: MDPI stays neutral with regard to jurisdictional claims in published maps and institutional affiliations.

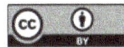

Copyright: © 2021 by the authors. Licensee MDPI, Basel, Switzerland. This article is an open access article distributed under the terms and conditions of the Creative Commons Attribution (CC BY) license (https://creativecommons.org/licenses/by/4.0/).

Abstract: Introduction and aim of the study: We aim to determine whether the changes in the spine in scoliogenesis of idiopathic scoliosis (IS), are primary/inherent or secondary. There is limited information on this issue in the literature. We studied the sagittal profile of the spine in IS using surface topography. Material and methods: After approval of the ethics committee of the hospital, we studied 45 children, 4 boys and 41 girls, with an average age of 12.5 years (range 7.5–16.4 years), referred to the scoliosis clinic by our school screening program. These children were divided in two groups: A and B. Group A included 17 children with IS, 15 girls and 2 boys. All of them had a trunk asymmetry, measured with a scoliometer, greater than or equal to 5 degrees. Group B, (control group) included 26 children, 15 girls and 11 boys, with no trunk asymmetry and scoliometer measurement less than 2 degrees. The height and weight of children were measured. The Prujis scoliometer was used in standing Adam test in the thoracic (T), thoraco-lumbar (TL) and lumbar (L) regions. All IS children had an ATR greater than or equal to 5 degrees. The Cobb angle was assessed in the postero-anterior radiographs in Group A. A posterior truncal surface topogram, using the "Formetric 4" apparatus, was also performed and the distance from the vertebra prominence (VP) to the apex of the kyphosis (KA), and similarly to the apex of the lumbar lordosis (LA) was calculated. The ratio of the distances (VP-KA) for (PV-LA) was calculated. The averages of the parameters were studied, and the correlation of the ratio of distances (VP-KA) to (VP-KA) with the scoliometer and Cobb angle measurements were assessed, respectively (Pearson corr. Coeff. r), in both groups and between them. Results: Regarding group A (IS), the average height was 1.55 m (range 1.37, 1.71), weight 47.76 kg (range 33, 65). The IS children had right (Rt) T or TL curves. The mean T Cobb angle was 24 degrees and 26 in L. In the same group, the kyphotic apex (KA (VPDM)) distance was −125.82 mm (range −26, −184) and the lordotic apex (LA (VPDM)) distance was −321.65 mm (range −237, −417). The correlations of the ratio of distances (KA (VPDM))/(LA (VPDM)) with the Major Curve Cobb angle measurement and scoliometer findings were non-statistically significant (Pearson r = 0.077, −0.211, *p*: 0.768, 0.416, respectively. Similarly, in the control group, KA (VPDM)/(LA (VPDM) was not significantly correlated with scoliometer findings (Pearson r = −0.016, −*p*: 0.939). Discussion and conclusions: The lateral profile of the spine was commonly considered to be a primary aetiological factor of IS due to the fact that the kyphotic thoracic apex in IS is located in a higher thoracic vertebra (more vertebrae are posteriorly inclined), thus creating conditions of greater rotational instability and therefore greater vulnerability for IS development. Our findings do not confirm this hypothesis, since the correlation of the (VP-KA) to (VP-KA) ratio with the truncal asymmetry, assessed with the scoliometer and Cobb angle measurements, is non-statistically significant, in both groups A and B. In addition, the aforementioned ratio did not differ significantly between the two groups in our sample

(0.39 ± 0.11 vs. 0.44 ± 0.08, *p*: 0.134). It is clear that hypokyphosis is not a primary causal factor for the commencing, mild or moderate scoliotic curve, as published elsewhere. We consider that the small thoracic hypokyphosis in developing scoliosis adds to the view that the reduced kyphosis, facilitating the axial rotation, could be considered as a permissive factor rather than a causal one, in the pathogenesis of IS. This view is consistent with previously published views and it is obviously the result of gravity, growth and muscle tone.

Keywords: idiopathic scoliosis; scoliometer; truncal asymmetry; lateral spinal profile; surface topography; aetiology

1. Introduction

Idiopathic scoliosis (IS) is defined as a three-dimensional (3D) structural deformity of the spine and is associated with asymmetries of the trunk and the extremities [1]. The aetiology of this deformity is not yet clear, because there is no established theory of scoliogenesis. Adolescent idiopathic scoliosis (AIS) is the most common type of IS, and begins in early puberty. The incidence of AIS is 1–4% in adolescents and affects mainly females [2]. The frontal plane spinal curvature in IS is commonly assessed in the postero-anterior standing radiographs using the Cobb angle [3]. Similarly, the thoracic kyphosis is commonly assessed in the lateral standing radiographs using the Cobb method, usually from T4 to T12 vertebrae.

A major question in the study of IS aetiology is whether the growth changes in the spine in initiating and mild cases, are primary/inherent or secondary. There is no clear answer and there is limited information on this issue in the peer review literature. Some maintain that pathology begins within the spine [4], while others argue that changes in the spine are secondary [5]. The research approach to shed some light in this issue is multidimensional, with the study of the various anatomical components of the deformity, such as the thoracic cage and the lateral vertebral profile.

As concerns the thoracic cage in IS, and especially in adolescents, there is the view that the rib length asymmetry in apical region is a secondary event to the scoliosis deformity and not a protagonist in the aetiopathogenesis [6,7]. The opponents of this view claim that in the chain of the pathological deformations leading to scoliosis, the ribs deform first and then the spine follows [8,9]. The rib cage deformity can be traditionally assessed radiographically using the rib vertebra angles (RVAs), mainly in early onset scoliosis, if it is developed before 10 years of age. A prognostic indicator for the progression of the curve is the difference of the concave minus the convex apical thoracic RVA (RVAD), if this is more than 20 degrees [10,11].

Regarding the frontal plane (FP), it was revealed by [12], that the scoliotic spine first deforms at the level of the intervertebral disc (IVD), not the vertebrae. These findings were confirmed three years later by [13]. Moreover, it was published that the histological abnormalities in the IVD in AIS are secondary to an altered mechanical environment [14–18]. These findings were based on the CTs of AIS patients, which showed that the IVDs contribute more to anterior spinal length compared to the contribution by the vertebrae, and suggested that the curve progression is not a primary vertebra growth disorder; rather, it is the result of altered mechanical loading.

The lateral spinal profile (LSP) and its significance in IS scoliogenesis is a topic that was discussed by many researches for many years, e.g., [19–39].

An answer to the question of whether emerging IS changes during growth are endogenous to or outside the vertebrae may be provided comparing the morphology of the growing spine during the early stages of IS development to normal peers' spines.

It can be determined whether developmental changes in the spine are intrinsic or secondary by studying the various elements of the morphology of the growing spine during the early stages of IS development and correlating them with each other. This study may reveal the real role of the LSP in IS patho-biomechanics. Moreover, it may be helpful for tailoring an aetiological rather than symptomatic treatment, which is currently the case. This could be a medical treatment leaving the spine mobile and unfused.

Thus, the aim of this study is to address the above question by studying the sagittal profile of the onset and mild IS, using the radiography, the surface topography and the scoliometer readings of children with IS, examined in the scoliosis clinic of our department. We compared findings of these different examination methods and assessed their agreement or disagreement.

2. Materials and Methods

We performed a retrospective study of children and adolescents (16 years and younger), referred to the scoliosis clinic of our hospital by our school scoliosis screening (SSS) program, between January 2013 and December 2019. During this period, 2512 children attending schools located in the district of our hospital were screened.

In order to proceed with the study, we obtained approval by the hospital's ethical committee (excerpt from the 24th on 6 October 2021 Ethical committee meeting) to conduct a retrospective study of radio-morphology of the spine, the scoliometer readings and the surface topography of patients attending our hospital scoliosis clinic.

Informed consent was also obtained by the parents of children for the examination.

2.1. The Examined Children

We studied two groups which included 43 children, 13 (30.2%) boys and 30 (69.8%) girls, with an average age of 12.7 ± 1.9 years (range 8.4–16.4 years).

The group A (IS group) included 17 children with IS, 15 girls and 2 boys. All of them had a trunk asymmetry, measured with a scoliometer, greater than or equal to 5 degrees, and Cobb angle more than 10 degrees in postero-anterior radiographs.

The group B (control group) included 26 children, 15 girls and 11 boys, with no trunk asymmetry, scoliometer measurement equal or less than 2 degrees, and straight spines in 4D Formetric.

2.2. The Measurements

The height and weight of children were measured. The Prujis scoliometer was used to examine the children in standing forward bending position (Adam test) in thoracic (T), thoraco-lumbar (TL) and lumbar (L) regions. The Cobb angle in the scoliotic children was assessed in the postero-anterior radiographs. The posterior truncal surface topogram, using the "Diers-Formetric 4" apparatus, was also performed.

The lateral truncal projection produced with the Diers 4D Formetric topogram is demonstrated in Figure 1. The lateral projection corresponds to the midline of the spine in the lateral view. This curve forms the 3D reconstruction of the spinal midline on conjunction with the frontal projection. The continuous green curve represents the external back profile (i.e., the symmetry line in the lateral view). The symmetry lines and anatomical landmarks are displayed in addition to the profiles. The symmetry line divides each profile into two halves with minimal lateral asymmetry. It approximates the line of the spinal process. In a healthy individual, the symmetry line is a straight line through VP (Vertebra Promines) and DM (Dimple Middle). The kyphotic apex is marked KA and the lordotic apex LA as seen in the diagram in lateral projection in Figures 1 and 2.

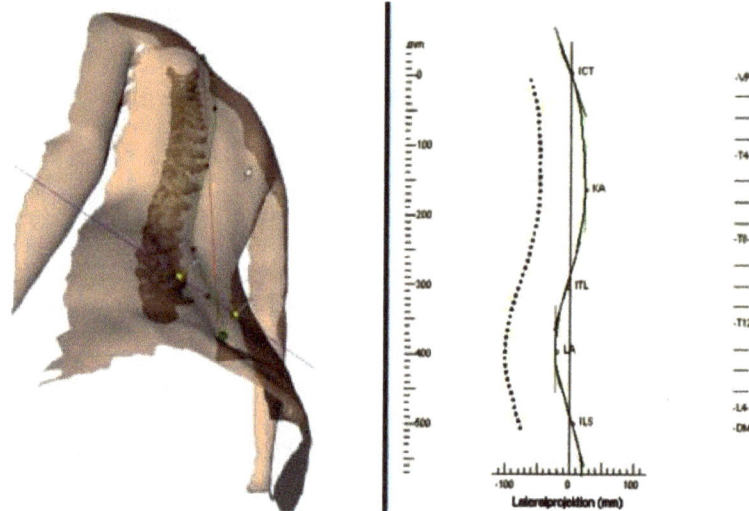

Figure 1. ICT or VP = vertebra prominence, KA = Kyphotic Apex, LA = Lordotic Apex, DM = Dimple Middle.

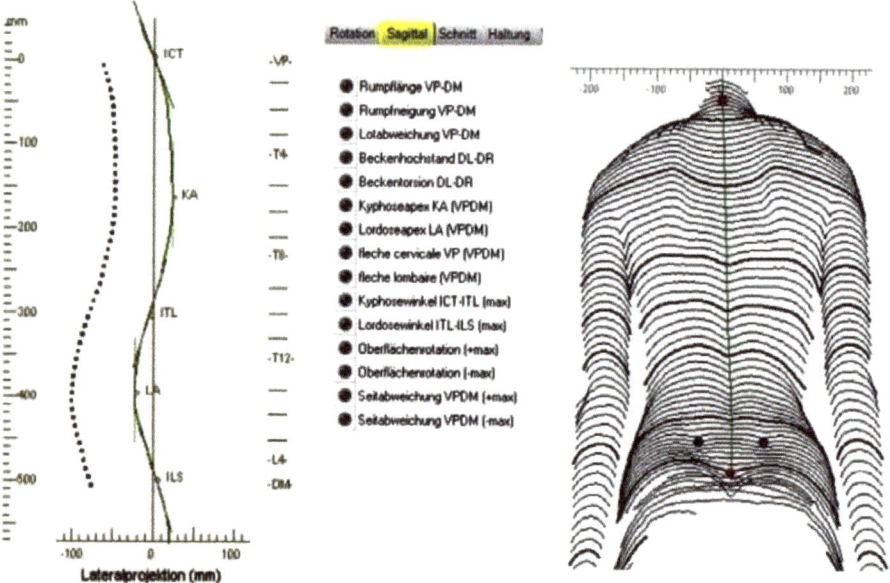

Figure 2. VP = Vertebra prominence, this corresponds to ICT (zero 0 mm), KA = Kyphotic Apex, LA = Lordotic Apex. If the (VP-KA) distance is shorter, that is, if the IS thoracic vertebra corresponding to KA is higher at the thoracic spine, then the value of the distances' ratio (VP-KA)/(VP-LA) turns smaller, because the nominator of the quotient is smaller, (shorter VP-KA) distance. If this ratio were statistically significantly correlated with the Cobb angle and the truncal asymmetry, this would imply that this morphology (higher KA in IS) would be a primary aetiological factor for the commencement of IS. But this is not the case!

Using the ruler on the left of the projection of the lateral profile, the distances VP up to KA and VP up to LA are measured in mm. Then a quotient is formed with numerator VP-KA and denominator VP-LA.

The distance from the vertebra prominence (VP) to the apex of the kyphosis (KA) and similarly to the apex of the lumbar lordosis (LA) was calculated on the topograms. The quotient of the distances (VP to KA) divided by (PV to LA) was also calculated.

The distance of the apparatus from the examined child was set at 2 m, the temperature of the examined room is the standard indoors temperature of 23–24 degrees Celsius, with a normal humidity of 36–38% so that the child was comfortable. To reduce error caused by potential movement of the child during the examination, the apparatus was designed to shut eight pictures in 10 s and the final result was the mean of all these captures.

2.3. Statistical Analysis

Power analysis was performed in order to assess significant differences in the variable of interest (Kyphotic Apex KA/Lordotic Apex LA) higher than 0.1 with a standard deviation of 0.1.

The averages of the parameters were studied, and the correlation of the ratio of distances (VP-KA) to (VP-LA) with the scoliometer and Cobb angle measurements was assessed respectively (Pearson corr. Coeff. r).

3. Results

Power analysis showed that in order to assess significant differences in the variable of interest (Kyphotic Apex KA/Lordotic Apex LA) higher than 0.1 with a standard deviation of 0.1, a sample size of at least 17 individuals in each study group (control and experimental) would be needed in order to achieve statistical power of 80% at a significance level (alpha) of 0.05. Descriptive statistics by group of interest and by gender are shown in Table 1.

Table 1. Descriptive statistics by group.

	Group							
	Controls				IS			
	Gender				Gender			
	Boys		Girls		Boys		Girls	
	Mean	SD	Mean	SD	Mean	SD	Mean	SD
Age (years)	13.03	2.09	12.16	1.72	15.25	1.65	12.43	1.63
Height (cm)	165.14	16.36	155.55	10.28	168.50	3.54	154.00	8.47
Weight (kg)	55.64	22.43	45.55	8.86	56.50	0.71	46.60	8.93
Major Curve Cobb angle					28.00	11.31	30.33	9.22
Scoliometer	0.73	1.01	0.27	0.70	12.50	3.54	7.47	3.76
Kyphotic apex KA(VPDM)	−150.00	32.21	−140.93	35.90	−118.00	26.87	−126.87	36.48
Lordotic apex LA (VPDM)	−350.82	43.91	−313.07	48.61	−395.50	30.41	−311.80	37.20
Kyphotic Apex KA/Lordotic Apex LA	0.43	0.07	0.45	0.09	0.30	0.09	0.41	0.11

3.1. Group A (IS)

The mean age of the girls was 12.4 (range: 8.4–14.3 years) with seven Major T curves (five right and two left) and eight Major TL, eight of which were double curves. The average height was 1.54 m (range: 1.37–1.64) and the average weight was 46.6 kg (range: 33–65). The mean T Cobb angle measurement was 29.28 degrees (range: 23–38 degrees) and TL 31.25 degrees (range: 21–37 degrees).

The mean scoliometer measurement was 7.47 ± 3.76 degrees.

The mean age of the boys was 15.3 (range:14.1–16.4 years) with a right Major T curve with a TL and a left TL curve. The average height was 1.69 m (range:1.66–1.71) and the average weight was 56.5 kg (range: 56–57). The Cobb angle measurements were T 36 degrees and TL 20 degrees. The mean scoliometer measurement was 12.5 ± 3.54 degrees.

Regarding the whole group, the mean (VP-KA) distance was 125.82 mm (range: 26–184) and the mean (VP-LA) distance was 321.7 mm (range: 237–417).

3.2. Group B (Controls)

The mean age of the girls was 12.2 (range: 9.3–15.2 years). The average height was 1.56 m (range: 1.39–1.73) and the average weight was 45.6 kg (range: 33–59).

The mean age of the boys was 13 (range: 9.9–15.6 years). The average height was 1.65 m (range: 1.38–1.84) and the average weight was 55.6 kg (range: 29–105).

Regarding the whole group, the mean (VP-KA) distance was 144.77 mm (range: 77–226) and the mean (VP-LA) distance was 329.038 mm (range: 282–426).

The ratio did not differ significantly between the two groups in our sample (0.39 ± 0.11 vs. 0.44 ± 0.08, p: 0.134). In the control group, KA (VPDM))/(LA (VPDM) was not significantly correlated with scoliometer findings (Pearson r = −0.016, −p: 0.939). The correlations of the ratio of distances (KA (VPDM))/(LA (VPDM)) with the measurement and scoliometer findings were non-statistically significant (Pearson r = 0.077, −0.211, p: 0.768, 0.416, respectively).

4. Discussion

As regards the radiological examination of the asymmetric children referred to our scoliosis clinic, it is noted that according to our recent practice policy, we do not prescribe radiological examination in younger asymmetric referrals (hump less than 4–5 degrees and children younger than 12–13 years of age). In these cases, we usually base our assessment on the surface topography picture. Radiological examination is only prescribed if the child's asymmetry increases in the next visit to the scoliosis clinic [35].

It has been suggested that in IS, hypokyphosis is aetiological to the development of the deformity. The apex of the hypokyphosis is located in a vertebra located in a more cephalad level. In other words, the quotient numerator (VP-KA) decreases, and the quotient has a lower value. In that case, if the hypokyphosis were aetiologically responsible for the development of scoliosis, then the value of the quotient would have a negative statistically significant correlation with the Cobb angle and with the thoracic hump, too.

The results of the present report indicate that there is a negative correlation of the value of the ratio (VP-KA)/(VP-KA) with the scoliometer and Cobb angle measurements; yet it is not non-statistically significant (Pearson −0.356238) with a poor correlation coefficient. Similarly, the correlation with the scoliometer measurements is non-statistically significant (Pearson r = −0.2261). This means that both the transverse plane deformity of the thorax as expressed by the scoliometer measurements and the sagittal profile of the spine are not correlated with the Cobb angle, in mild and moderate scoliosis.

Additionally, this ratio did not differ significantly between the two groups in our sample (0.39 ± 0.11 vs. 0.44 ± 0.08, p: 0.134).

The opinion of the authors is that in initiating and mild scoliosis, the patho-biomechanics are probably dissimilar from the biomechanics when the curve is severe. This issue was studied in an earlier research project of our group in scoliotic children, and provided a clue to the question whether there is an intrinsic vertebral body growth disorder or not in mild/moderate IS. It was found that the sagittal profile of these IS curves do not differ significantly from the profile of normal peers, see: [36]. In other words, the growth potential in mild/moderate IS in the sagittal plane (the lateral spinal profile), is similar to that of peers having normal spines, in both vertebral bodies and the intervertebral discs (IVDs).

Regarding the role of hypokyphosis and its importance in IS aetiology, we stated earlier that in this report the minor hypokyphosis of the thoracic spine and its minimal differences observed in the small curves studied compared with that of non-scoliotics.

This adds to the view that the reduced kyphosis, by facilitating axial rotation, could be viewed as being permissive, rather than as aetiological, in the pathogenesis of idiopathic scoliosis [36]. In other words, a straight (not bended) beam is more easily rotated than a curved one!

It may be stated that the study could be framed as a new scientific research of high clinical interest. Nevertheless, as a limitation it might be stated that for many years researches have been carried out in this sense and even if specific research features are present they are not the exclusive prerogative of this study which among other things used an evaluation parameter, (the surface topography), that is always carefully managed in scientific works, as although not invasive (total absence of radiation) in the application it often results to have variables that can subvert the study, as among other things admitted in the comparisons with other methods by the same authors.

5. Conclusions

This study indicates that hypokyphosis is not a primary causal factor for the commencing, mild or moderate scoliotic curve, as published elsewhere. We consider that the small thoracic hypokyphosis in developing scoliosis is considered as a permissive factor, rather than a causal one, in the pathogenesis of IS. This view is consistent with views previously published [5].

Author Contributions: Conceptualization, T.B.G.; Data curation, G.V., M.C., C.M. (Christina Mazioti), D.P. and A.M.; Formal analysis, T.B.G. and C.M. (Constantinos Mihas); Investigation, T.B.G.; Project administration, T.B.G.; Writing—original draft, T.B.G.; Writing—review and editing, T.B.G. All authors have read and agreed to the published version of the manuscript.

Funding: The authors received no funding for this research.

Institutional Review Board Statement: This study was conducted in accordance with the approval of the "Tzaneio" hospital's Ethical Committee (Excerpt of the 24th on 6 October 2021 Ethical committee meeting).

Informed Consent Statement: Informed consent was obtained.

Acknowledgments: The authors express their appreciation to Paediatric outpatient department and Scoliosis Clinic staff nurses of the Tzaneio Hospital of Piraeus for their help.

Conflicts of Interest: The authors declare no conflict of interest and nothing to declare.

References

1. Grivas, T.B. *SOSORT 2014—4th Educational Courses*; SOSORT Educational Committee: Wiesbaden, Germany, 2014; pp. 38–43.
2. Cheng, J.C.; Castelein, R.M.; Chu, W.C.; Danielsson, A.J.; Dobbs, M.B.; Grivas, T.B.; Gurnett, C.A.; Luk, K.D.; Moreau, A.; Newton, P.O.; et al. Adolescent idiopathic scoliosis. *Nat. Rev. Dis.* **2015**, *1*, 15030. [CrossRef] [PubMed]
3. Cobb, J. Outline for the Study of Scoliosis. *Instr. Course Lect.* **1948**, *5*, 261–275.
4. Zhu, F.; Chu, W.C.W.; Sun, G.; Zhu, Z.Z.; Wang, W.J.; Cheng, J.C.Y.; Qiu, Y. Rib length asymmetry in thoracic adolescent idiopathic scoliosis: Is it primary or secondary? *Eur. Spine J.* **2011**, *20*, 254–259. [CrossRef]
5. Burwell, R.G.; Cole, A.A.; Cook, T.A.; Grivas, T.B.; Kiel, A.W.; Moulton, A.; Thirlwall, A.S.; Upadhyay, S.S.; Webb, J.K.; Wemyss-Holden, S.A.; et al. Pathogenesis of idiopathic scoliosis. The Nottingham concept. *Acta Orthop. Belg.* **1992**, *58* (Suppl. S1), 33–58.
6. Qiu, Y.; Sun, G.Q.; Zhu, F.; Wang, W.J.; Zhu, Z.Z. Rib length discrepancy in patients with adolescent idiopathic scoliosis. *Stud. Health Technol. Inform.* **2010**, *158*, 63–66. [PubMed]
7. Schlager, B.; Krump, F.; Boettinger, J.; Jonas, R.; Liebsch, C.; Ruf, M.; Beer, M.; Wilke, H.J. Morphological patterns of the rib cage and lung in the healthy and adolescent idiopathic scoliosis. *J. Anat.* **2021**, *240*, 120–130. [CrossRef] [PubMed]
8. Sevastik, J.A. Dysfunction of the autonomic nerve system (ANS) in the aetiopathogenesis of adolescent idiopathic scoliosis. *Stud. Health Technol. Inform.* **2002**, *88*, 20–23. [PubMed]
9. Sevastik, J.; Burwell, R.G.; Dangerfield, P.H. A new concept for the etiopathogenesis of the thoracospinal deformity of idiopathic scoliosis: Summary of an electronic focus group debate of the IBSE. *Eur. Spine J.* **2003**, *12*, 440–450. [CrossRef] [PubMed]
10. Mehta, M. The rib-vertebra angle in the early diagnosis between resolving and progressive scoliosis. *J. Bone Jt. Surg.* **1972**, *54*, 230. [CrossRef]
11. Ballhause, T.M.; Moritz, M.; Hättich, A.; Stücker, R.; Mladenov, K. Serial casting in early onset scoliosis: Syndromic scoliosis is no contraindication. *BMC Musculoskelet. Disord.* **2019**, *20*, 554. [CrossRef]

12. Grivas, T.B.; Vasiliadis, E.; Malakasis, M.; Mouzakis, V.; Segos, D. Intervertebral disc biomechanics in the pathogenesis of idiopathic scoliosis. *Stud. Health Technol. Inform.* **2006**, *123*, 80–83.
13. Will, R.E.; Stokes, I.A.; Qiu, X. Cobb angle progression in adolescent scoliosis begins at the intervertebral disc. *Spine* **2009**, *34*, 2782–2786. [CrossRef]
14. Roberts, S.; Menage, J.; Eisenstein, S.M. The cartilage end-plate and intervertebral disc in scoliosis: Calcification and other sequelae. *J. Orthop. Res.* **1993**, *11*, 747–757. [CrossRef] [PubMed]
15. Antoniou, J.; Arlet, V.; Goswami, T.; Aebi, M.; Alini, M. Elevated synthetic activity in the convex side of scoliotic intervertebral discs and endplates compared with normal tissues. *Spine* **2001**, *26*, E198–E206. [CrossRef] [PubMed]
16. Burger, E.L.; Noshchenko, A.; Patel, V.V.; Lindley, E.M.; Bradford, A.P. Ultrastructure of Intervertebral Disc and Vertebra-Disc Junctions Zones as a Link in Etiopathogenesis of Idiopathic Scoliosis. *Adv. Orthop. Surg.* **2014**, *2014*, 23. [CrossRef]
17. Shu, C.C.; Melrose, J. The adolescent idiopathic scoliotic IVD displays advanced aggrecanolysis and a glycosaminoglycan composition similar to that of aged human and ovine (sheep) IVDs. *Eur. Spine J.* **2018**, *27*, 2102–2113. [CrossRef] [PubMed]
18. Brink, R.C.; Schlosser, T.P.C.; Colo, D. Anterior Spinal Overgrowth is the Result of the Scoliotic Mechanism and is Located in the Disc. *Spine* **2017**, *42*, 818–822. [CrossRef] [PubMed]
19. Adams, W. *Lectures on the Pathology and Treatment of Lateral and Other Forms of Curvature of the Spine*; Churchill: London, UK, 1865.
20. Meyer, H. Die Mechanik der Skoliose. *Virchows Arch. Pathol. Anat.* **1866**, *35*, 125.
21. Staffel, F. *Die Menschlichen Haltungstypen und Ihre Beziehungen zn den Ruckgrats Verkrummungen*; Inktank Publishing: Wiesbaden, Germany, 1889.
22. Albert, E. Zur Anatomie der scoliose. *Wien. Klin. Wochenschr.* **1889**, *9*, 159.
23. Nicoladoni, C. *Anatomie und Mechanismns der Skoliose*; Erwin Nagele, Stuttgart: Leipzig, Germany, 1904.
24. Roaf, R. The basic anatomy of scoliosis. *J. Bone Jt. Surg.* **1966**, *48*, 786–792. [CrossRef]
25. Sommerville, E.W. Rotational lordosis: The development of the single curve. *J. Bone Jt. Surg.* **1952**, *34*, 421–427. [CrossRef]
26. Mehta, M.H. Growth as a corrective force in the early treatment of progressive infantile scoliosis. *J. Bone Jt. Surg. Br.* **2005**, *87*, 1237–1247. [CrossRef] [PubMed]
27. Deane, G.; Duthie, R.B. A new projectional look at articulated scoliotic spine. *Acta Orthop. Scand.* **1973**, *44*, 351–356. [CrossRef]
28. Perdriolle, R. *La Scoliose Son Etude Tridimensionelle*; Maloine: Paris, France, 1979.
29. Dickson, R.A.; Lawton, J.O.; Archer, I.A.; Butt, W.P. The pathogenesis of idiopathic scoliosis; biplanar spinal asymmetry. *J. Bone Jt. Surg.* **1984**, *66*, 8–15. [CrossRef] [PubMed]
30. Propst-Proctor, S.L.; Bleck, E.E. Radiographic determination of lordosis and kyphosis in normal and scoliotic children. *J. Pediatr. Orthop.* **1983**, *3*, 344–346. [CrossRef]
31. Lonstein, J.E.; Carlson, J.M. The prediction of curve progression in untreated idiopathic scoliosis during growth. *J. Bone Jt. Surg.* **1984**, *66*, 1061–1071. [CrossRef]
32. Bnnnell, W.P. The natural history of idiopathic scoliosis before skeletal maturity. *Spine* **1986**, *11*, 773–776. [CrossRef]
33. Dickson, R.A.; Stirling, A.J.; Whitaker, I.A.; Howell, F.R.; Mahood, J. Prognosis of early idiopathic scoliosis. In *Prognostic Factors Derived from Screening Studies*; Siegler, D., Harrison, D., Edgar, M., Eds.; Prognosis in Scoliosis: London, UK, 1988.
34. Vercauteren, M. Dorso-Lumbale Curvendistributie en Etiopathogene van de Scoliois Adolecentium. Ph.D. Thesis, Ghent University, Gent, Belgium, 1980.
35. Grivas, T.B.; Vasiliadis, E.S.; Mihas, C.; Savvidou, O. The effect of growth on the correlation between the spinal and rib cage deformity: Implications on idiopathic scoliosis pathogenesis. *Scoliosis* **2007**, *2*, 11. [CrossRef]
36. Grivas, T.B.; Dangas, S.; Samelis, P.; Maziotou, C.; Kandris, K. Lateral spinal profile in school-screening referrals with and without late onset idiopathic scoliosis 10 degrees-20 degrees. *Stud. Health Technol. Inform.* **2002**, *91*, 25–31. [PubMed]
37. Bayerl, S.H.; Pöhlmann, F.; Finger, T.; Franke, J.; Woitzik, J.; Vajkoczy, P. The sagittal spinal profile type: A principal precondition for surgical decision making in patients with lumbar spinal stenosis. *J. Neurosurg. Spine* **2017**, *27*, 552–559. [CrossRef]
38. Pasha, S.; Baldwin, K. Preoperative Sagittal Spinal Profile of Adolescent Idiopathic Scoliosis Lenke Types and Non-Scoliotic Adolescents: A Systematic Review and Meta-Analysis. *Spine* **2019**, *44*, 134–142. [CrossRef] [PubMed]
39. Homans, J.F.; Schlösser, T.P.C.; Pasha, S.; Kruyt, M.C.; Castelein, R.M.; Spine, J. Variations in the sagittal spinal profile precede the development of scoliosis: A pilot study of a new approach. *Spine J.* **2021**, *21*, 638–641. [CrossRef] [PubMed]

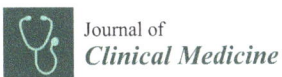

Comment

Comment on Grivas et al. Morphology, Development and Deformation of the Spine in Mild and Moderate Scoliosis: Are Changes in the Spine Primary or Secondary? *J. Clin. Med.* 2021, *10*, 5901

Steven de Reuver [1], Tom P. C. Schlösser [1], Moyo C. Kruyt [1], Keita Ito [1,2] and René M. Castelein [1,*]

[1] Department of Orthopaedic Surgery, University Medical Center Utrecht, 3584 CX Utrecht, The Netherlands; s.dereuver-4@umcutrecht.nl (S.d.R.); t.p.c.schlosser@umcutrecht.nl (T.P.C.S.); m.c.kruyt@umcutrecht.nl (M.C.K.); k.ito@tue.nl (K.I.)

[2] Department of Biomedical Engineering, Eindhoven University of Technology, 5600 MB Eindhoven, The Netherlands

* Correspondence: r.m.castelein-3@umcutrecht.nl; Tel.: +31-88-75-5555

With great interest, we have read the article entitled "Morphology, Development and Deformation of the Spine in Mild and Moderate Scoliosis: Are Changes in the Spine Pri-mary or Secondary?" by Grivas et al., an incredibly interesting read [1]. This study covers the important but divided topic of sagittal spinal alignment as a causal factor in the etiology of idiopathic scoliosis, and we would like to compliment the authors on their work. The purpose was to study *"the sagittal profile of the onset and mild idiopathic scoliosis, using the radiography, the surface topography and the scoliometer readings of children with idiopathic scoliosis"*. The data presented in this study contribute to the discussion; however, we believe it should be interpreted with caution since there are substantial methodological limitations, and these results should not seek to provide a definitive answer.

1. The authors try to translate their data towards a definitive answer on whether sagittal spinal alignment is a primary etiological factor of idiopathic scoliosis. In contrast to the defined aim, they studied the sagittal profile of patients with already established idiopathic scoliosis (mean Cobb angle of 28 and 30 degrees) cross-sectionally and without radiographic sagittal measurements. It has been widely described that the apical deformation in idiopathic scoliosis is characterized by apical lordosis and alters the regional and global sagittal profile [2]. Additionally, the cross-sectional nature of these data can only suggest a relationship; the only way to discriminate between cause and effect would be a prospective longitudinal study.

2. The authors summarize the theoretical background and state that the *"lateral spinal profile"* was commonly considered to be a primary etiological factor of idiopathic scoliosis, because the thoracic kyphosis apex is located in a higher thoracic vertebra (therefore, more vertebrae are posteriorly inclined), which creates conditions of greater rotational instability and, therefore, increases vulnerability for idiopathic scoliosis development. We appreciate this simplification; however, it misses an important nuance: A longer posteriorly inclined segment was previously shown to be associated with thoracic scoliosis, but not necessarily with (thoraco) lumbar scoliosis. For the latter, in fact, a shorter but more steep posteriorly inclined segment with a more distal kyphotic apex may be much more relevant [3,4]. From the scoliosis patients included in the study, 9 out of 17 had a primary (thoraco) lumbar curve, and the primary thoracic curves were not analyzed separately. This actually counterbalances the outcome parameter of this study, since only for thoracic scoliosis, this apex is expected to be higher.

Citation: de Reuver, S.; Schlösser, T.P.C.; Kruyt, M.C.; Ito, K.; Castelein, R.M. Comment on Grivas et al. Morphology, Development and Deformation of the Spine in Mild and Moderate Scoliosis: Are Changes in the Spine Primary or Secondary? *J. Clin. Med.* 2021, *10*, 5901. *J. Clin. Med.* 2022, *11*, 1160. https://doi.org/10.3390/jcm11051160

Academic Editor: Hiroyuki Katoh

Received: 22 December 2021
Accepted: 17 February 2022
Published: 22 February 2022

Publisher's Note: MDPI stays neutral with regard to jurisdictional claims in published maps and institutional affiliations.

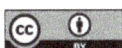

Copyright: © 2022 by the authors. Licensee MDPI, Basel, Switzerland. This article is an open access article distributed under the terms and conditions of the Creative Commons Attribution (CC BY) license (https:// creativecommons.org/licenses/by/ 4.0/).

3. The efforts of the authors to provide a sample-size calculation is appreciated, and since the calculated $n = 17$ for the cases (total of thoracic and (thoraco) lumbar curves) are precisely met, they are confident that the non-significant difference of 0.39 ± 0.11 in scoliosis vs. 0.44 ± 0.08 in controls ($p = 0.134$) is not a type II error. The type of power analysis and whether the test was one or two sided is not mentioned. The 0.1 standard deviation seems to have been well chosen looking at the results; however, the rationale for a 0.1 margin was not given. A 0.1 margin for equivalence seems rather broad, since in the controls, the mean difference between boys and girls is only 0.02, and it is likely that slight, not drastic, inter-individual sagittal spinal alignment variability predisposes for scoliosis development. If this study used a smaller margin, this would sharply increase the required sample size [5].

4. There is a fair chance of selection bias as only two of the 17 scoliosis patients were boys (which is expected given the epidemiology of idiopathic scoliosis), while the sex distribution of the controls was more even with 15 girls and 11 boys. Moreover, the age distribution of the controls and scoliosis series does not match, and they include juveniles as well as adolescents. The mean VP-KA/VP-LA ratio in the controls was higher in girls, representing a relatively lower kyphotic apex than boys, which indicates a sex difference. Therefore, the scoliosis group, which mostly consisted of girls, is biased to have a higher ratio. Interestingly, the ratio was still lower in the scoliosis group compared to controls, although not significant. This is important, since a trend towards a smaller VP-KA/VP-LA ratio (i.e., higher kyphotic apex) in idiopathic scoliosis, probably corresponds to a relatively longer posteriorly inclined segment, which is opposite to the authors' conclusion but in line with other hypotheses in the literature [3].

5. In addition to comparing the two groups, the authors demonstrate that the VP-KA/VP-LA ratio did not significantly correlate with the scoliometer trunk asymmetry measurements ($r = 0.211$, $p = 0.416$). Therefore, the authors conclude that the hypothesis of a larger posteriorly inclined spinal segment being a primary etiological factor for idiopathic scoliosis is not confirmed. This study did not include a power analysis for this specific test, possibly introducing a type II error. However, most importantly, the correlation with curve severity is not relevant for the sagittal spinal alignment, since it has been hypothesized to influence scoliosis risk, not severity. Scoliosis severity is probably mostly correlated with time from onset, not the sagittal profile.

6. Throughout the manuscript, the authors interchange the terms 'posteriorly inclined segment' and 'hypokyphosis'; however, we would like to emphasize that these are distinct. Based on previous findings and the results presented, we agree that hypokyphosis is not likely the primary causal factor in idiopathic scoliosis, rather a passive result of the combined effect of the rotation and anterior opening of the apical intervertebral disc spaces [6]. However, the individual posteriorly inclined spine, specifically the relative length and inclination of that segment, is hypothesized to be a risk factor for scoliosis development, which is supported by recently published prospective data [4].

In conclusion, the statistical limitations, interchange of distinct terminology and the cross-sectional nature of this study, in our mind, may lead to a less conclusive statement that sagittal alignment has no place in idiopathic scoliosis etiology. If anything, we feel that the hypothesis rejected by the authors, that the posteriorly inclined segment is larger in scoliosis patients, is actually suggested in their data but masked by poor group selection of both the scoliosis and the control group. Regardless of the shortcomings related to these types of studies, we commend the authors for their efforts in exploring the sagittal spinal alignment in relation to idiopathic scoliosis etiology, and we look forward to their future contributions.

Author Contributions: Conceptualization, S.d.R., T.P.C.S., M.C.K., K.I. and R.M.C.; methodology, S.d.R., T.P.C.S., M.C.K., K.I. and R.M.C.; writing—original draft preparation, S.d.R.; writing—review and editing, T.P.C.S., M.C.K., K.I. and R.M.C.; supervision, K.I. and R.M.C. All authors have read and agreed to the published version of the manuscript.

Funding: This research received no external funding.

Conflicts of Interest: The authors declare no conflict of interest.

References

1. Grivas, T.B.; Vynichakis, G.; Chandrinos, M.; Mazioti, C.; Papagianni, D.; Mamzeri, A.; Mihas, C. Morphology, Development and Deformation of the Spine in Mild and Moderate Scoliosis: Are Changes in the Spine Primary or Secondary? *J. Clin. Med.* **2021**, *10*, 5901. [CrossRef] [PubMed]
2. Deacon, P.; Flood, B.; Dickson, R. Idiopathic scoliosis in three dimensions. A radiographic and morphometric analysis. *J. Bone Jt. Surg. Br.* **1984**, *66*, 509–512. [CrossRef] [PubMed]
3. Schlösser, T.P.C.; Shah, S.A.; Reichard, S.J.; Rogers, K.; Vincken, K.L.; Castelein, R.M. Differences in early sagittal plane alignment between thoracic and lumbar adolescent idiopathic scoliosis. *Spine J.* **2014**, *14*, 282–290. [CrossRef] [PubMed]
4. Homans, J.F.; Schlösser, T.P.C.; Pasha, S.; Kruyt, M.C.; Castelein, R.M. Variations in the sagittal spinal profile precede the development of scoliosis: A pilot study of a new approach. *Spine J.* **2021**, *21*, 638–641. [CrossRef] [PubMed]
5. Chow, S.-C.; Shao, J.; Wang, H. *Sample Size Calculations in Clinical Research*, 2nd ed.; Biostatistics Series; Chapman & Hall/CRC: Boca Raton, FL, USA, 2008.
6. Brink, R.C.; Schlösser, T.P.C.; van Stralen, M.; Vincken, K.L.; Kruyt, M.C.; Hui, S.C.N.; Viergever, M.A.; Chu, W.C.W.; Cheng, J.C.Y.; Castelein, R.M. Anterior-posterior length discrepancy of the spinal column in adolescent idiopathic scoliosis-a 3D CT study. *Spine J.* **2018**, *18*, 2259–2265. [CrossRef] [PubMed]

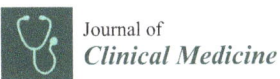

Journal of
Clinical Medicine

Reply

Reply to de Reuver et al. Comment on "Grivas et al. Morphology, Development and Deformation of the Spine in Mild and Moderate Scoliosis: Are Changes in the Spine Primary or Secondary? *J. Clin. Med.* 2021, 10, 5901"

Theodoros B. Grivas [1,*], George Vynichakis [1], Michail Chandrinos [1], Christina Mazioti [2], Despina Papagianni [3], Aristea Mamzeri [4] and Constantinos Mihas [5]

1. Department of Orthopedics & Traumatology, "Tzaneio" General Hospital of Piraeus, 185 36 Piraeus, Greece; vini_gio@windowslive.com (G.V.); chandrinosmichail@gmail.com (M.C.)
2. Health Visitor, "Tzaneio" General Hospital of Piraeus, 185 36 Piraeus, Greece; maziotix@gmail.com
3. School Nurse—Health Visitor, Special Primary School of Rafina, 190 09 Rafina, Greece; papdes2009@hotmail.com
4. Health Visitor, TOMY Attica Square, 104 45 Athens, Greece; mamzeri_aristea@hotmail.com
5. Department of Internal Medicine, Kymi General Hospital—Health Centre, 340 03 Kymi, Greece; gas521@yahoo.co.uk
* Correspondence: tgri69@otenet.gr

Citation: Grivas, T.B.; Vynichakis, G.; Chandrinos, M.; Mazioti, C.; Papagianni, D.; Mamzeri, A.; Mihas, C. Reply to de Reuver et al. Comment on "Grivas et al. Morphology, Development and Deformation of the Spine in Mild and Moderate Scoliosis: Are Changes in the Spine Primary or Secondary? *J. Clin. Med.* 2021, 10, 5901". *J. Clin. Med.* **2022**, *11*, 2049. https://doi.org/10.3390/jcm11072049

Academic Editor: Hiroyuki Katoh

Received: 1 February 2022
Accepted: 31 March 2022
Published: 6 April 2022

Publisher's Note: MDPI stays neutral with regard to jurisdictional claims in published maps and institutional affiliations.

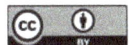

Copyright: © 2022 by the authors. Licensee MDPI, Basel, Switzerland. This article is an open access article distributed under the terms and conditions of the Creative Commons Attribution (CC BY) license (https://creativecommons.org/licenses/by/4.0/).

With great interest we have read the "Letter to the editor by de Reuve et al. concerning "Morphology, Development and Deformation of the Spine in Mild and Moderate Scoliosis: Are Changes in the Spine Primary or Secondary?" by Grivas et al. [1]".

We appreciate their compliments on our work and we would like to thank them for their kind words [2]. Moreover, we should thank the authors who have studied the publication so thoroughly, providing us with a great opportunity to controvert the arguments put forward by a group of colleagues world-renowned for their studies on the aetiology of idiopathic scoliosis. The authors of the letter state that "The data presented in this study contribute to the discussion", and they claim, "however, we believe it should be interpreted with caution since there are substantial methodological limitations, and these results should not seek to provide a definitive answer". However, the comments by de Reuve, et al. generally apply to scoliosis cases that are more severe than the subjects examined in our series.

Furthermore, it would be useful to have a look at the definitions of the severity of scoliosis. There is not full agreement on what is mild and moderate idiopathic scoliosis. Mild idiopathic scoliosis is characterized by a Cobb angle of more than 10 and less than 30 degrees [3], of more than 10 but less than 25 degrees [4], and of more than 10 but less than 20 degrees [5]. Moderate IS is characterized by a Cobb angle of 25–40 degrees, which is indicated for non-operative treatment [6,7], and a Cobb angle greater than 21 to 35 degrees [5]. We consider as mild curves those with a Cobb angle of greater than 10 but less than 20 degrees and as moderate those with a Cobb angle of greater than 21 to 35–40 degrees. In our material, only one patient had a Cobble angle greater than 40 degrees, which is practically not affecting the mean Cobb angle.

In these curves, especially in the mild ones, the rotation of the apical vertebrae is not large [8,9]; this morphology is very important for the measurements of a true sagittal profile, which is minimally affected. This fact results in more reliable contacted measurements, and it is very important for our study.

Our response point by point to authors' comments is presented below.

In comment number 1, the authors of the letter notice that "the study is cross-sectional and without radiographic sagittal measurements". This research is indeed a cross-sectional one and not a longitudinal study. It could not have been a longitudinal design because we studied mild and moderate scoliosis, and it is not an attempt to establish the definite causality of IS. All these children were presented in the scoliosis clinic and diagnosed with IS for the first time; as a result, they had not had any previous imaging examination for IS. Moreover, we only used the data of diagnosis at presentation, as this was the aim of the study. Therefore, we did not aim to conduct a longitudinal study.

The letter's authors state that "the study was done without radiographic sagittal measurements". We do have lateral radiographs for all the IS children included in the study because this imaging is asked for, based on our protocol, during the first examination and assessment. However, the sagittal profile using surface topography (ST) is correlated to the sagittal profile to radiographic imaging with a strong correlation coefficient, not only for the surface apparatus we utilized but also for other systems of ST as well [10–15]. Therefore, for this reason, it was not deemed necessary to study the lateral radiographs of IS children. Consequently, the results of the study were not affected.

Moreover, the reference of Deacon et al. 1984 stating "that the apical deformation in IS is characterized by apical lordosis and alters the regional and global sagittal profile", which is quite true, cannot be used for mild or moderate IS. All of Deacon's scoliotic spines are severely deformed up to 184 Cobb degrees, except for one of 18 degrees, with a significant/severe rotation, which is not the case, as mentioned above, for mild or moderate IS. Mild IS children were analyzed in the study by Grivas et al. [16,17]; thus, a comparison to severe scoliosis is not advisable.

At this point, we are given the opportunity to reiterate and emphasize our view, which is also expressed in our publication, that is "at initiating and mild scoliosis, the patho-biomechanics are probably dissimilar from the biomechanics when the curve is severe". Furthermore, we consider that at initiating and mild IS cases, genetics, epigenetics, and biology have the dominant/protagonistic aetiological role; however, we should not overlook the non-protagonistic role of patho-biomechanics, which later become dominant for progressive IS.

In comment number 2 in the letter, the authors claim: "A longer posteriorly inclined segment was previously shown to be associated with thoracic scoliosis, but not necessarily with (thoraco)lumbar scoliosis. For the latter in fact, a shorter but more steep posteriorly inclined segment with a more distal kyphotic apex may be much more relevant. [5,6]" We would like to note that in the study, we included no children with lumbar IS curve, as was the case in Schlösser et al. 2014 [16]; this publication did not include any thoracolumbar curve, either. Therefore, the comment on the morphology of lumbar curves is not applicable to our study.

In comment number 3 in the letter, the authors claim: "The type of power analysis and whether the test was one or two-sided is not mentioned".

It should be stated that it was an a priori, one-sided power analysis. The types of power analyses and the selection of the margins were both based on our previously unpublished data, due to lack of sufficient published results for this specific marker (ratio of distances). Although we acknowledge the fact that, in controls, the mean difference proved lower than the expected one, it should be noticed that the main comparison of interest was between scoliosis patients and controls, rather than a gender-based comparison. However, a larger sample size would make the margin lower and thus make the whole study more robust to gender and other potentially confounding effects.

In comment number 4 in the letter, the authors claim: "the age distribution of the controls and scoliosis series do not match and they include juveniles as well as adolescents".

In Group A (IS), the mean age of the girls was 12.4 (range: 8.4–14.3 years). The mean age of the boys was 15.3 (range:14.1–16.4 years). In Group B (Controls), the mean age of the girls was 12.2 (range: 9.3–15.2 years). The mean age of the boys was 13 (range: 9.9–15.6 years).

It is stated by the authors of the letter that "The mean VP-KA/VP-LA ratio in the controls was higher in girls, representing a relatively lower kyphotic apex than boys, which indicates a sex difference. Therefore, the scoliosis group which mostly consisted of girls, is biased to have a higher ratio. Interestingly, the ratio was still lower in the scoliosis group compared to controls, although not significant. This is important, since a trend towards a smaller VP-KA/VP-LA ratio (i.e., higher kyphotic apex) in idiopathic scoliosis, probably corresponds to a relatively longer posteriorly inclined segment, which is opposite to the authors conclusion but in line with other hypotheses in the literature [5]". This argument is rather weak and of no use because no matter the non-statistical variations of VP-KA/VP-LA ratio among the groups, the main finding—which was not emphasized and taken into consideration by the authors of the letter—is that all of these ratios were not correlated to Cobb angle and the truncal asymmetry measured using the scoliometer. In other words, in the studied group suffering mild and moderate IS, the sagittal profile is not associated with coronal and transverse plane deformity.

In comment number 5, the authors claim, "Besides comparing the two groups, the authors demonstrate that the VP-KA/VP-LA ratio did not significantly correlate to the scoliometer trunk asymmetry measurements ($r = 0.211$, $p = 0.416$). Therefore, the authors conclude that the hypothesis of a larger posteriorly inclined spinal segment being a primary etiological factor for idiopathic scoliosis is not confirmed. This study was not powered for this analysis, possibly introducing a type II error".

As far as the power analysis concerns the introduction of a type II error, it is plausible given the fact that the power analysis in our study was—as usual—performed for the purposes of the main comparison. However, the large deviation from a significance level close to 0.05 increases the probability of a real correlation.

Additionally, the authors of the letter mention the following: "But most importantly, the correlation with curve severity is not relevant for the sagittal spinal alignment, since it has been hypothesized to influence scoliosis risk, not severity. Scoliosis severity is probably mostly correlated to time from onset, not the sagittal profile".

We did not aim to study severe curves or the prediction of which curve will become severe.

In comment number 6, the authors write: "Throughout the manuscript, the authors interchange the terms 'posteriorly inclined segment' and 'hypokyphosis', however, we would like to emphasize that these are distinct".

The terms 'posteriorly inclined segment' and 'hypokyphosis' in a linguistic sense are completely distinct, but in IS, they are anatomically considered strictly interconnected and justifiably may be used both describing the same entity. The reason for this consideration may be described below.

When the decrease in the normal spinal thoracic kyphosis angle (T4–T12 or T1–T12) changes below a cutoff point, then this kyphosis is termed hypokyphosis. The normal kyphotic angle can only be decreased if the kyphotic apex is placed more cephalad, and then the posteriorly inclined segment of the kyphosis is increased. This can only occur if the number of the so-called "declived vertebrae", in other words, the number of the posterior inclined vertebrae—comprising the posteriorly inclined segment—are increased, and consequently, the "proclive" segment (the segment with the number of vertebrae inclined anteriorly) is decreased, so the total thoracic vertebrae number will always be 12.

The terms "declive" and "proclive" vertebra in kyphosis were introduced by Prof. RG Burwell 31 years ago [18–20].

The authors also write: "Based on previous findings and the results presented, we agree that hypokyphosis is not likely the primary causal factor in idiopathic scoliosis, rather a passive result of the combined effect of rotation and anterior opening of the apical intervertebral disc spaces [21]". We agree with this fact—that hypokyphosis is not likely the primary causal factor—and we mention the following in the publication: "Regarding the role of hypokyphosis and its importance in IS aetiology, we stated earlier that the minor hypokyphosis of the thoracic spine and its minimal differences observed in the small curves studied compared with that of non-scoliotics, this adds to the view that the reduced kyphosis, by facilitating axial rotation, could be viewed as being permissive, rather than as aetiological, in the pathogenesis of IS [17]". In other words, a straight (not bended) beam is more easily rotated than a curved one.

The authors next write: "However, the individual posteriorly inclined spine, specifically the relative length and inclination of that segment, is hypothesized to be a risk factor for scoliosis development and supported by recently published prospective data [22]".

For our response, see our statement above.

In contrast to the proposition that sagittal alignment has no place in the aetiology of IS, we mention in our article that the minor hypokyphosis of the thoracic spine and its minimal differences observed in the small curves studied compared with that of non-scoliotics adds to the view that the reduced kyphosis, by facilitating axial rotation, could be viewed as being permissive, rather than as aetiological, in the pathogenesis of idiopathic scoliosis [17].

In conclusion, we would honestly like to thank the authors for their kindness in dealing with our article. With their comments, we were given the great opportunity to productively and positively expand and augment our arguments and discussion on such an interesting topic as that of the sagittal profile in relation to the aetiology of IS.

We are looking forward to future research contributions from other groups studying the aetiology of IS and further insights about the effect of the sagittal profile. Since the topic is very much under discussion, we might think about proceeding with the study and including more patients to increase its power. If contact to the patients is feasible, a follow-up might be possible, e.g., after growth completion.

Funding: This research received no external funding.

Conflicts of Interest: The authors declare no conflict of interest.

References

1. Grivas, T.B.; Vynichakis, G.; Chandrinos, M.; Mazioti, C.; Papagianni, D.; Mamzeri, A.; Mihas, C. Morphology, Development and Deformation of the Spine in Mild and Moderate Scoliosis: Are Changes in the Spine Primary or Secondary? *J. Clin. Med.* **2021**, *10*, 5901. [CrossRef]
2. de Reuver, S.; Schlösser, T.P.C.; Kruyt, M.C.; Ito, K.; Castelein, R.M. Comment on Grivas et al. Morphology, Development and Deformation of the Spine in Mild and Moderate Scoliosis: Are Changes in the Spine Primary or Secondary? *J. Clin. Med.* 2021, 10, 5901. *J. Clin. Med.* **2022**, *11*, 1160. [CrossRef]
3. Cheung, M.-C.; Yip, J.; Lai, J.S.K. Biofeedback Posture Training for Adolescents with Mild Scoliosis. *BioMed Res. Int.* **2022**, *2022*, 1–8. [CrossRef] [PubMed]
4. Monticone, M.; Ambrosini, E.; Cazzaniga, D.; Rocca, B.; Ferrante, S. Active self-correction and task-oriented exercises reduce spinal deformity and improve quality of life in subjects with mild adolescent idiopathic scoliosis. Results of a randomised controlled trial. *Eur. Spine J.* **2014**, *23*, 1204–1214. [CrossRef] [PubMed]
5. Negrini, S.; Donzelli, S.; Aulisa, A.G.; Czaprowski, D.; Schreiber, S.; De Mauroy, J.C.; Diers, H.; Grivas, T.B.; Knott, P.; Kotwicki, T.; et al. 2016 SOSORT guidelines: Orthopaedic and rehabilitation treatment of idiopathic scoliosis during growth. *Scoliosis Spinal Disord.* **2018**, *13*, 3. [CrossRef] [PubMed]
6. Weinstein, S.L.; Dolan, L.A.; Wright, J.G.; Dobbs, M.B. Effects of bracing in adolescents with idiopathic. *N. Engl. J. Med.* **2013**, *369*, 1512–1521. [CrossRef] [PubMed]
7. Kuznia, A.L.; Hernandez, A.K.; Lee, L.U. Adolescent Idiopathic Scoliosis: Common Questions and Answers. *Am. Fam. Physician* **2020**, *101*, 19–23. [PubMed]
8. Courvoisier, A.; Drevelle, X.; Dubousset, J.; Skalli, W. Transverse plane 3D analysis of mild scoliosis. *Eur. Spine J.* **2013**, *22*, 2427–2432. [CrossRef] [PubMed]
9. Grivas, T.B.; Vasiliadis, E.; Malakasis, M.; Mouzakis, V.; Segos, D. Intervertebral disc biomechanics in the pathogenesis of idiopathic scoliosis. *Stud. Health Technol. Inform.* **2006**, *123*, 17108407.
10. Frerich, J.M.; Hertzler, K.; Knott, P.; Mardjetko, S. Comparison of Radiographic and Surface Topography Measurements in Adolescents with Idiopathic Scoliosis. *Open Orthop. J.* **2012**, *6*, 261–265. [CrossRef] [PubMed]
11. Knott, P.; Sturm, P.; Lonner, B.; Cahill, P.; Betsch, M.; McCarthy, R.; Kelly, M.; Lenke, L.; Betz, R. Multicenter Comparison of 3D Spinal Measurements Using Surface Topography with Those from Conventional Radiography. *Spine Deform.* **2016**, *4*, 98–103. [CrossRef] [PubMed]
12. Pino-Almero, L.; Mínguez-Rey, M.F.; De Anda, R.M.C.-O.; Salvador-Palmer, M.R.; Sentamans-Segarra, S. Correlation between Topographic Parameters Obtained by Back Surface Topography Based on Structured Light and Radiographic Variables in the Assessment of Back Morphology in Young Patients with Idiopathic Scoliosis. *Asian Spine J.* **2017**, *11*, 219–229. [CrossRef] [PubMed]

13. Pino-Almero, L.; Mínguez-Rey, M.F.; Sentamans-Segarra, S.; Salvador-Palmer, M.R.; De Anda, R.M.C.-O. Quantification of topographic changes in the surface of back of young patients monitored for idiopathic scoliosis: Correlation with radiographic variables. *J. Biomed. Opt.* **2016**, *21*, 116001. [CrossRef] [PubMed]
14. Pino-Almero, L.; Mínguez-Rey, M.F.; Rodríguez-Martínez, D.; de Anda, R.M.C.-O.; Salvador-Palmer, M.R.; Sentamans-Segarra, S. Clinical application of back surface topography by means of structured light in the screening of idiopathic scoliosis. *J. Pediatr. Orthop. B* **2017**, *26*, 64–72. [CrossRef] [PubMed]
15. Applebaum, A.; Cho, W.; Nessim, A.; Kim, K.; Tarpada, S.P.; Yoon, S.H.; Pujar, B.; Kim, D.; Kim, S.Y. Establishing the validity of surface topography for assessment of scoliosis: A prospective study. *Spine Deform.* **2021**, *9*, 685–689. [CrossRef] [PubMed]
16. Schlösser, T.P.C.; Shah, S.A.; Reichard, S.J.; Rogers, K.; Vincken, K.L.; Castelein, R.M. Differences in early sagittal plane alignment between thoracic and lumbar adolescent idiopathic scoliosis. *Spine J.* **2014**, *14*, 282–290. [CrossRef] [PubMed]
17. Grivas, T.; Dangas, S.; Samelis, P.; Maziotou, C.; Kandris, K. Lateral spinal profile in school-screening referrals with and without late onset idiopathic scoliosis 10 degrees-20 degrees. *Stud. Health Technol. Inform.* **2002**, *91*, 25–31. [PubMed]
18. Kiel, A.W.; Bunvell, R.G.; Jacobs, K.J.; Moulton, A.; Purdue, M.; Webb, J.K.; Wojcik, A.S. Sagittal spinal curvatures in idiopathic thoracic scoliosis: A kyphotic angulation in the thoracolumbar region suggesting a relation to the mortice joint of Davis. *Clin. Anat.* **1990**, *3*, 67.
19. Kiel, A.W.; Bunvell, R.G.; Cattle, J.; Jacobs, K.J.; Moulton, A.; Webb, J.K.; Wojcik, A.S. A segmental analysis of the lateral profile of the spine revealing changes in the thoracolumbar region of thoracic curves. *J. Bone Joint. Surg.* **1990**, *72*, 333.
20. Kiel, A.W.; Burwell, R.G.; Moulton, A.; Purdue, M.; Webb, J.K.; Wojcik, A.S. Segmental patterns of sagittal spinal curvatures in children screened for scoliosis: Kyphotic angulation at the thoracolumbar region and the mortice joint. *Clin. Anat.* **1992**, *5*, 353–371. [CrossRef]
21. Brink, R.C.; Schlösser, T.P.; van Stralen, M.; Vincken, K.L.; Kruyt, M.C.; Hui, S.C.; Viergever, M.A.; Chu, W.C.; Cheng, J.C.; Castelein, R.M. Anterior-posterior length discrepancy of the spinal column in adolescent idiopathic scoliosis—A 3D CT study. *Spine J.* **2018**, *18*, 2259–2265. [CrossRef] [PubMed]
22. Homans, J.F.; Schlösser, T.P.C.; Pasha, S.; Kruyt, M.C.; Castelein, R.M. Variations in the sagittal spinal profile precede the development of scoliosis: A pilot study of a new approach. *Spine J.* **2021**, *21*, 638–641. [CrossRef] [PubMed]

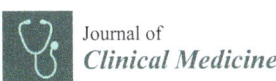

Article

Evaluation of Brace Treatment Using the Soft Brace Spinaposture: A Four-Years Follow-Up

Christian Wong [1,*] and Thomas B. Andersen [2]

[1] Department of Orthopedics, Hvidovre Hospital, Kettegaards Alle 30, 2650 Hvidovre, Denmark
[2] Department of Orthopedics, National University Hospital, Blegdamsvej 9, 2100 Copenhagen, Denmark; thomas.borbjerg.andersen@regionh.dk
* Correspondence: cwong0002@regionh.dk; Tel.: +45-38-62-66-69

Abstract: The braces of today are constructed to correct the frontal plane deformity of idiopathic adolescent scoliosis (AIS). The Spinaposture brace© (Spinaposture Aps, Copenhagen, Denmark) is a soft-fabric brace for AIS and is designed to enhance rotational axial stability by inducing a sagittal plane kyphotic correction. This prospective observational study evaluated the brace in fifteen patients with AIS. The initial average CA was 16.8° (SD: 2.8). They were followed prospectively every 3 to 6 months during their brace usage until skeletal maturity of 25 months and at long-term follow-up of 44 months. In- and out-of-brace radiographs were performed in six subjects at inclusion. This resulted in an immediate in-brace correction of 25.3 percent in CA (14.3°→10.8°) and induced a kyphotic effect of 14.9 percent (40.8°→47.9°). The average in-brace improvement at first follow-up was 4.5° in CA, and the CA at skeletal maturity was 11° (SD: 7.4°) and long-term 12.0° (SD: 6.8°). In conclusion, the Spinaposture brace© had an immediate in-brace deformity correction and a thoracic kyphotic effect. At skeletal maturity, the deformities improved more than expected when compared to that of the natural history/observation and similar to that of other soft braces. No long-term deformity progression was seen. To substantiate these findings, stronger designed studies with additional subjects are needed.

Keywords: spinal deformities; idiopathic scoliosis; bracing; pathobiomechanics; follow-up study

1. Introduction

Idiopathic adolescent scoliosis (AIS) is a structural spinal disorder that sometimes requires the intervention of either bracing or surgery due to the magnitude of or progression in the spinal deformity [1,2]. The bracing of today has a governing principle of three points pressure-mediated correction in the frontal plane supplemented by derotation to prevent curve progression using a hard brace of polyethene [1–6]. Such hard braces can have a negative psychological impact, which subsequently leads to decreased compliance and thereby diminished correctional effect [3,7,8]. The efficacy of the current treatment of bracing has been debated [9–11]. It has been claimed that omitting bracing is inconsequential [11]. However, the efficacy of bracing was tested in a rigorous scientifically design, and it minimizes the need for corrective surgery [3]. Doubts still loom concerning the efficacy of bracing despite the meticulous scientific effort [9]. Earlier studies have introduced soft braces, which consist of, for example, correctional elastic ribbons [12]. This seems to have a correctional effect, but it is not as effective as hard bracing (especially not in the period of pubertal growth) [12,13]. An insufficient correction in the sagittal profile in the first soft braces has been considered as a reason for the lack of correction [14]. Bracing concepts have now evolved to include not only restoring the frontal plane deformity but also focusing on correction in the sagittal alignment with seemingly promising results [12,15,16]. The Spinaposture© brace is a soft brace focused on sagittal alignment which consists of two parts. The first part is a soft 'suit' that is custom made to fit the individual anthropometric measures using the measures from a whole trunk optical 3D scan of the individual patient. The brace is sewn using Sensotex, a special elastic fabric of Neopren and Sensotex Lycra, and has a 'memory effect' (with the ability to return to its original shape). The brace is designed to induce a kyphotic effect. This is induced both by the tactile response to the elastic component of the fabric and incorporated into the design of the 'suit'. The brace has a second part, namely a hard shield with 'fingers' to be placed in a 'pocket' of the soft fabric placed posterior at the thoracic level. This induces a further kyphotic effect. The hard shield is introduced secondarily if the frontal plane deformity is progressing (increased CA) or if initial correction is insufficient. Figure 1 displays the 'suit' and the 'hard shield' of the Spinaposture brace©.

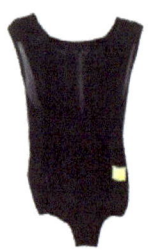 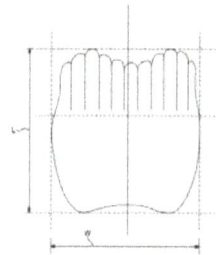 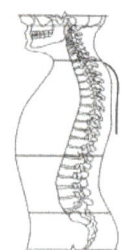 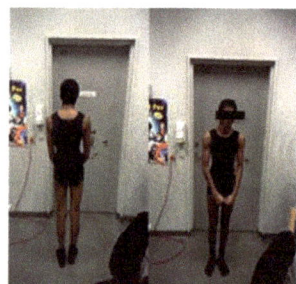

Figure 1. The 'suit' of the Spinaposture brace (**left**), a schematic diagram of the 'shield with fingers' and placement of the shield (**middle**) and the Spinaposture brace© worn by a subject (**right**).

The brace is intended to augment axial stability by inducing a sagittal plane thoracic kyphotic effect and, if needed, a derotation in the spine depending on the individual curve pattern. The brace is intentionally built to induce minor to no direct frontal plane correction, and to realign or restore the thoracic kyphosis by inducing an inherently proprioceptive 'hyper-kyphotic strive'. The strive is induced utilizing the principle of autocorrection derived from physiotherapeutic practice [17]. Specifically, the aim is to realign the temporary, naturally occurring thoracic hyperkyphosis occurring during the normal growth in adolescence [18]. This is considered to have a role in the initial development of thoracic AIS [19]. AIS is typically associated with the adolescent female. AIS has been perceived as developing as a consequence of the spine growing into a mechanically unstable column and might progress in a self-sustaining 'vicious cycle' due to the effect of gravity and asymmetric loads in a growth-modulating buckling-like manner. The spinal growth spurt for both sexes coincides with adolescence, but adolescent females distinguish themselves from males by a significantly increased and earlier thoracic growth. These factors coincide with a temporal sagittal flattening of thoracic vertebrae for adolescent females. This contributes to rotational instability of the spine. The brace is aimed to improve or reestablish axial stability by the sagittal plane correction/realignment. The intended purpose is to prevent curve progression without being as strenuous as the conventional hard braces. The brace is designed as an advanced t-shirt/body stocking, and the discomfort of the brace is closer to regular clothing than a hard brace, which we perceive as beneficial for promoting compliance and subsequent treatment efficacy [8]. Being less strenuous whilst probably having a less frontal plane correctional effect, justified bracing smaller curves, and early intervention also has a better correctional effect [20]. Thus, we braced AIS with Cobb's angle (CA) between 15° and 25° [21]. This study evaluated the correctional effect of the Spinaposture brace© with in- and out-of-brace radiographs for patients with AIS, and in a prospective follow-up study, we evaluated the initial correction when the brace was discontinued at skeletal maturity and long-term at approximately four years.

2. Materials and Methods

2.1. Inclusion, Bracing and Strengthening Exercises

The subjects were patients referred with AIS from our hospital service area and included as a convenience sample. At the first visit, the including doctor diagnosed them with AIS, and if having a thoracic or thoracolumbar AIS with a CA between 15° and 25°, they were included after informed consent. The subjects and caregivers were specifically told that longitudinal radiological follow-up without bracing was the 'gold standard' treatment. Exclusion criteria were subjects with primary lumbar scoliosis, previous brace treatment or inability to cope with bracing in general, or if MRI-verified intraspinal pathology was present. If the subjects had a correction of approximately one-fourth in the frontal plane deformity after three months, when using the brace, this was continued. If the correction was less than one-fourth then the 'hard shield' was introduced. If the subjects had a correction of approximately one-fourth in the frontal plane deformity after another three months, when using the brace, then this was continued. Otherwise, the subjects were excluded. The 'body stocking' part of the brace was worn in the daytime (<16 h and defined as part-time) to counteract the effect of gravity on the spine and was not worn at night [13,22]. We allowed them not to wear the brace when performing sports and when the subjects were too hot in the brace. We considered the brace as a passive correctional measure [19], thus we advised them to perform strengthening exercises either through a home exercise program, formal physiotherapy and/or participate in sports such as crawl swimming [23]. We allowed all forms of physical exercises at the patient's discretion throughout the study.

2.2. Initial in-Brace Radiographs

At study initiation, the subjects were asked to volunteer to have performed initial in-brace radiographs (both anteroposterior and lateral projections).

2.3. Outpatient Follow-Up

The subjects were followed prospectively with anteroposterior out-of-brace radiographs every six months in general. However, the initial radiographs were taken every three months as a precaution since we had no previous experience using the brace [12]. The subjects were instructed not to wear the brace one day before the follow-up. We used a local developed low-dose anteroposterior radiological examination [24]. Figure 2 shows a typical radiographic follow-up using the low dose radiographic technique.

The brace was worn until skeletal maturity. Skeletal maturity was determined by having at least Risser 4, duration of menstruation of 2 years for girls, and a skeletal hand age of 14 years and 16 years for girls and boys (Sanders stage 8), respectively. The follow-up was continued for an additional three to six months with a final radiographical and clinical evaluation. The subjects were recalled for one long-term radiographic follow-up.

2.4. Study Assessments and Statistical Analyses

The primary outcome was Cobb's angle for the primary curves at skeletal maturity. A change of five degrees or more was considered either a progression or regression [13,25]. If the CA remained within five degrees of the initial measurement before the brace treatment was initiated, we considered them as 'stable'. We compared the course of the spinal deformity when using the brace with comparison to the expected outcomes in relation to the Risser classification at brace initiation [13]. At skeletal maturity, 42 percent of AIS is expected to improve or remain stable for Risser 0–1 and 71 percent of AIS is expected to improve or remain stable for Risser 0–2 [13]. In this study, we considered an improvement or remaining stable as a good outcome. For observation only, the expected outcome is 50% (CI: 44–56%) [13].

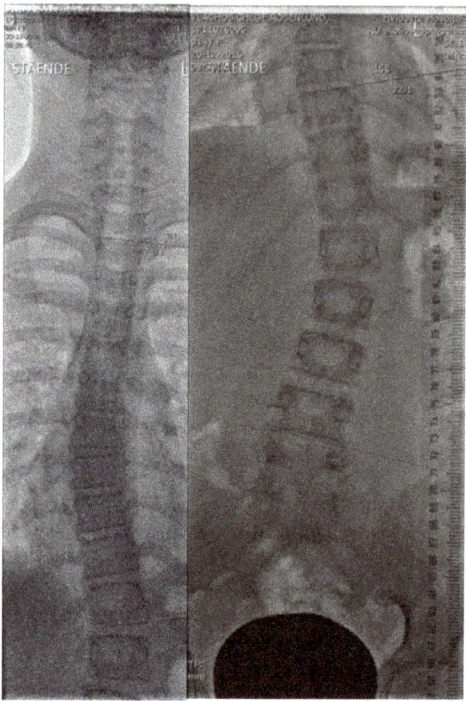

Figure 2. An example of radiographs using the low dose technique.

Secondary parameters were radiographic and evaluated as categorical variables of changed or unchanged. The parameters were the descriptive categorization of scoliosis according to the Moe-Kettleson classification [26], changes in the level of the apex vertebrae (if more than two levels difference), Nash and Moe's classification (if rotation changed more than one segment) at the apex vertebrae, change in rib vertebrae angle differences/Metha angle (if more than 20° difference), and change in CA of the secondary curves if any.

The evaluators were two doctors of pediatric orthopaedic and spinal surgery with 26 and 20 years of experience, respectively. All measurements were performed separately and blinded using the Synedra View Personal 19 (Ver. 19.0.0.2, Innsbruck, Austria) and the PACS system (Impax 6.4.0, Agfa® HealthCare, Mortsel, Belgium) on a three-megapixel viewing station. For statistical analyses, we performed an inter-class correlation for inter-observer variability between the evaluators. The chi-square cross-tabulation test and the Spearman correlation test were performed for differences between subjects and drop-outs. All tests were performed using IBM SPSS Statistics, Version 25 (IBM, Richmond, VA, USA). A post hoc power analysis was performed using GPower (Ver 3.0.10, Aichach, Germany).

The study was conducted according to the guidelines of the Declaration of Helsinki II. The local ethical committee evaluated this study as a clinical observational follow-up series (reference number H-17014162). Informed consent was obtained from all involved subjects. This research received no external funding.

3. Results

3.1. Population

Twenty-two patients were screened. Seven patients were excluded from the study at first evaluation. Two subjects had CA larger than 25° and previous brace treatment, three subjects were not included due to syrinx or anisomelia, and two subjects received the brace but never used it. Fifteen subjects were included with no prior treatment, except for observation. Five subjects dropped out. Two subjects, after joining a formal Schroth therapy, acquired the Chêneau Gensigen brace by their own accord. This was encouraged by their private physiotherapists. One subject had back pain without improvement by bracing, one changed to Rolfing structural integration therapy, and one did not attend the follow-ups. All three subjects discontinued bracing. Two subjects did not attend the long-term follow-up. One subject was too busy with school work and we were unable to recall one. We considered them as drop-outs. Otherwise, there were no subjects lost in follow-up or withdrawals. Figure 3 shows a flow chart of the history of the subject's participation, exclusion, and drop-out.

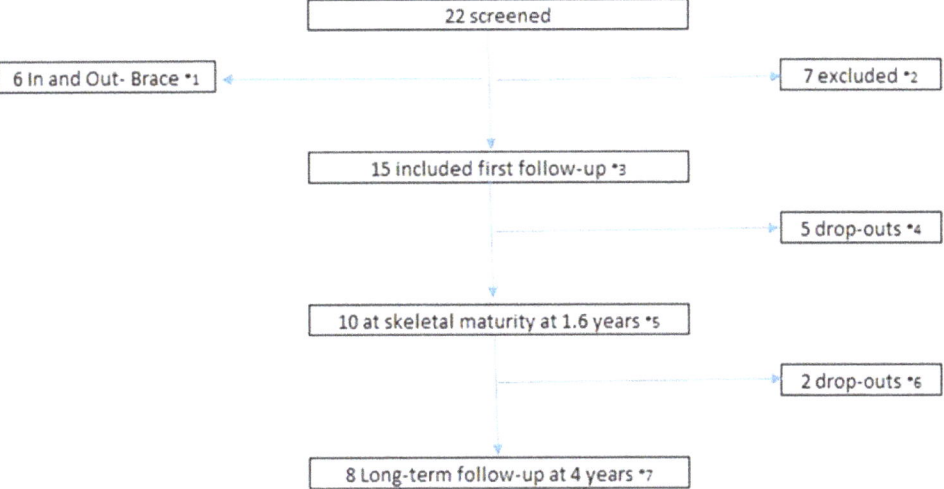

Figure 3. Timeline of the subject's participation. *[1] Six patients had initial in and out-of-brace radiographs as part of the inclusion process. *[2] Seven patients did not fulfil the inclusion and exclusion criteria, thus were excluded. *[3] Fifteen subjects were included with an improvement of one-fourth in Cobb's angle. *[4] Five subjects dropped out due to change to other brace strategies by their own accord. *[5] Evaluation at skeletal maturity and when the soft brace was discontinued. *[6] Two subjects did not participate in the follow-up at four years. *[7] Evaluation at follow-up at four years.

For the ten subjects at skeletal maturity in the follow-up study, the average age at brace initiation was 12.26 (SD: 2.76) years. The clinical characteristics of the subjects and relevant medical history are summarized in Table 1.

3.2. In-Brace Correction

Six subjects were examined for the in-brace correction with radiographs in the anteroposterior and lateral projections. The frontal plane correction and kyphotic effect were measured by comparing the CA measured at the same levels on the in- and out-of-bracing radiographs. The in-brace correction of the primary curve in the frontal plane was 25.3 percent (14.3° to 10.8°). The in-brace thoracic kyphosis in the sagittal plane increased 14.9 percent (40.8° to 47.9°). Figure 4 shows an example of the radiographic in-brace correction.

Table 1. Patient Characteristics. *[1] Patient ID. *[2] Age when diagnosed (years). *[3] Gender (fem = female, male = male). *[4] Age of menarche (years). *[5] Not relevant since male. *[6] Pre-menarche. *[7] Type of scoliosis (C, single curve; ju, juvinil; de, dextrokonvex; si, sinistrokonvex; TS, thoracic; TLS, thoracolumbar; s-s, combined curve). *[8] AIS related events. *[9] MRI of columna. *[10] intermittent back pain, which was relieved by the brace, and the brace was omitted temporarily at the beginning of 2017 since her spine was straight, but radiographic monitoring is continued. *[11] anisomelia of 1.3 cm, but still had radiologic diagnosed AIS after leg length correction (after hip fracture). *[12] back pain after using the Spinaposture brace and whilst using the Chêneau light brace. *[13] normal MRI. *[14] improvement at First Visit. *[15] improvement at Skeletal Maturity. *[16] improvement at Long-Term.

Pt *[1]	Age *[2]	Sex *[3]	Risser	Mena *[4]	Type of Scoliosis *[7]	AIS Events *[8]	MR col. *[9]	CA FV *[14]	CA SM *[15]	CA LT *[16]
1	14.6	male	2	- *[5]	high de-TS	-	-	9.6	6.85	9.1
2	9.1	fem	0	12.2	high de-TS	Back pain *[10]	MR ia *[13]	10.85	16.5	14.9
3	14.8	fem	1	15.7	s-s de-TLS	Anisomelia *[11]	-	1.3	3.7	0.65
4	13.9	male	1	- *[5]	de-TLS	-	-	7.4	−0.7	−2.3
5	10.9	fem	1	12	s-s de-TLS	-	-	1.45	4.95	6.05
6	15.2	male	2	- *[5]	low de-TLS	-	-	3.75	-	-
7	9.7	fem	0	pm *[6]	s-s de-TLS	-	-	4.2	4.4	−0.35
8	13.5	fem	0	14.4	s-s de-TLS	Back pain *[12]	MR ia *[13]	0.8	-	-
9	15.1	fem	1	15.3	low de-TS	-	-	2.45	-	-
10	14.6	fem	2	15.5	low de-TS	-	-	2.7	3.8	-
11	7.2	fem	0	pm *[6]	s-s ju-deTLS	-	-	3.5	1.4	-
12	12.8	fem	0	13.6	s-s de-TLS	-	-	4.45	−3.8	−0.1
13	11.5	fem	0	13	C si-TLS	-	-	2.2	−0.4	−3.25
14	7	male	0	- *[5]	C ju-deTLS	-	-	14.4	-	-
15	15.2	fem	2	14.8	s-s de-TLS	Back pain	MR *[13]	4.9	-	-

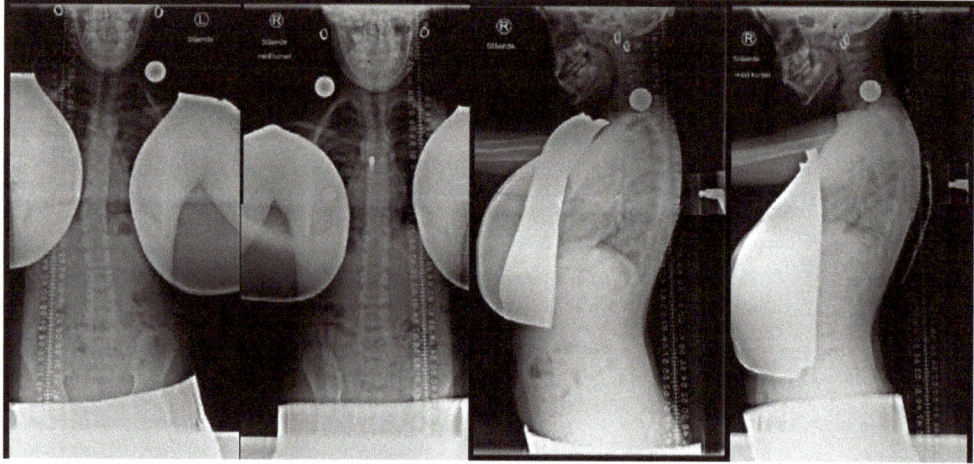

Figure 4. In-brace (picture two and four from left) and out-of-brace (picture one and three from left) of the frontal and sagittal radiographic examinations of a 10-year-old girl. The brace can be identified by the zipper at chest level in picture two and the 'fingers' are seen in picture four.

3.3. Follow-Up Study

In the prospective follow-up, the average CA when starting bracing was 16.8° (SD: 2.8°). The average correction in CA at the first follow-up was 4.5° (SD: 3.2°). Initially, four subjects (4/15) improved in CA with more than 5 dg. and eleven (11/15) remained stable. The average bracing period was 21 months (range: 12.4–37.63 months; SD: 9.5 months). The average CA at the end of bracing was 11.0° (SD: 7.2°). At end of bracing, six subjects (6/10) had straight spines with a CA less than ten degrees and four (4/10) remained stable. In accordance with Costa et al. (2021), the expected outcome for bracing at skeletal maturity was 6/11 and 9/15 for the Risser stage 0–1 and 0–2 at brace initiation, respectively [13]. The achieved outcome was 11/11 and 15/15 for the Risser stage 0–1 and 0–2, respectively, when using the brace. The expected outcome for observation is 50% (CI 44–56%) [13]. Thus, approximately 8/15 was expected to improve or be stable by observation/natural history. In the long term, none of the subjects deteriorated. When extrapolating the expected outcome from Costa et al. (2021), the expected outcome for bracing long-term was 4/9 and 7/10 for the Risser stage 0–1 and 0–2 at brace initiation, respectively [13]. The achieved outcome was 9/9 and 10/150 for the Risser stage 0–1 and 0–2, respectively, when using the brace. The last follow-up was at 24 months (SD: 7.5 months). The average CA at the last follow-up was 10.0° (SD: 6.8). The average long-term follow-up was at 44 months (SD: 9.3 months). The average CA at the long-term follow-up was 12.0° (SD: 6.8°). Three subjects (3/8) had straight spines and five (5/8) remained stable. The individual curve developments are shown in the Supplementary Materials. Figure 5 shows the average changes over time (left-A) and Table 2 displays the achieved and expected outcomes (right-B).

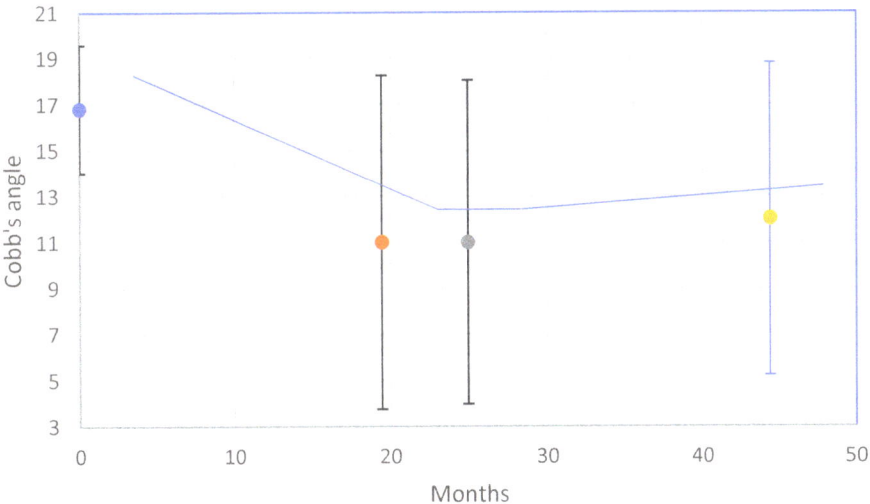

Figure 5. Average changes in Cobb's angle (±one standard deviation) over time in the follow-up from the brace initiation to the long-term follow-up. (Upper-A).

Table 2. The achieved and expected outcomes after using the soft brace at skeletal maturity. * expected outcome in accordance to Costa et al. (2021) [13] (Lower-B).

Risser	N	Achieved in the Present Study			Expected Number of "Improved/Straight" or "Stable" *
		Improved/Straight	Stable	Improved/Straight or Stable	
0–1	11	5	6	11	6 (42%)
0–2	15	6	9	15	9 (71%)

Secondary radiographic parameters in the follow-up study were evaluated according to if changed and are illustrated in Table 3.

Table 3. Secondary radiographic parameters. *¹ Patient ID. *² Time in the brace (in months). *³ changes in descriptive morphology/classification (straight = developed from initial curve straight, → = changed to, otherwise unchanged/Type of scoliosis (C, single curve; ju, juvenile; de, dextrokonvex; si, sinistrokonvex; TS, thoracic; TLS, thoracolumbar; s-s, combined curve). *⁴ Level of apex vertebrae for the primary curve (→ = changed to, otherwise unchanged). *⁵ Difference in Metha angle at apex vertebra. *⁶ change in Nash and Moe's classification at apex vertebra for the primary curve (→ = changed to, otherwise unchanged).

Pt *¹	Time in Brace *²	DM/C *³	A.Ver. *⁴	Metha.A. *⁵	NashMoe *⁶
1	12.3	→straight	Th3→Th12	13.4	0→0
2	36.6	→straight	Th4→Th5	5.9	0→0
3	28.8	→straight	Th5	6.2	0→0
4	13.7	deTLS	Th12→Th11	14.9	0→0
5	22.3	→straight	Th12→Th11	11.4	0→0
6	6.8	low de-TLS	Th8→Th10	4.5	0→0
7	24.7	→straigh	Th9	1.5	0→0
8	8.3	s-s TL	Th9	7.3	1→1
9	7.1	low dTS	Th10	11	0→1
10	16.7	low dTS	Th9	11.3	0→0
11	12.6	→straight	Th9→Th10	19.5	0→0
12	12.8	s-s de-TLS	Th12	10.4	0→0
13	34	C si-TLS	Th10	21.2	0→1
14	4.5	C ju-deTLS	Th12→Th11	27.8	0→1
15	8.1	s-s de-TLS	Th10	13.4	0→0

3.4. Brace Compliance and Events

The compliance of brace usage and events were evaluated by open questioning at every follow-up where the subjects and caregivers were encouraged to disclose non-compliance and discomfort when using the brace in an open-minded dialogue. Non-compliance and brace events were seen in periods of warm weather and the subjects often had subsequently deformity progression at the next follow-up. This motivated the subjects to a more rigorous brace usage motivated by the deterioration (see supplement S1). Two subjects had heat sensors embedded in their braces. This is considered an objective way of measuring brace wear compliance by body heat [27]. The heat sensor would register an increase in temperature when the brace was worn. The compliance for those two subjects seemed to be fulfilled. Figure 6 (Upper-A) shows an example of the monitoring with spikes of increased temperature when the brace was worn, and Table 4 (Lower-B) illustrates the events and bracing history.

When performing analysis for interobserver variation, the two doctors had an excellent inter-class correlation of 0.85 [25].

When performing a posthoc power analysis, the power (1-β, α = 0.05) for the first follow-up with 15 subjects was 0.98, at skeletal maturity 0.88 for ten subjects and long-term 0.79 for eight subjects.

When performing the Chi-square cross-tabulation, none of the parameters of gender, age, Risser stage, and initial CA between subjects and dropouts was statistically significant (z < 1.96). The Spearman correlation for dropout found a positive and negative association between initial CA ($p < 0.001$) and the duration of bracing ($p < 0.01$), respectively.

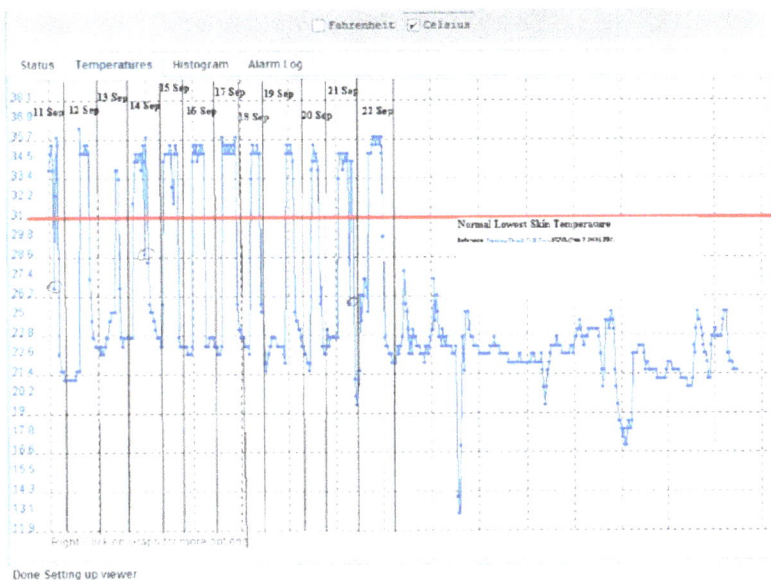

Figure 6. An example of a period with daytime and nighttime use of the brace. The heat sensor would register the temperature rise when the brace was worn. A period of brace use is seen on the left-hand side of the figure (compliance) and a period of non-compliance is seen on the right-hand side of the figure. (Upper-A).

Table 4. Brace events and brace history. [1] Patient ID. [2] Brace events and clinical comments. [3] Types of physiotherapy (- = ordinary strengthening spine muscle exercises). [4] omitted the brace during periods due to hot weather and had a subsequent progression in CA, which regressed again using the brace. [5] irritation in the crotch, which was amended partly by modification of the brace. [6] intermittent back pain, which was relieved by the brace, and the brace was omitted temporarily at the beginning of 2017 since her spine was straight, but radiographic monitoring is continued. [7] back pain after using the Spinaposture brace and whilst using the Chêneau light brace. [8] change brace to Chêneau light. [9] change brace to providence in a short period and afterwards Chêneau light. [10] Excluded. [11] Straight spine and the brace was omitted. (Lower-B).

Pt [1]	Brace events [2]	Brace Change	Exercise [3]
1	-	-	schroth
2	Sum [4] & Irr [5] & BP [6]	-	schroth
3	Sum [4] & Irr [5]	-	schroth
4	-	-	-
5	-	-	-
6	E [10]	-	-
7	-	-	-
8	BP [7] & E [10]	chea [8]	schroth
9	Irr [5] & E [10]	prov/chea [9]	schroth
10	-	-	schroth
11	OM [11]	-	-
12	-	-	-
13	-	-	-
14	E [10] & OM [11]	-	Roofing
15	E [10]	-	-

4. Discussion

In this study, we examined a new brace for adolescent idiopathic scoliosis. When testing for immediate correction by in- and out-of-brace radiographs, the proprioceptive-mediated 'strive' of the brace induced a thoracic sagittal kyphotic effect. This led to an immediate thoracic frontal plane correction of the AIS deformity. This suggests that there can be an interrelationship between the frontal and sagittal plane spinal curves of the spine which is described as 'coupled motions' by Panjabi and White [28]. To our knowledge, this has not been demonstrated in vivo in humans. In the follow-up study, there was a deformity correction of one-fourth at the first follow-up visit. At skeletal maturity, all subjects either improved or remained stable in their frontal plane deformity. When compared to the expected outcome for observation only (50% success rate) or other soft braces (62.5% success rate) [13], more subjects were improving or remaining stable when using the soft brace when stratified to the Risser stage 0–1 and 0–2 at brace initiation. In the long term, none of the subjects deteriorated. Based on these findings, the correctional effect or brace efficacy for this soft brace was better than those of previous studies with soft bracing and observation only. One can argue that more subjects are needed to detect an effect (especially long-term) but as a precautious measure, only a small cohort of subjects was included. In conclusion, our results for the Spinaposture brace are comparable to those of previous studies with soft braces when used part-time and for small curve AIS.

When interpreting our results, we had the following deliberations. In the initial evaluations of the subjects, we performed in- and out-of-brace radiographs and closer follow-ups with three months intervals in the initial period of brace wearing as well. The in and out-of-brace radiographs were voluntary for the subjects since this induced additional radiation [29]. We refrained from in and out-of-brace radiographs throughout the study for this reason. The initial closer follow-up was carried out as a precautious measure. We justified the more frequent follow-up and excess radiation [30] by using a local developed low dose radiographic technique [24]. This exposed the subjects to eight-fold lower radiation doses than the standard posteroanterior radiographs. In this study, only a small cohort of subjects was included as a precautious measure when testing a new brace, and since this study was a clinical follow-up study, we performed a posthoc power analysis that determined our findings as adequately powered at skeletal maturity. However, we acknowledge the impediments of posthoc power analysis [31]. Our subjects were chosen as a convenience sample, and thus our study could be influenced by selection bias. However, there were no differences in demography of gender and age distribution when compared to previous studies [3,32], thus indicating that our subjects were comparable. Our study could also be influenced by selection bias due to our exclusions and drop-outs. Five of the seven initial exclusions were due to the encouragement of private therapists using different braces and exercise therapies despite neither of the subjects progressing in deformity before converting to other treatments motivating this change. Non-compliance to any spine-related intervention was another cause of exclusion and the subsequent drop-outs during the study were either due to being unable to contact them or being too busy to attend the follow-up. We were unable to identify specific parameters that caused the drop-outs since there were no significant differences between subjects and dropouts when comparing the parameters. However, we found an association between the initial corrective effect of the brace and the duration of brace treatment and dropout.

The purpose of examining the brace was two-fold, namely to discover if the hypnotized frontal plane deformity would be correctable using a sagittal plane strive and to determine if the brace was effective at skeletal maturity and long-term. The hard braces used today are strenuous, causing pressure marks, pain/soreness, and general discomfort with low compliance to follow [2,7,8]. The Spinaposture brace© was designed to be less strenuous and to be a supplement to our current non-operative treatment of watchful follow-up and physiotherapy. We acknowledge that using temperature monitoring for all subjects are needed for adequate and quantified brace compliance evaluation [3]. However, this first study has not discouraged that the brace can be used as an option of early intervention in AIS for the smaller thoracic and thoracolumbar curves with a CA between 15° and 25°. However, to substantiate this, additional studies are needed such as a stronger prospective randomized design with a control group and a larger number of subjects [13]. These studies should entail quantifiable monitoring of brace compliance, a more detailed evaluation for skeletal maturity, and a more detailed stratification of outcome than using the initial Risser stage.

5. Conclusions

In conclusion, this prospective observational study demonstrated an immediate in-brace correction of the frontal deformity of AIS in six subjects. In follow-up, there was an immediate correction of one-fourth of the deformity. At skeletal maturity, the deformities improved more than expected when compared to that of the natural history/observation and similar to that of other soft braces. No long-term deformity progression was seen.

Supplementary Materials: The following supporting information can be downloaded at: https://www.mdpi.com/article/10.3390/jcm11010264/s1, Supplement S1, Development in Cobb' angle for the 15 patients with AIS 1.

Author Contributions: The authors have made substantial contributions to Conceptualization: C.W.; methodology: C.W. and T.B.A.; formal analysis: C.W. and T.B.A.; investigation: C.W. and T.B.A.; resources: C.W.; writing—original draft preparation: C.W. and T.B.A.; writing—review and editing: C.W. and T.B.A.; visualization: C.W.; project administration: C.W.; funding acquisition: C.W. All authors have drafted the work or substantively revised it and has approved the submitted version and agrees to be personally accountable for the author's contributions and for ensuring that questions related to the accuracy or integrity of any part of the work, even ones in which the author was not personally involved, are appropriately investigated, resolved, and documented in the literature. All authors have read and agreed to the published version of the manuscript.

Funding: This research received no external funding.

Institutional Review Board Statement: Ethical review and approval were waived for this study. The local ethical committee evaluated this study as a clinical follow-up (reference number H-17014162).

Informed Consent Statement: Informed consent was obtained from all subjects involved in the study.

Data Availability Statement: Data from this study can be requested from the corresponding author.

Acknowledgments: We acknowledge Bandagist Jan Nielsen for technical support.

Conflicts of Interest: The first author is part owner of the company with the patent for the Spinaposture brace. This company had no role in the design of the study; in the collection, analyses, or interpretation of data; in the writing of the manuscript, or in the decision to publish the results.

References

1. Negrini, S.; Minozzi, S.; Bettany-Saltikov, J.; Chockalingam, N.; Grivas, T.B.; Kotwicki, T.; Maruyama, T.; Romano, M.; Zaina, F. Braces for idiopathic scoliosis in adolescents. *Cochrane Database Syst. Rev.* **2015**, *6*, CD006850. [CrossRef]
2. Weiss, H.-R. Is there a body of evidence for the treatment of patients with Adolescent Idiopathic Scoliosis (AIS)? *Scoliosis* **2007**, *2*, 19. [CrossRef]
3. Weinstein, S.L.; Dolan, L.; Wright, J.G.; Dobbs, M.B. Effects of Bracing in Adolescents with Idiopathic Scoliosis. *N. Engl. J. Med.* **2013**, *369*, 1512–1521. [CrossRef]
4. Nachemson, A.L.; Peterson, L.E. Effectiveness of treatment with a brace in girls who have adolescent idiopathic scoliosis. A prospective, controlled study based on data from the Brace Study of the Scoliosis Research Society. *J. Bone Jt. Surg. Am.* **1995**, *77*, 815–822. [CrossRef]
5. Wiley, J.W.; Thomson, J.D.; Mitchell, T.M.; Smith, B.G.; Banta, J.V. Effectiveness of The Boston Brace in Treatment of Large Curves in Adolescent Idiopathic Scoliosis. *Spine* **2000**, *25*, 2326–2332. [CrossRef] [PubMed]
6. Negrini, S.; Grivas, T.B. Introduction to the "Scoliosis" Journal Brace Technology Thematic Series: Increasing existing knowledge and promoting future developments. *Scoliosis* **2010**, *5*, 2–6. [CrossRef] [PubMed]
7. Rivett, L.; Rothberg, A.; Stewart, A.; Berkowitz, R. The relationship between quality of life and compliance to a brace protocol in adolescents with idiopathic scoliosis: A comparative study. *BMC Musculoskelet. Disord.* **2009**, *10*, 5. [CrossRef]
8. Reichel, D.; Schanz, J. Developmental psychological aspects of scoliosis treatment. *Pediatr. Rehabil.* **2003**, *6*, 221–225. [CrossRef] [PubMed]

9. Dolan, L.A.; Wright, J.G.; Weinstein, S.L. Correspondence: Effects of Bracing in Adolescents with Idiopathic Scoliosis. *N. Engl. J. Med.* **2014**, *370*, 680–681. [CrossRef]
10. Davies, E.; Norvell, D.; Hermsmeyer, J. Efficacy of bracing versus observation in the treatment of idiopathic scoliosis. *Evid. Based Spine Care J.* **2011**, *2*, 25–34. [CrossRef] [PubMed]
11. Goldberg, C.J.; Moore, D.P.; Fogarty, E.E.; Dowling, F.E. Adolescent Idiopathic Scoliosis: The effect of brace treatment on the incidence of surgery. *Spine* **2001**, *26*, 42–47. [CrossRef] [PubMed]
12. Weiss, H.-R.; Werkmann, M. Soft braces in the treatment of Adolescent Idiopathic Scoliosis (AIS)—Review of the literature and description of a new approach. *Scoliosis* **2012**, *7*, 11, Retraction: *Scoliosis* **2013**, *8*, 7. [CrossRef]
13. Costa, L.; Schlosser, T.P.C.; Jimale, H.; Homans, J.F.; Kruyt, M.C.; Castelein, R.M. The Effectiveness of Different Concepts of Bracing in Adolescent Idiopathic Scoliosis (AIS): A Systematic Review and Meta-Analysis. *J. Clin. Med.* **2021**, *10*, 2145. [CrossRef] [PubMed]
14. Weiss, H.-R. SpineCor vs. natural history—Explanation of the results obtained using a simple biomechanical model. *Stud. Health Technol. Inform.* **2008**, *140*, 133–136. [PubMed]
15. van Loon, P.J.M.; Kühbauch, B.A.G.; Thunnissen, F.B. Forced Lordosis on the Thoracolumbar Junction Can Correct Coronal Plane Deformity in Adolescents with Double Major Curve Pattern Idiopathic Scoliosis. *Spine* **2008**, *33*, 797–801. [CrossRef]
16. Weiss, H.-R.; Tournavitis, N.; Seibel, S.; Kleban, A. A Prospective Cohort Study of AIS Patients with 40° and More Treated with a Gensingen Brace (GBW): Preliminary Results. *Open Orthop. J.* **2017**, *11*, 1558–1567. [CrossRef] [PubMed]
17. Negrini, S.; Fusco, C.; Minozzi, S.; Atanasio, S.; Zaina, F.; Romano, M. Exercises reduce the progression rate of adolescent idiopathic scoliosis: Results of a comprehensive systematic review of the literature. *Disabil. Rehabil.* **2008**, *30*, 772–785. [CrossRef] [PubMed]
18. Adams, W. *Lectures on the Pathology and Treatment of Lateral and Other Forms of Curvature of the Spine*; Churchill: London, UK, 1882, 2nd ed. Available online: https://wellcomecollection.org/works/qc5xzydx (accessed on 1 December 2021).
19. Wong, C. Mechanism of right thoracic adolescent idiopathic scoliosis at risk for progression; a unifying pathway of development by normal growth and imbalance. *Scoliosis* **2015**, *10*, 1–5. [CrossRef]
20. Donzelli, S.; Zaina, F.; Negrini, S. End growth results analysis related to Risser score, Cobb degrees, and curve types at the beginning of the treatment. *Scoliosis* **2013**, *8*, O10. [CrossRef]
21. Coillard, C.; Circo, A.B.; Rivard, C.H. A prospective randomized controlled trial of the natural history of idiopathic scoliosis versus treatment with the SpineCor brace. Sosort Award 2011 winner. *Eur. J. Phys. Rehabil. Med.* **2014**, *50*, 479–487. [CrossRef]
22. Kouwenhoven, J.-W.M.; Smit, T.H.; van der Veen, A.J.; Kingma, I.; van Dieën, J.H.; Castelein, R.M. Effects of Dorsal Versus Ventral Shear Loads on the Rotational Stability of the Thoracic Spine: A biomechanical porcine and human cadaveric study. *Spine* **2007**, *32*, 2545–2550. [CrossRef]
23. Lomax, M.; Tasker, L.; Bostanci, O. An electromyographic evaluation of dual role breathing and upper body muscles in response to front crawl swimming. *Scand. J. Med. Sci. Sports* **2014**, *25*, e472–e478. [CrossRef]
24. Wong, C.; Adriansen, J.; Jeppsen, J.; Balslev-Clausen, A. Intervariability in radiographic parameters and general evaluation of a low-dose fluoroscopic technique in patients with idiopathic scoliosis. *Acta Radiol. Open* **2021**, *10*. [CrossRef]
25. Langensiepen, S.; Semler, O.; Sobottke, R.; Fricke, O.; Franklin, J.; Schönau, E.; Eysel, P. Measuring procedures to determine the Cobb angle in idiopathic scoliosis: A systematic review. *Eur. Spine J.* **2013**, *22*, 2360–2371. [CrossRef]
26. Moe, J.H.; Kettleson, D.N. Idiopathic scoliosis. Analysis of curve patterns and the preliminary results of Milwau-kee-brace treatment in one hundred sixty-nine patients. *J. Bone Jt. Surg. Am.* **1970**, *52*, 1509–1533. [CrossRef]
27. Rahman, T.; Borkhuu, B.; Littleton, A.G.; Sample, W.; Moran, E.; Campbell, S.; Rogers, K.; Bowen, J.R. Electronic monitoring of scoliosis brace wear compliance. *J. Child. Orthop.* **2010**, *4*, 343–347. [CrossRef]
28. Panjabi, M.M.; Brand, R.A., Jr.; White, A.A., 3rd. Mechanical properties of the human thoracic spine as shown by three-dimensional load-displacement curves. *J. Bone Jt. Surg. Am.* **1976**, *58*, 642–652. [CrossRef]
29. Simony, A.; Hansen, E.J.; Christensen, S.B.; Carreon, L.Y.; Andersen, M.Ø. Incidence of cancer in adolescent idiopathic scoliosis patients treated 25 years previously. *Eur. Spine J.* **2016**, *25*, 3366–3370. [CrossRef] [PubMed]
30. Knott, P.; Pappo, E.; Cameron, M.; Demauroy, J.C.; Rivard, C.; Kotwicki, T.; Zaina, F.; Wynne, J.; Stikeleather, L.; Bettany-Saltikov, J.; et al. SOSORT 2012 consensus paper: Reducing X-ray exposure in pediatric patients with scoliosis. *Scoliosis* **2014**, *9*, 4. [CrossRef]
31. Zhang, Y.; Hedo, R.; Rivera, A.; Rull, R.; Richardson, S.; Tu, X.M. Post hoc power analysis: Is it an informative and meaningful analysis? *Gen. Psychiatry* **2019**, *32*, e100069. [CrossRef]
32. Soucacos, P.N.; Zacharis, K.; Gelalis, J.; Soultanis, K.; Kalos, N.; Beris, A.; Xenakis, T.; Johnson, E.O. Assessment of curve progression in idiopathic scoliosis. *Eur. Spine J.* **1998**, *7*, 270–277. [CrossRef] [PubMed]

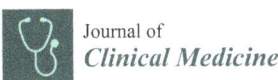

Article

Intensive Postural and Motor Activity Program Reduces Scoliosis Progression in People with Rett Syndrome

Alberto Romano [1,2,3,*], Elena Ippolito [4], Camilla Risoli [5], Edoardo Malerba [6], Martina Favetta [2], Andrea Sancesario [2], Meir Lotan [7,8] and Daniel Sender Moran [1]

1. Department of Health System Management, Ariel University, Ariel 4070000, Israel; danielm@ariel.ac.il
2. Movement Analysis and Robotics Laboratory, Intensive Neurorehabilitation and Robotics Department, Bambino Gesù Children's Hospital, 00165 Rome, Italy; martina.favetta@opbg.net (M.F.); andrea.sancesario@opbg.net (A.S.)
3. Centro AIRETT Ricerca e Innovazione (CARI), Research and Innovation AIRETT Center, 37122 Verona, Italy
4. SMART Learning Center, 20133 Milan, Italy; elena.ippolito@centrosmart.it
5. Department of Radiological Functions, Radiology Unit, Guglielmo da Saliceto Hospital, 29121 Piacenza, Italy; camilla.risoli11@gmail.com
6. Poliambulatorio Health Medical, 29122 Piacenza, Italy; edoardo.malerba11@gmail.com
7. Department of Physiotherapy, Ariel University, Ariel 4070000, Israel; meirlo@ariel.ac.il
8. Israeli Rett Syndrome National Evaluation Team, Ramat Gan 5200100, Israel
* Correspondence: alberto.romano01@ateneopv.it

Abstract: Background: A scoliosis prevalence of 94% was reported in the population with Rett syndrome (RTT), with an annual progression rate of 14 to 21° Cobb which may result in pain, loss of sitting balance, deterioration of motor skills, and lung disfunction. This paper describes the efficacy of an intensive conservative individualized physical and postural activity program in preventing scoliosis curvature progression in patients with RTT. Methods: Twenty subjects diagnosed with RTT and scoliosis were recruited, and an individualized intensive daily physical activity program was developed for each participant. Each program was conducted for six months by participants' primary caregivers in their daily living environment. Fortnightly remote supervision of the program implementation was provided by an expert therapist. Pre- and post-intervention radiographs and motor functioning were analyzed. Results: An averaged progression of +1.7° ± 8.7° Cobb, over one year (12.3 ± 3.5 months) was observed in our group, together with motor function improvements. A relation between curve progression and motor skill improvement was observed. Conclusions: The intervention prevented scoliosis progression in our group. The achievement of functional motor improvements could enable better body segment control and muscle balancing, with a protective effect on scoliosis progression. The intervention was effective for individuals with RTT across various ages and severity levels. Individual characteristics of each participant and the details of their activity program are described.

Keywords: Rett syndrome; scoliosis; motor skills; telerehabilitation; physical therapy modalities; home exercise program

1. Introduction

Rett syndrome (RTT) is a severe neurodevelopmental disease caused by a mutation in the MECP2 gene located on the X chromosome [1], affecting about 1/10,000 females worldwide [2–4]. Scoliosis is the most common orthopedic comorbidity in RTT [5–7], showing a prevalence of up to 94% [7–11]. Reported median age of scoliosis onset in RTT is at 9.8 years, with 25% of subjects affected by the age of 6 years, about 79% by the age of 13 years, and 85% by the age of 16 years or older [7,9,12,13]. Scoliosis in RTT is neurogenic in origin and can result in pain, loss of sitting balance, deterioration of motor skills, and progressive restrictive lung disease development [14]. Diminished early development, inability to sit and walk without support, the onset of puberty, and enhanced clinical severity are also associated with developing scoliosis at an early age [11,13,15].

The case literature suggests a fast mean curve progression in this population, ranging from 14 to 21° Cobb per year, accompanied by an acceleration in the progression at puberty with an average age of 13 years [11,14,16]. Moreover, in a large cohort study analyzing radiographs of 128 girls and women with RTT followed for two years (three radiographs for each subject), the magnitude of scoliosis was found to generally increase with age with a yearly 0.438-unit increase in the square root of the baseline Cobb's angle (95% confidence interval 0.374–0.503) [17].

A corset is usually suggested to individuals with RTT with Cobb's angle greater than 20–25°, and spinal fusion is considered if Cobb's angle progresses over 40–50° [12,15,18].

Spinal surgery is considered the definitive management of neuromuscular scoliosis [19]. In most cases, posterior-only spinal fusion is performed [20]. However, if an anteroposterior surgery is required, a single-stage approach is preferable to reduce anesthetic and surgical complications [12]. Fixation to the pelvis is indicated in non-ambulant children with pelvic obliquity [12] and in the presence of a preceding rapid decline in neurological function with a lethargic presentation and uncontrolled, treatment-resistant daily seizures [21]. Surgery should not be delayed until skeletal maturity has been achieved. Barney and colleagues suggested the need for RTT-specific post-operative pain management [22]. The authors reported that, after spinal fusion, patients with RTT received fewer total doses of opioids compared to girls with cerebral palsy and idiopathic scoliosis. With modern technology, severe curves can be safely treated [21] and positive outcomes following spinal surgery were reported [23–26]. Even so, the decision to perform the operation is challenging for the family due to anxiety about their daughter undergoing such a complex procedure [8,24]. Moreover, a large cohort study reported that 18.5% of subjects with RTT and scoliosis had spinal instrumentation [15], showing that the vast majority of this group of clients will not undergo surgery and therefore will rely on non-surgical, conservative treatment. Therefore, the development and evaluation of such programs are critical for individuals with RTT.

Available conservative interventions for scoliosis include observation and monitoring, bracing, orthotics, and physical therapy [27–29]. As specific guidelines for the management of scoliosis for people with RTT were published [12], the available treatments for scoliosis were here described in the light of such guidelines. The scoliosis monitoring for these patients should start before the diagnosis of scoliosis. Before-diagnosis monitoring strategies for people with RTT include genetic testing, parental teaching on the characteristic aspects of scoliosis, and physical assessment upon the diagnosis of RTT and at least every six months after that [12]. After diagnosing scoliosis, yearly spine radiographs are suggested to monitor the curve progression. The collection of radiographs every six months is recommended if the Cobb's angle progresses over 25° before the skeletal maturity. The maintenance of physical examinations every six months is advised after the scoliosis diagnosis [12]. Bracing strategies were suggested in the literature for neuromuscular scoliosis management among its conservative treatments. A recent literature review identified 23 typologies of braces proposed to care for scoliosis curves of different types ("C" or "S" shaped), levels (thoracic, lumbar, and thoracolumbar), and entities, using different approaches (passive and active correction) [30]. Indications for bracing are stronger in younger children and more controversial in adolescents. Bracing aims to contain the curve until skeletal maturity [31] and regain the sitting position [32]. However, the role of bracing in patients with neuromuscular scoliosis is contentious and there is no compelling evidence supporting the use of braces to prevent the deformity progression in neuromuscular scoliosis [19,32]. There is no consensus among experts on RTT that bracing is beneficial in reducing the scoliosis progression in this population [12]. Nevertheless, bracing may be found valuable if support is needed in a sitting position (usually for very hypotonic children who find it difficult to maintain an erect posture for long periods) or to delay the necessity of surgery [12,33,34].

When considering conventional interventions regarding scoliosis, there is a consensus among experts that efforts should be made to maintain the ability to walk and increase duration and distance walked to counteract the curve progression [19,27,35]. However, the capacity of physical therapy treatments to reduce scoliosis or prevent mild scoliosis from rapidly progressing has, to date, received mild consideration in the literature [35]. Although, so far, physical therapy interventions have not been found to improve etiological factors for neuromuscular scoliosis or prevent progression of established scoliosis, they were reported as helpful in avoiding any adverse effects, such as prolonged brace use, prevention or prolonging onset of joint contractures, and maintenance of both chest mobility and respiratory excursion [27,32]. The implementation of physical therapy for scoliosis must be based on the particular spinal deformity characteristics and requires specifically trained therapists and clinicians [28].

To our knowledge, only one anti-scoliotic physical therapy intervention explicitly directed to patients with RTT was noted in the literature [35]. This is a specific physical therapy regimen comprised of an intensive program of postural positioning and enhanced activity level carried out in joint cooperation with the participant's family members and caregivers (within the educational facility). The intervention was conducted with a 5-year-old girl with RTT whose Cobb's angle reduced from 30 to 20° over an 18-month treatment period, through the use of positioning equipment, postural strategies (activating automatic equilibrium reactions, which oppose the natural scoliotic curve), and a motor activity program (walking or standing) during waking hours. Similar programs were found helpful to increase the motor function of five girls with RTT in Ireland [36], and 17 girls and women with RTT in Italy [37], providing evidence of feasibility and acceptability of this treatment in a broader age and functional range of participants. Yet, to date, no anti-scoliotic, conventional, physical regime was evaluated for a cohort of participants with Rett syndrome.

The present paper aims to describe the efficacy of such a physical activity program in preventing the scoliosis curvature progression in a group of patients with RTT and analyzing the variables that can affect the intervention efficacy. The proposed intervention is ecological and intensive; it was carried out by primary caregivers within the participants' daily living environment and was planned and remotely supervised fortnightly by therapists with expertise in carrying out motor rehabilitation treatments for people with RTT. The proposed intervention was developed based on the one proposed by Lotan and colleagues [35].

2. Materials and Methods

2.1. Study Design

A single-subject A-B-A design was applied.

The dependent variable was the Cobb's angle changes before (T1) and after (T2) the intervention, 12.3 ± 3.5 months apart.

The independent variable was the implementation of a six-month individualized motor and postural activity program carried out by participants' parents and care providers within the participants' daily living environment for one hour a day, five days a week.

2.2. Participants

Twenty Italian girls and women with genetically confirmed classic RTT and diagnoses of scoliosis participated in this research. Participants were recruited from the Italian Rett Association (AIRett) database. All participants lived at home with their parents. One subject was waiting for scoliosis surgery at enrolment (T1). Descriptive statistics of participants' age, RTT severity level, and daily physical activity level are presented in Table 1.

Table 1. Descriptive statistics of participants' ages, RARS total and subscale scores, and m-BAR scores.

		Mean (SD)	Median	Range
	Age	15.6 (8.4)	13.2	3.8–38.3
RARS	Cognitive	13.4 (2.8)	13.5	9–18.5
	Sensory	3.2 (1.1)	3.0	2–5.5
	Motor	10.4 (2.1)	10.3	5.5–13
	Emotional	3.2 (0.8)	3.0	2–5
	Independence	10.7 (1.8)	11.3	4.5–12
	Rett characteristics	23.8 (4.5)	24.3	15–33
	Total	64.7 (9.5)	66.0	45.5–81.5
m-BAR		92.8 (26.1)	93.5	52–145

Abbreviation list: SD = Standard Deviation; RARS = Rett Assessment Rating Scale; m-BAR = modified Bouchard activity record.

2.3. Outcome Measures

2.3.1. RTT Severity Level

The Rett Assessment Rating Scale (RARS) was used to assess the severity of clinical manifestation of RTT [38]. The RARS was established by a standardization procedure, proving that the instrument is statistically valid and reliable [39].

2.3.2. Activity Level

Participants' parents completed the modified Bouchard activity record (m-BAR) to evaluate their daughter's physical activity level [40,41]. Previous studies demonstrated good reliability of the m-BAR as a daily activity level measure for individuals with RTT [40,41]. The m-BAR was collected at T1 to help the researchers figure out how active participants were during their typical day.

2.3.3. Motor Functioning

The motor functioning level was scored at T1 and T2 using the Rett Syndrome Motor Evaluation Scale (RESMES) [39,42]. This RTT-specific gross motor evaluation scale showed optimal inter-rater agreement among clinicians and strong internal consistency [42].

2.3.4. Scoliosis Severity

A clinical score for the scoliosis severity was given to each participant at T1 to help understand the curve's characteristics. The scoliosis severity level was coded with a 0 to 3 ordinal score (0: no scoliosis; 1: mild scoliosis, curve visible only on thorough examination in forward bending; 2: moderate scoliosis, obvious curve in both upright and forward bending; 3: severe scoliosis, pronounced curve preventing upright position without external support) as suggested for individuals with RTT by Rodocanachi and colleagues [43].

Participants' coronal Cobb's angles were digitally measured by two independent assessors through manual use of the RadiAnt DICOM Viewer software (version 2020.2.1—Medixant, Poznan, Poland) "Cobb's angle" tool on the participants' anterior–posterior radiograph images. The Cobb angle is a standard quantification value of scoliosis certified by the Scoliosis Research Society. This study has adopted it as an objective measure, to quantify state of scoliosis at T1 and change in scoliosis, based on the radiograph images [44]. The manual measurement of Cobb's angle required determining the upper/lower end vertebras (UEV/LEV) on the participants' whole spine antero–posterior radiograph images and drawing two lines corresponding to the upper and lower end vertebra endplate lines (UEVEL; LEVEL). Then, two lines respectively perpendicular to the UEVEL and LEVEL are drawn. The angle included between the two perpendicular lines represents the Cobb's angle. Visual explanation of Cobb's angle measurement procedure is available in Figure 1. Each participant's radiographs were collected at T1 and T2 at the same facility, in the same posture, and by the same technician following international guidelines [12]. If a double curve was present, the bigger curvature was considered.

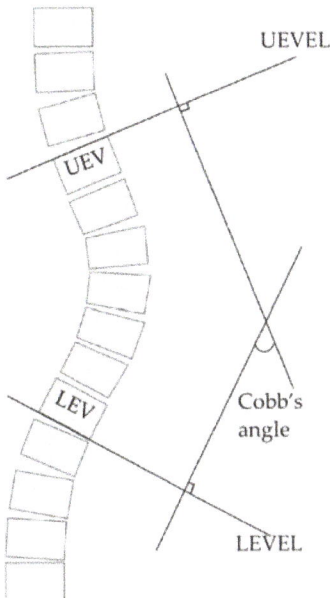

Figure 1. Visual explanation of the method used to measure the Cobb's angle. Upper and lower end vertebra endplate lines (UEVEL; LEVEL).

Detailed clinical descriptions of motor functioning changes between T1 and T2 due to the present intervention program will be presented in a future article.

2.4. Procedure

The present research was conducted following the Declaration of Helsinki principles and approved by the Ariel University Institutional Review Board (AU-HEA-ML-20190326-1). Before starting the intervention, informed consent for participation and study publication was collected for all participants from their legal guardians. Each participant was then clinically evaluated at her home by two therapists experienced in treating people with RTT (pre-intervention evaluation meeting—T1). At T1, the levels of RTT severity, daily physical activity, motor functioning, and scoliosis severity were assessed, and relevant information related to participants' clinical conditions (such as the presence of comorbidities typically associated with RTT), daily activities, routines, and living environments were collected. Participants' parents and referred rehabilitation professionals (when available) participated in this meeting.

At the end of the T1 meeting, a draft of individualized motor activities and the postural program was prepared relying on the collected information. The draft was then discussed with participants' parents and referred therapists until consensus on activity characteristics and their execution timetable was reached. Each program included 4–7 (median: 5) therapeutic activities that parents could perform at home and that could be easily integrated into the participant's daily routine. Those activities were based on passive (hypercorrective) [35,45] and active (causing the participant to use balance reactions while sitting, standing, and walking, working asymmetrically and harder with the extensors and side flexors of the convexity side of her body, against the natural pull of scoliosis) [35,46] postural strategies and on the performance of motor tasks that strengthened the trunk muscles. A full description of each activity included in each program is available as

Supplementary Material (see "Text file—Supplementary material", which illustrates each participant's activities carried out during the intervention). Each activity in the program was shown and taught to the participants' parents, other involved caregivers (e.g., babysitters and teachers), and therapists in vivo during the first evaluation meeting where possible, and through video call and digital material sharing (such as figures and videos) in the other cases. Each participant was required to perform the programmed activities for at least one non-consecutive hour per day, five days a week, for six months. The progress of each program was supervised fortnightly for the first three months of the intervention by one of the therapists who had created the programs via video call with the involved caregivers. The supervision meetings lasted for one hour each and were aimed to support the program execution, answering caregivers' questions, adapting the program to the emerged needs, solving problems, rearranging timetables, adapting the suggested exercises, and, if needed, setting new activities. At the end of the intervention, participants' motor functioning level was assessed again, and the post-intervention spine radiographs were collected (T2).

2.5. Statistical Analysis

As the obtained results were not normally distributed, non-parametric statistics were used for the data analysis. Wilcoxon signed-rank test was conducted to compare the participants' Cobb's angles and RESMES total scores collected at T1 and T2. If a statistical difference was found within the above-reported comparisons, the size of the effect was calculated using the matched-pairs rank-biserial correlation [47,48]. The effect size can be defined as the degree to which a null hypothesis is false or the degree to which the phenomenon is present in the population [49]. Cohen [50] proposed widely used interpretative guidelines for the effect size, considering it small if between 0.200 and 0.500, medium between 0.500 and 0.800, and large if above 0.800. However, a meaningful interpretation of the magnitude of a treatment effect requires a comparison of the result to a frame of reference, such as previous findings [51]. Accordingly, Cohen suggested that his interpretative framework should only be used when the discipline lacks specific guidelines [50,52]. Therefore, for the present study, the effect size interpretation followed the empirically derived guidelines proposed by Kinney and colleagues [53] for rehabilitation studies. Accordingly, the effect size was considered small if between 0.140 and 0.310, medium if between 0.310 and 0.610, and large if above 0.610 [53].

Relations between Cobb's angles changes with participant's age, Cobb's angles at T1, level of RTT severity, daily physical activity at T1, motor function at T1, and the variation of motor functional levels that occurred between T1 and T2 were explored using Spearman's rank correlation coefficient. This non-parametric test assesses how well a monotonic function can describe the relationship between two variables and is equal to using the Pearson correlation between the rank values of two variables. The threshold for significance for the comparisons above has been assumed as $\alpha = 0.05$. No correction for multiple comparisons was applied [54].

3. Results

All our participants carried out their individualized program for its entire duration (six months). The descriptive statistics of Cobb's angles measured at T1 and T2 and the difference between Cobb's angles measured at the two evaluations are collected in Table 2.

Table 2. Descriptive statistics of participants' Cobb's angles at T1 and T2 divided between those whose scoliosis worsened, those whose curve improved, and all participants together. Delta (Δ) Cobb's angles represent the simple difference between Cobb's angle measured at T2 and T1. Positive values represent a worsening, while negative values represent an improvement in the scoliotic curve.

		Worsening	Improving	All
	No. (%)	12 (60%)	8 (40%)	20 (100%)
Cobb's angles T1 (°)	Mean (SD)	23.6 (13.8)	27.9 (12.5)	25.3 (13.2)
	Median	21.5	29.2	23.3
	Range	8–56	10–41	8–56
Cobb's angles T2 (°)	Mean (SD)	30.8 (16.5)	21.5 (14.8)	27.1 (16.1)
	Median	25.6	24.4	25.6
	Range	14–65	0–39	0–65
Δ Cobb's angles (°)	Mean (SD)	7.2 (6.5)	−6.4 (4.1)	1.7 (8.7)
	Median	5.0	−4.8	2.1
	Range	1–23	−13—2.5	−13–23

Abbreviation list: SD = Standard Deviation; T1 = pre-intervention evaluation meeting; T2 = post-intervention evaluation meeting.

Figure 2 shows Cobb's angles of each participant at T1 and T2. Four of the eight participants (50%) who reduced their Cobb's angle improved their curve for at least five degrees. On the other hand, a worsening of more than 5° Cobb was observed in 6 out of 12 subjects (50%) who worsened their curves. Considering as a curve progression a Cobb's angle increment of more than 5°, the scoliosis of 70% of participants did not deteriorate at T2.

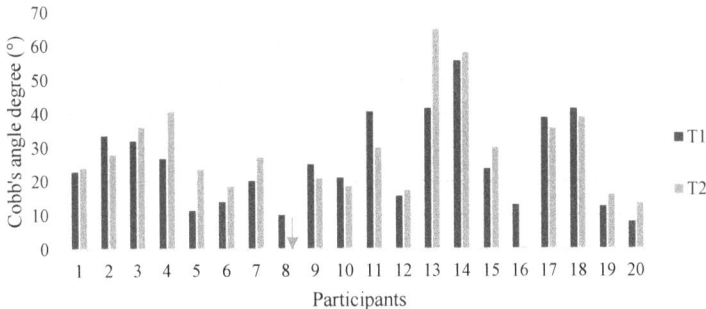

Figure 2. Cobb's angles of each participant at T1 and T2. Gray arrow (participant no. 8) represents the absence of scoliosis at T2.

The Wilcoxon signed-rank test showed no statistical difference between Cobb's angles collected at T1 and T2 ($p = 0.400$). Descriptive statistics of RESMES total and subscales results collected at T1 and T2, and corresponding p-values and size effects, are collected in Table 3. On average, the motor function of participants in our group improved at the end of the intervention. Statistically significant improvements were found for the transitions and stair-climbing RESMES subscales but without a size effect. On the other hand, the total RESMES score showed a statistically significant reduction after the intervention (representing an improvement in global motor functioning) with a large size effect.

Table 3. Descriptive statistics and corresponding *p*-value and effect size of participants' RESMES total and subscales scores.

			Mean (SD)	Median	Range	*p*-Value	Effect Size
RESMES Subscales	Standing	T1	3.2 (4)	1	0–11	0.098	\
		T2	2.6 (3.5)	0	0–10		
	Sitting	T1	1 (2.3)	0	0–9	0.066	\
		T2	0.4 (1)	0	0–3		
	Transition	T1	14.6 (6.7)	16	0–24	0.034 *	0.138
		T2	14.1 (6.7)	13.5	0–24		
	Walking	T1	7.6 (7)	5.5	0–18	0.094	\
		T2	7.1 (6.7)	4.5	0–18		
	Running	T1	4 (0)	4	4–4	1.000	\
		T2	4 (0)	4	4–4		
	Stairs	T1	6.5 (1.8)	6.5	2–8	0.038 *	0.071
		T2	6.1 (1.9)	6	2–8		
RESMES Total		T1	36.8 (19.3)	32.5	6–70	<0.001 *	0.648
		T2	34.3 (18.1)	28.5	6–66		

Abbreviation list: SD = Standard Deviation; RESMES = Rett Syndrome Motor Evaluation Scale; T1 = pre-intervention evaluation meeting; T2 = post-intervention evaluation meeting. *: $p < 0.05$.

A moderate positive correlation ($p = 0.008$; $\rho = 0.574$) was found between the Cobb's angles variation and functional motor level variation (evaluated with RESMES) between T1 and T2. No other correlations were found between the Cobb's angle changes at T2 and the other investigated variables. Participants' individual data are available as Supplementary Material (see Tables S1–S3 in "Tables—Supplementary material", which illustrates each participant's age, genetic mutation, RARS scores, daily physical activity level, scoliosis severity, Cobb's angles, and RESMES scores measured at T1 and T2).

4. Discussion

This paper presented the effect of a six-month remotely supervised individualized motor and postural activity program carried out by parents, therapists, and primary caregivers (when available) with their daughters and clients with RTT. The results suggest that the proposed intervention effectively prevented the participants' scoliosis progression as 70% of participants did not worsen their curves. The available literature reported the absence of progression in 0–17% of cases. [11,16,55] One study reported that 62% of the 21 included participants (age range= 4.3–18 years) did not worsen their curve [56], but this result was never replicated. This finding is significant for the population with RTT that shows a high prevalence of scoliosis (up to 94%). According to a large observational study, only 18.5% of people with RTT and scoliosis undergo spinal surgery [15]. Therefore, most subjects with RTT rely on non-surgical, conservative intervention, such as the one suggested within the current intervention program, to cope with the scoliosis progression. As of today, the existing literature regarding conservative treatments for scoliosis is limited, and the current article presents the first evidence on the established efficacy of a conservative intervention coping with scoliosis progression in people with RTT. The case series available in the literature reported an average annual curve progression ranging from 14–21° Cobb with an acceleration in the progression during adolescence [11,14,16]. Compared to them, participants in our group have shown a much lower progression rate (average Cobb's angle change= $+1.7° \pm 8.7°$ in 12.3 ± 3.5 months) even though the average age of the current intervention program's participants was mid-puberty (15.6 years). Moreover, the participants' motor functional level improved at T2 with a large effect size when considering the global motor function. As the intervention was focused on daily physical activities, this result suggests that the daily performance of such activities had a positive effect also on the participants' global motor functioning. Furthermore, even though no statistical differences or significant effect size were found, a positive trend was identifiable in all the RESMES subscales (except the "running" subscale). The findings of the current intervention program agree with previous reports, suggesting an improvement in functional abilities in RTT after two months of a daily treadmill training program [57]. Similar programs (remote supervision of intensive activity programs for individuals with RTT) performed in different groups and at different locations (Ireland and Italy) have also presented similar results [36,37,58,59]. The correlation between Cobb's angles and RESMES total score variations suggests that a greater improvement in motor functioning is related to a more significant benefit to the scoliotic curve. These findings can be explained by the fact that higher-level functional abilities necessitated more complex dynamical control of the body that requires better integration of sensory information and increased core muscle strength and usage, leading to a better balance in back muscle strength. In support of this consideration, our group statistically improved stair climbing ability, which was related in previous research to better scoliosis outcomes in this population [60]. Moreover, these considerations echo a previous report of Bisgaard and colleagues describing a negative relation between scoliosis entity and motor functioning in adults with RTT [61]. The authors highlighted the need for lifelong rehabilitation and promotion of an active lifestyle to maintain physical health and functional level, which the authors of the current article wholeheartedly support.

Furthermore, when looking at the individual results, in two cases (participants no. 8 and 16) showing unstructured flexible scoliosis, the intervention was able to eliminate the scoliotic curve completely. This result is highly significant as no spontaneous scoliosis curve regression was ever reported in people with RTT. These participants were the youngest in our group and the only two who also learned to walk independently during the intervention. Walking ability development, maintenance, and promotion for as long as possible are strongly recommended by the guidelines for scoliosis management in RTT [12] and were found to be associated with a reduced risk of severe scoliosis development in this population [15,62]. Participant no. 8's case description and pre- and post-intervention radiographs are available in Figure 3.

On the other hand, the curve of two participants (no. 4 and 13) progressed for at least 14° despite the intervention. In both cases, between T1 and T2, the researchers recognized a progressive reduction in mobility. In one case (participant no. 4), this reduction was driven by the scoliosis progression that made it harder and harder for her to move. In the other case (participant no. 13), the increased immobility could be attributed to progressive and painful supination of the right foot that prevented her from standing and walking for a long duration. Therefore, the authors would like to reiterate the importance of starting the intervention at an early age and of the continuative promotion of the motor skills (walking in particular) of people with RTT, as was repeatedly suggested by experts in the field of RTT [63,64].

The absence of correlations between Cobb's angle variations and the other investigated variables, together with the wide range of participants' age and RTT severity level, suggests that the proposed intervention can effectively limit the scoliosis progression of people with RTT at any age and severity level. Interestingly, among the four participants older than 20 years in our group (no. 2, 3, 11, and 18), three reduced their curve (in one case, by 11°—subject no. 11—Figure 4).

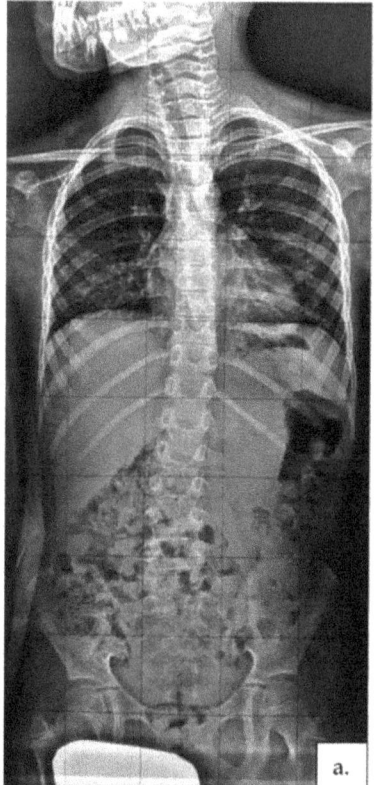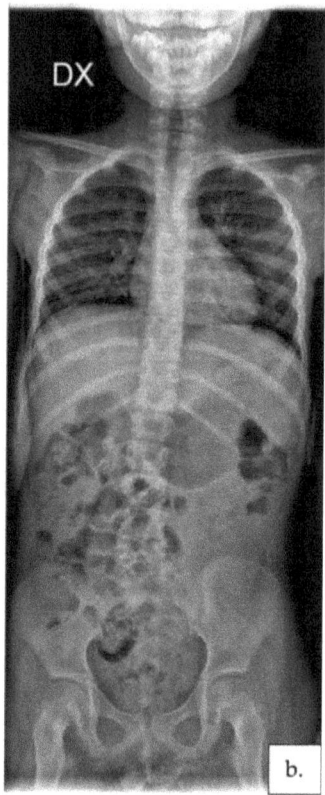

Figure 3. Participant no. 8's X-rays collected before (**a**) and after (**b**) the intervention. She was 6.5 years old at T1. At baseline, she could walk for more than 10 steps supported by one hand and independently stand for 30 s. Lack of efficient balance reaction was recognized at T1. Therefore, her program included intensive balance training and asymmetrical posture maintenance. At the end of the intervention, she could walk for more than 10 steps and stand for more than one minute independently. An improvement of 10° Cobb was recognized at T2.

Moreover, the only subject showing a severe manifestation of RTT (RARS score >81—subject no. 17) also improved her curve of three degrees Cobb (showing the absence of progression). She used to lie down or be fully supported throughout her waking hours. Therefore, in her case and others, the activity program led to a considerable increment in her daily abilities (standing and walking activity with support), bringing positive results for her scoliosis. The above presented cases, as well as others presented within the scope of the present article, reiterate the fact that physical activity is extremely important to those with RTT continuously from a young age and that improvements in functional abilities can be achieved by this group of clients at all severity levels and at all ages.

The main limitation of the present research is that the study design limits the generalization of the results. A randomized controlled trial with a more solid baseline and follow-up is required to verify the robustness of the results. Moreover, the small sample size and the absence of a control group limit the presented results' external validity and robustness. Future studies with larger samples and control groups are needed to establish the cause/effect relationship between the proposed intervention and the obtained results and compare the intervention benefit with other treatment options (such as standard care or bracing regimens). However, the presented investigation demonstrated the feasibility of this type of intervention, proving its effectiveness, in a group of 20 participants with RTT. Another limitation relates to the lack of kyphosis and pelvic obliquity data collection. This information could provide more insight into the participants' full clinical pictures and highlight possible treatment effects on such conditions. Finally, even though one participant qualified as a surgery candidate, the absence of data on the pre-intervention progression trajectory of scoliosis development impeded the evaluation of the proposed treatment efficacy in preventing the surgical intervention.

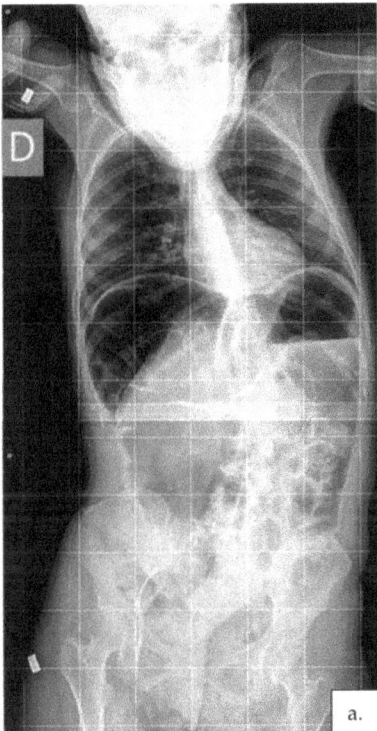 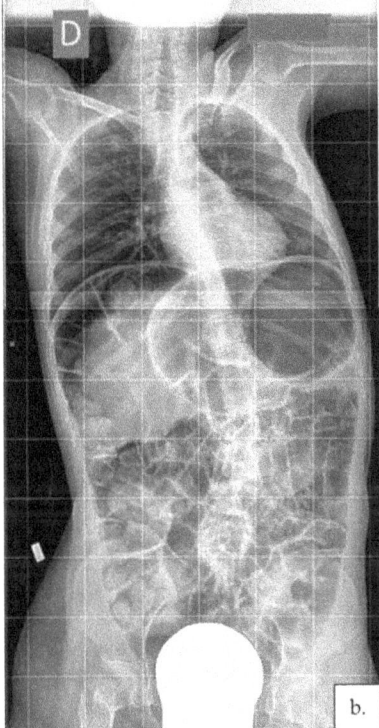

Figure 4. Participant no. 11's radiographs collected before (**a**) and after (**b**) the intervention. She was 31.6 years old at T1 and used to sit with trunk supported for most of her waking hours. She was able to stand and walk only with significant support given at the trunk from behind. During the intervention, she started a daily program of unsupported asymmetrical sitting, walking on a treadmill, and overcorrecting passive posture maintenance. At the end of the intervention, she was able to walk more than 10 steps and stand for more than one minute with support given to the distal section of both hands. An improvement of 11° Cobb was recognized at T2.

5. Conclusions

The present article proposes an effective intervention to prevent scoliosis progression of people with RTT, a population with no established conservative treatments for spinal asymmetries until now. The proposed program was found to be feasible for people with RTT across a wide range of ages and severity levels and can represent a valid strategy to prevent or delay the need for a complex surgery such as spinal fusion. A detailed description of each participant's characteristics and the therapeutic program was presented and can be found online as Supplementary Materials.

Supplementary Materials: The following are available online at https://www.mdpi.com/article/10.3390/jcm11030559/s1, Text file S1: List of proposed activities for each participant, Tables—Supplementary material: Participant's age, genetic mutation, RARS scores, daily physical activity level, scoliosis severity, Cobb's angles, and RESMES scores measured at T1 and T2.

Author Contributions: Conceptualization, A.R. and M.L.; data curation, A.R., M.L. and D.S.M.; formal analysis, A.R., C.R., E.M. and A.S.; funding acquisition, M.L.; investigation, A.R., E.I., M.F. and M.L.; methodology, A.R. and M.L.; project administration, A.R. and M.L.; resources, A.R. and M.L.; supervision, D.S.M.; validation, M.L. and D.S.M.; visualization, E.I., C.R., E.M., M.F. and A.S.; writing—original draft, A.R.; writing—review and editing, A.R., M.L. and D.S.M. All authors have read and agreed to the published version of the manuscript.

Funding: This research was funded by the International Rett Syndrome Foundation, within the HeART grant number 3610.

Institutional Review Board Statement: The study was conducted according to the guidelines of the Declaration of Helsinki and approved by the Institutional Review Board of Ariel University (AU-HEA-ML-20190326-1).

Informed Consent Statement: Informed consent was obtained from all subjects involved in the study. Written informed consent has been obtained from the patients' legal guardians to publish this paper.

Data Availability Statement: Data available as Supplementary Material (see "Tables—Supplementary material").

Acknowledgments: We would like to thank the International Rett Syndrome Association for financially supporting this research project. We would also like to thank the Italian Rett Syndrome Association (AIRett) and the head of the organization, Lucia Dovigo, for supporting this project, connecting researchers and involved families, and constantly supporting the experimentation of therapeutic strategies based on telerehabilitation. Finally, we would also like to thank the parents and individuals with RTT involved in this project.

Conflicts of Interest: The authors declare no conflict of interest. The funders had no role in the design of the study; in the collection, analyses, or interpretation of data; in the writing of the manuscript; or in the decision to publish the results.

References

1. Amir, R.E.; Van den Veyver, I.B.; Wan, M.; Tran, C.Q.; Francke, U.; Zoghbi, H.Y. Rett syndrome is caused by mutations in X-linked MECP2, encoding methyl-CpG-binding protein 2. *Nat. Genet.* **1999**, *23*, 185–188. [CrossRef]
2. Fombonne, E.; Simmons, H.; Ford, T.; Meltzer, H.; Goodman, R. Prevalence of pervasive developmental disorders in the British nationwide survey of child mental health. *Int. Rev. Psychiatry* **2003**, *15*, 158–165. [CrossRef] [PubMed]
3. Skjeldal, O.H.; Von Tetzchner, S.; Aspelund, F.; Herder, G.A.; Lofterød, B. Rett syndrome: Geographic variation in prevalence in Norway. *Brain Dev.* **1997**, *19*, 258–261. [CrossRef]
4. Pini, G.; Milan, M.; Zappella, M. Rett syndrome in Northern Tuscany (Italy): Family tree studies. *Clin. Genet.* **1996**, *50*, 486–490. [CrossRef] [PubMed]
5. Logan, S.W.; Huang, H.H.; Stahlin, K.; Galloway, J.C. Modified ride-on car for mobility and socialization: Single-case study of an infant with down syndrome. *Pediatr. Phys. Ther.* **2014**, *26*, 418–4269. [CrossRef] [PubMed]
6. Hagberg, B.; Witt-Engerström, I.; Opitz, J.M.; Reynolds, J.F. Rett Syndrome: A suggested staging system for describing impairment profile with increasing age towards adolescence. *Am. J. Med. Genet.* **1986**, *25*, 47–59. [CrossRef] [PubMed]
7. Bassett, G.S.; Tolo, V.T. The Incidence and Natural History of Scoliosis in Rett Syndrome. *Dev. Med. Child Neurol.* **1990**, *32*, 963–966. [CrossRef] [PubMed]
8. Ager, S.; Downs, J.; Fyfe, S.; Leonard, H. Parental experiences of scoliosis management in Rett syndrome. *Disabil. Rehabil.* **2009**, *31*, 1917–1924. [CrossRef] [PubMed]
9. Ager, S.; Fyfe, S.; Christodoulou, J.; Jacoby, P.; Schmitt, L.; Leonard, H. Predictors of scoliosis in Rett syndrome. *J. Child Neurol.* **2006**, *21*, 809–813. [CrossRef] [PubMed]
10. Riise, R.; Brox, J.I.; Sorensen, R.; Skjeldal, O.H. Spinal deformity and disability in patients with Rett syndrome. *Dev. Med. Child Neurol.* **2011**, *53*, 653–657. [CrossRef]
11. Lidström, J.; Stokland, E.; Hagberg, B. Scoliosis in rett syndrome clinical and biological aspects. *Spine* **1994**, *19*, 1632–1635. [CrossRef] [PubMed]

12. Downs, J.; Bergman, A.; Carter, P.; Anderson, A.; Palmer, G.M.; Roye, D.; Van Bosse, H.; Bebbington, A.; Larsson, E.L.; Smith, B.G.; et al. Guidelines for management of scoliosis in rett syndrome patients based on expert consensus and clinical evidence. *Spine* **2009**, *34*, E607–E617. [CrossRef] [PubMed]
13. Percy, A.K.; Lee, H.S.; Neul, J.L.; Lane, J.B.; Skinner, S.A.; Geerts, S.P.; Annese, F.; Graham, J.; McNair, L.; Motil, K.J.; et al. Profiling scoliosis in rett syndrome. *Pediatr. Res.* **2010**, *67*, 435–439. [CrossRef] [PubMed]
14. Huang, T.J.; Lubicky, J.P.; Hammerberg, K.W. Scoliosis in Rett syndrome. *Orthop. Rev.* **1994**, *23*, 931–937. [CrossRef]
15. Killian, J.T.; Lane, J.B.; Lee, H.S.; Skinner, S.A.; Kaufmann, W.E.; Glaze, D.G.; Neul, J.L.; Percy, A.K. Scoliosis in Rett Syndrome: Progression, Comorbidities, and Predictors. *Pediatr. Neurol.* **2017**, *70*, 20–25. [CrossRef]
16. Harrison, D.J.; Webb, P.J. Scoliosis in the rett syndrome: Natural history and treatment. *Brain Dev.* **1990**, *12*, 154–156. [CrossRef]
17. Downs, J.; Torode, I.; Wong, K.; Ellaway, C.; Elliott, E.J.; Christodoulou, J.; Jacoby, P.; Thomson, M.R.; Izatt, M.T.; Askin, G.N.; et al. The natural history of scoliosis in females with rett syndrome. *Spine* **2016**, *41*, 856–863. [CrossRef]
18. Neul, J.L.; Fang, P.; Barrish, J.; Lane, J.; Caeg, E.B.; Smith, E.O.; Zoghbi, H.; Percy, A.; Glaze, D.G. Specific mutations in methyl-CpG-binding protein 2 confer different severity in Rett syndrome. *Neurology* **2008**, *70*, 1313–1321. [CrossRef]
19. Mehta, J.S.; Gibson, M.J. The Treatment of Neuromuscular Scoliosis. *Curr. Orthop.* **2003**, *17*, 313–321. [CrossRef]
20. Westerlund, L.E.; Gill, S.S.; Jarosz, T.S.; Abel, M.F.; Blanco, J.S. Posterior-only unit rod instrumentation and fusion for neuromuscular scoliosis. *Spine* **2001**, *26*, 1984–1989. [CrossRef]
21. Rocos, B.; Zeller, R. Correcting Scoliosis in Rett Syndrome. *Cureus* **2021**, *13*, e15411. [CrossRef]
22. Barney, C.C.; Merbler, A.M.; Quest, K.; Byiers, B.J.; Wilcox, G.L.; Schwantes, S.; Roiko, S.A.; Feyma, T.; Beisang, A.; Symons, F.J. A case-controlled comparison of postoperative analgesic dosing between girls with Rett syndrome and girls with and without developmental disability undergoing spinal fusion surgery. *Pediatr. Anaesth.* **2017**, *27*, 290–299. [CrossRef]
23. Larsson, E.L.; Aaro, S.; Ahlinder, P.; Normelli, H.; Tropp, H.; Öberg, B. Long-term follow-up of functioning after spinal surgery in patients with Rett syndrome. *Eur. Spine J.* **2009**, *18*, 506–511. [CrossRef]
24. Downs, J.; Young, D.; de Klerk, N.; Bebbington, A.; Baikie, G.; Leonard, H. Impact of scoliosis surgery on activities of daily living in females with Rett syndrome. *J. Pediatr. Orthop.* **2009**, *29*, 369–374. [CrossRef]
25. Downs, J.; Torode, I.; Wong, K.; Ellaway, C.; Elliott, E.J.; Izatt, M.T.; Askin, G.N.; Mcphee, B.I.; Cundy, P.; Leonard, H.; et al. Surgical fusion of early onset severe scoliosis increases survival in Rett syndrome: A cohort study. *Dev. Med. Child Neurol.* **2016**, *58*, 632–638. [CrossRef]
26. Kerr, A.M.; Webb, P.; Prescott, R.J.; Milne, Y. Results of surgery for scoliosis in Rett syndrome. *J. Child Neurol.* **2003**, *18*, 703–708. [CrossRef] [PubMed]
27. Roberts, S.B.; Tsirikos, A.I. Factors influencing the evaluation and management of neuromuscular scoliosis: A review of the literature. *J. Back Musculoskelet. Rehabil.* **2016**, *29*, 613–623. [CrossRef] [PubMed]
28. Weiss, H.R.; Negrini, S.; Rigo, M.; Kotwicki, T.; Hawes, M.C.; Grivas, T.B.; Maruyama, T.; Landauer, F. Indications for conservative management of scoliosis (guidelines). *Scoliosis* **2006**, *1*, 5. [CrossRef] [PubMed]
29. Kotwicki, T.; Jozwiak, M. Conservative management of neuromuscular scoliosis: Personal experience and review of literature. *Disabil. Rehabil.* **2008**, *30*, 792–798. [CrossRef] [PubMed]
30. Karimi, M.; Rabczuk, T. Scoliosis conservative treatment: A review of literature. *J. Craniovertebral Junction Spine* **2018**, *9*, 3. [CrossRef]
31. Haleem, S.; Nnadi, C. Scoliosis: A review. *Pediatr. Child Health* **2018**, *28*, 209–217. [CrossRef]
32. Ferrari, A.; Ferrara, C.; Balugani, M.; Sassi, S. Severe scoliosis in neurodevelopmental disabilities: Clinical signs and therapeutic proposals. *Eur. J. Phys. Rehabil. Med.* **2010**, *46*, 563–579.
33. Downs, J.; Torode, I.; Ellaway, C.; Jacoby, P.; Bunting, C.; Wong, K.; Christodoulou, J.; Leonard, H. Family satisfaction following spinal fusion in Rett syndrome. *Dev. Neurorehabil.* **2016**, *19*, 31–37. [CrossRef] [PubMed]
34. Olafsson, Y.; Saraste, H.; Al-Dabbagh, Z. Brace treatment in neuromuscular spine deformity. *Stud. Health Technol. Inform.* **1999**, *59*, 332–335. [CrossRef]
35. Lotan, M.; Merrick, J.; Carmeli, E. Managing scoliosis in a young child with Rett syndrome: A case study. *ScientificWorldJournal*. **2005**, *5*, 264–273. [CrossRef]
36. Lotan, M.; Downs, J.; Elefant, C. A Pilot Study Delivering Physiotherapy Support for Rett Syndrome Using a Telehealth Framework Suitable for COVID-19 Lockdown. *Dev. Neurorehabil.* **2021**, 429–434. [CrossRef]
37. Romano, A.; Di Rosa, G.; Tisano, A.; Fabio, R.A.; Lotan, M. Effects of a remotely supervised motor rehabilitation program for individuals with Rett syndrome at home. *Disabil. Rehabil.* **2021**, 1–11. [CrossRef]
38. Fabio, R.A.; Martinazzoli, C.; Antonietti, A. Development and standardization of the "rars" (Rett assessment rating scale). *Life Span Disabil.* **2005**, *8*, 257–281.
39. Romano, A.; Caprì, T.; Semino, M.; Bizzego, I.; Di Rosa, G.; Fabio, R.A. Gross Motor, Physical Activity and Musculoskeletal Disorder Evaluation Tools for Rett Syndrome: A Systematic Review. *Dev. Neurorehabil.* **2020**, *23*, 485–501. [CrossRef]
40. Stahlhut, M.; Hill, K.; Bisgaard, A.M.; Jensen, A.K.; Andersen, M.; Leonard, H.; Downs, J. Measurement of Sedentary Behaviors or "downtime" in Rett Syndrome. *J. Child Neurol.* **2017**, *32*, 1009–1013. [CrossRef]
41. Lor, L.; Hill, K.; Jacoby, P.; Leonard, H.; Downs, J. A validation study of a modified Bouchard activity record that extends the concept of "uptime" to Rett syndrome. *Dev. Med. Child Neurol.* **2015**, *57*, 1137–1142. [CrossRef] [PubMed]

42. Rodocanachi Roidi, M.L.; Isaias, I.U.; Cozzi, F.; Grange, F.; Scotti, F.M.; Gestra, V.F.; Gandini, A.; Ripamonti, E. A New Scale to Evaluate Motor Function in Rett Syndrome: Validation and Psychometric Properties. *Pediatr. Neurol.* **2019**, *100*, 80–86. [CrossRef] [PubMed]
43. Rodocanachi Roidi, M.L.; Isaias, I.U.; Cozzi, F.; Grange, F.; Scotti, F.M.; Gestra, V.F.; Gandini, A.; Ripamonti, E. Motor function in Rett syndrome: Comparing clinical and parental assessments. *Dev. Med. Child Neurol.* **2019**, *61*, 957–963. [CrossRef]
44. Horng, M.-H.; Kuok, C.-P.; Fu, M.-J.; Lin, C.-J.; Sun, Y.-N. Cobb angle measurement of spine from X-ray images using convolutional neural network. *Comput. Math. Methods Med.* **2019**, *2019*, 6357171. [CrossRef]
45. Hanks, S.B. Motor disabilities in the rett syndrome and physical therapy strategies. *Brain Dev.* **1990**, *12*, 157–161. [CrossRef]
46. Uyanik, M.; Bumin, G.; Kayihan, H. Comparison of different therapy approaches in children with Down syndrome. *Pediatr. Int.* **2003**, *45*, 68–73. [CrossRef]
47. Tomczak, E. The need to report effect size estimates revisited. An overview of some recommended measures of effect size Language and cognition: L2 influence on conceptualization of motion and event construal. View project. *Trends Sport Sci.* **2014**, *21*, 19–25.
48. King, B.M.; Minium, E.W. *Statistical Reasoning in the Behavioral Sciences*, 7th ed.; John Wiley & Sons, Inc.: Hoboken, NJ, USA, 2008; ISBN 9780470134870.
49. Ottenbacher, K.J. Why Rehabilitation Research Does Not Work (As Well as We Think It Should). *Arch. Phys. Med. Rehabil.* **1995**, *76*, 123–129. [CrossRef]
50. Cohen, J. *Statistical Power Analysis for the Behavioral Sciences*, 2nd ed.; Lawrence Erlbaum Associates: New York, NY, USA, 1988; ISBN 0805802835.
51. Thompson, B. Effect sizes, confidence intervals, and confidence intervals for effect sizes. *Psychol. Sch.* **2007**, *44*, 423–432. [CrossRef]
52. Cohen, J. A power primer. *Psychol. Bull.* **1992**, *112*, 155–159. [CrossRef] [PubMed]
53. Kinney, A.R.; Eakman, A.M.; Graham, J.E. Novel Effect Size Interpretation Guidelines and an Evaluation of Statistical Power in Rehabilitation Research. *Arch. Phys. Med. Rehabil.* **2020**, *101*, 2219–2226. [CrossRef] [PubMed]
54. Armstrong, R.A. When to use the Bonferroni correction. *Ophthalmic Physiol. Opt.* **2014**, *34*, 502–508. [CrossRef]
55. Keret, D.; Bassett, G.S.; Bunnell, W.P.; Marks, H.G. Scoliosis in Rett syndrome. *J. Pediatr. Orthop.* **1988**, *8*, 138–142. [CrossRef]
56. Loder, R.T.; Lee, C.L.; Richards, B.S. Orthopedic aspects of Rett syndrome: A multicenter review. *J. Pediatr. Orthop.* **1989**, *9*, 557–562. [CrossRef] [PubMed]
57. Lotan, M.; Isakov, E.; Merrick, J. Improving functional skills and physical fitness in children with Rett syndrome. *J. Intellect. Disabil. Res.* **2004**, *48*, 730–735. [CrossRef]
58. Lotan, M.; Ippolito, E.; Favetta, M.; Romano, A. Skype Supervised, Individualized, Home-Based Rehabilitation Programs for Individuals With Rett Syndrome and Their Families—Parental Satisfaction and Point of View. *Front. Psychol.* **2021**, *12*, 3995. [CrossRef] [PubMed]
59. Lotan, M.; Stahlhut, M.; Romano, A.; Downs, J.; Elefant, C. Family-Centered Telehealth Supporting Motor Skills and Activity in Individuals With Rett Syndrome. In *Assistive Technologies for Assessment and Recovery of Neurological Impairments*; Stasolla, F., Ed.; IGI Global: Hershey, PA, USA, 2022; pp. 147–171.
60. Hagberg, B.; Anvret, M.; Wahlstrom, J. *Rett Syndrome—Clinical and Biological Aspects: Studies on 130 Swedish Females*; MacKeith Press Press: London, UK, 1993; ISBN 0521412838.
61. Bisgaard, A.M.; Wong, K.; Højfeldt, A.K.; Larsen, J.L.; Schönewolf-Greulich, B.; Rønde, G.; Downs, J.; Stahlhut, M. Decline in gross motor skills in adult Rett syndrome; results from a Danish longitudinal study. *Am. J. Med. Genet. Part A* **2021**, *185*, 3683–3693. [CrossRef] [PubMed]
62. McClure, M.K.; Battaglia, C.; McClure, R.J. The Relationship of Cumulative Motor Asymmetries to Scoliosis in Rett Syndrome. *Am. J. Occup. Ther.* **1998**, *52*, 196–204. [CrossRef] [PubMed]
63. Lotan, M.; Merrick, J.; Kandel, I.; Morad, M. Aging in persons with Rett syndrome: An updated review. *ScientificWorldJournal* **2010**, *10*, 778–787. [CrossRef] [PubMed]
64. Lotan, M.; Merrick, J. *Rett Syndrome: Therapeutic Interventions*; Nova Science Publishers Inc.: Hauppauge, NY, USA, 2011; ISBN 978-1-61728-080-1.

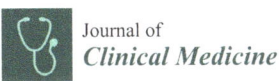

Article

Neurodynamic Functions and Their Correlations with Postural Parameters in Adolescents with Idiopathic Scoliosis

Agnieszka Stępień [1,2,*] and Beata Pałdyna [2]

1. Department of Rehabilitation, Józef Piłsudski University of Physical Education, 00-968 Warsaw, Poland
2. ORTHOS Functional Rehabilitation Centre, 02-793 Warsaw, Poland; beata.paldyna@gmail.com
* Correspondence: orthosas@wp.pl

Abstract: Knowledge about neurodynamic functions of the nervous system (NS) in patients with idiopathic scoliosis (IS) is limited. This study aimed to assess the mechanosensitivity of the NS structures (MNS) in adolescents with IS. The study included 69 adolescents with IS and 57 healthy peers aged 10–15 years. The Upper Limb Neurodynamic Test 1 (ULNT1), straight leg raise (SLR) test, and slump test (SLUMP) were used to assess MNS. The spinal curvatures in the sagittal plane and selected ranges of motion were measured. The data were analysed using the Mann–Whitney U test and Spearman's rank correlation. Increased MNS assessed by ULNT1 and SLUMP tests was observed in participants with IS. Values of the neurodynamic tests correlated significantly with the sagittal profile of the spine and the mobility of the spine and lower limbs in both groups. In conclusion, increased MNS occurs in adolescents with IS. Therefore, the examination of adolescents with IS should include an assessment of MNS with the neurodynamic tests. Future studies should investigate this issue to better understand the mechanisms that coexist with IS.

Keywords: idiopathic scoliosis; neurodynamic functions; assessment; pain; treatment

Citation: Stępień, A.; Pałdyna, B. Neurodynamic Functions and Their Correlations with Postural Parameters in Adolescents with Idiopathic Scoliosis. *J. Clin. Med.* **2022**, *11*, 1115. https://doi.org/10.3390/jcm11041115

Academic Editor: Theodoros B. Grivas

Received: 24 November 2021
Accepted: 17 February 2022
Published: 19 February 2022

Publisher's Note: MDPI stays neutral with regard to jurisdictional claims in published maps and institutional affiliations.

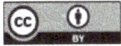

Copyright: © 2022 by the authors. Licensee MDPI, Basel, Switzerland. This article is an open access article distributed under the terms and conditions of the Creative Commons Attribution (CC BY) license (https://creativecommons.org/licenses/by/4.0/).

1. Introduction

Various co-existent abnormalities have been described in patients with idiopathic scoliosis (IS), but knowledge about the neurodynamic functions of the nervous system (NS) is still limited [1,2].

Neurodynamics is the science of the correlations between the mechanics and physiology of the nervous system, as well as between assessment and therapy [3–5]. This field of medicine has been developing intensively for several decades.

The literature indicates that tensile loading is necessary for mechanical adaptation and the normal functioning of neurons and nerves [3,4]. Various aspects of adverse neural mechanics have been presented in the past. It is known that mechanical disorders, such as disturbed tensile strength, nerve gliding disturbance (the limited movement of the neural structures relative to other tissues) or compression (pressure-induced deformation) of the nerve, may decrease neural tissue extensibility and cause irritation. In this case, these structures become sensitive to tensile forces [3]. Some authors of the neurodynamic concept strongly emphasised that many neural problems have their causes in the musculoskeletal system. They suggested that the structures of NS follow the body's movements and are mechanically loaded during daily activities [3].

Mechanosensitivity of the NS structures (MNS) can be detected with the neurodynamic tests. These tests are designed to apply tensile forces to the tissues of NS. Elongation is applied to the neural tissues by increasing the distance between the ends of the nerve tract [3]. Impaired MNS may be manifested by pain, reduced range of motion or sensory disturbances. The neurodynamic tests were used mainly to examine the patients with various impairments in the musculoskeletal system and evaluate the effects of the therapy.

Tensioning techniques were the first neurodynamic techniques applied to treat patients with neuropathies. Later, sliding techniques were developed [4]. The positive effect of neural mobilisation on neuromusculoskeletal conditions has been observed, especially its benefits for back and neck pain [6,7]. Current studies analysing tensioning techniques revealed neuroimmune, neurophysiological, and neurochemical effects in the structures of the nervous system [4].

Previous studies have demonstrated various tests such as (1) the upper limb neurodynamic test 1 (ULNT1), which assesses length and mobility of the peripheral NS in an upper limb [8,9], (2) the straight leg raise (SLR) test with ankle dorsiflexion, which is often used in patients with back and lower limb pain [10–13], or (3) the slump (SLUMP) test, which assess the correlations between the patient's symptoms and movement limitations in the pain-sensitive structures located in the spinal canal and intervertebral foramen [10,12]. The studies have proven the reliability of ULNT1 [14–16], SLR [13,17,18], and SLUMP tests [17,18]. Moreover, the ULNT1, SLR, and SLUMP tests have been used mainly to assess back and leg pain among adults [10,12]. However, the utility of the tests in individuals without symptoms has also been investigated [11,16,19].

A few studies revealed that a limited range of motion in the SLR test might also be applied during the period of childrens' growth [9]. The SLR test was also used in a study of children with cerebral palsy [20]. In addition, the modified long sitting slump test was applied to examine children with headaches compared to healthy controls [21]. However, no study has examined neurodynamic functions in adolescents with IS. There have been no analyses of correlations between neural tissue extensibility, alignment of spinal curvatures in the sagittal plane, angle of trunk rotation (ATR), or ranges of motion. Given that a three-plane change in the position of the spine axis alters the vectors of forces acting on the body, spinal misalignment in individuals with IS may theoretically affect MNS.

Current literature presents different opinions regarding back pain in adolescents with scoliosis. Some researchers have reported back pain in this population [22–25], but others have argued that pain is not the primary problem related to IS [26]. In establishing the goals of IS treatment, experts of the International Society on Scoliosis Orthopaedic and Rehabilitation Treatment (SOSORT) indicated aesthetics, quality of life, and disability as the most important. However, pain prevention and reduction were included as equally important goals. The SOSORT guidelines have not included recommendations for assessing neurodynamic functions in individuals with IS [2,27].

Given the lack of knowledge regarding the neurodynamic of the NS in individuals with spine deformity, this study aimed to assess MNS, expressed by ranges of motion in neurodynamic tests, in adolescents with IS. Moreover, the correlations between MNS and selected postural parameters were analysed. Finally, the results were compared with those obtained in a group of healthy peers.

2. Materials and Methods

The study was conducted after being approved by the Senate Bioethical Commission at the Józef Piłsudski University of Physical Education in Warsaw (SKE 01-30/2020). The participants were informed about the study aims during consultations in the physiotherapy centre specialising in postural disorders prevention and spinal deformities treatment.

Participants self-reported directly to physiotherapists without referrals from other specialists. In addition, legal guardians of children gave written consent to participate in the study.

2.1. Participants

The criteria for inclusion in the study group were as follows: girls and boys aged 10–15 years, single-curve (a left-sided lumbar/thoracolumbar curve) or double-curve (a right-sided thoracic curve and a left-sided lumbar/thoracolumbar curve) IS confirmed by radiological examination with Cobb angle value of more than 10°, absence of central nervous system disorders, chronic respiratory system diseases, metabolic or oncological diseases, injuries, and fractures within the previous 6 months. The control group included girls and boys aged 10–15 years without systemic diseases and with an angle of ATR of 0–5°, as measured by a Bunnell scoliometer.

2.2. Measures

The study was carried out during individual physiotherapeutic consultations in the rehabilitation centre. The participants were examined by two physiotherapists with over 25 and 15 years of experience treating patients with IS. Both physiotherapists completed manual therapy training, including examination with neurodynamic tests. They met three times before the beginning of the study to unify the study methodology and manner of performing the tests. The physiotherapists were not blinded to the existence of scoliosis when examining the participants, as symptoms of scoliosis are usually visible.

At the beginning of the study, basic information regarding IS, the type of treatment (physiotherapy, brace), the occurrence of pain in the last 3 months, and pain localisation was collected. The question of pain prevalence was general. The type of pain and its occurrence and severity were not assessed.

The study included the following measurements: (1) body height and mass, (2) the ranges of motion in ULNT1, SLR, and SLUMP on the left and right side of the body, (3) ATR, (4) spinal curvatures in the sagittal plane (cervicothoracic junction—C, thoracic upper—T1, thoracolumbar junction—T2, lumbosacral junction—LS), (5) ranges of cervical rotation (CR), (6) hip joint extension with flexion of the knee (HE), (7) hip joint flexion with the extension of the knee joint (HF), (8) and rotation mobility of the lumbo-pelvic-hip complex with trunk-pelvis-hip angle (TPHA) on both sides of the body, (9) the fingertip-to-floor (FTF) test, and (10) generalised joint hypermobility (JHM) using the Beighton scale.

The abbreviations of the tests used in this study are presented in Figure 1. In addition, the test methodology is described below.

Neurodynamic tests
- ULNT1   Upper Limb Neurodynamic Test
- SLR   Straight Leg Raise Test
- SLUMP   Slump Test

Postural parameters
- ATRT   Angle of Trunk Rotation Thoracic
- ATRL   Angle of Trunk Rotation Lumbar
- Sternum sternum inclination
- C   inclination of the cervicothoracic junction
- T1   inclination of the upperthoracic spine
- T2   inclination of the thoracolumbar junction
- LS   inclination of the lumbosacral junction

Ranges of motion / mobility
- FTF   Fingertip-To-Floortest
- CR   Cervical Rotation
- HE   Hip Extension
- HF   Hip Flexion with knee extension
- TPHA   Trunk-Pelvis-Hip Angle
- JHM   Joint Hypermobility (Beightonscale)

Figure 1. List of abbreviations for parameters used in this paper.

The ULNT1 test [14–16] was performed with a patient lying on a table with an upper limb abducted by 90° and the head in a neutral position. The physiotherapist stabilised the arm and elbow of the patient with one upper limb, while the opposite upper limb performed wrist dorsiflexion, finger extension, forearm supination, shoulder joint external rotation, and elbow extension until the first feeling of tension. Verification of the affected structure was performed by moving the head to the tested side. Decreased symptoms meant disturbed NS slides. The range of motion was measured with a goniometer by placing the rotational axis along the axis of the elbow joint (Figure 2A,B). Lower values of the ULNT1 ranges meant greater neural tissue extensibility.

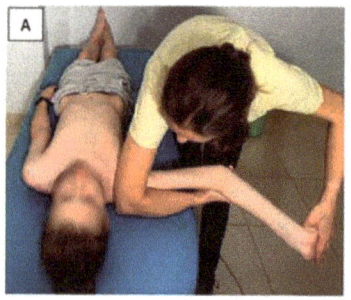 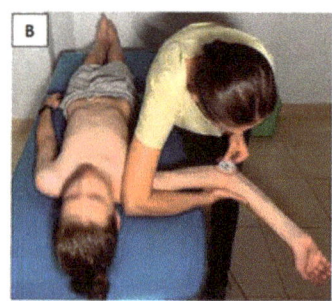

A. Upper Limb Neurodynamic Test (ULNT1)
B. ULNT1 measurement with a goniometer

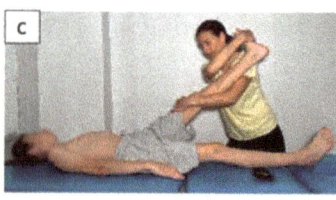 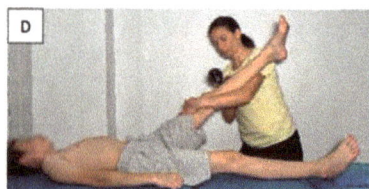

C. Straight Leg Raise test (SLR)
D. SLR measurement with the Rippstein plurimeter

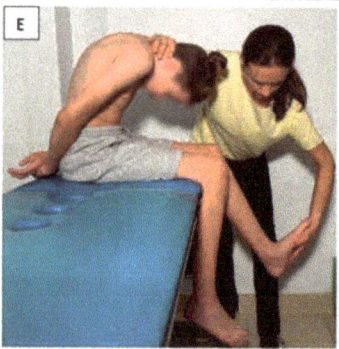 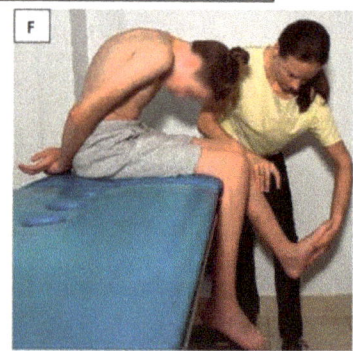

E. Slump test (SLUMP)
F. SLUMP measurement with the Rippstein plurimeter

Figure 2. Neurodynamic tests used in this study: (**A,B**) ULNT1, (**C,D**) SLR, (**E,F**) SLUMP.

The SLR test [11,13,19] was performed in a supine position. The physiotherapist initially arranged the patient's ankle joint in a neutral position, blocked the knee joint in extension, and then passively raised the lower limb until the first sign of tension. The patient's feelings were verified by plantar flexion in the ankle joint. Decreased symptoms meant disturbed peripheral NS slides. The measurement was performed with a Rippstein plurimeter zeroed horizontally and placed at the lower leg distally from the tibial tuberosity (Figure 2C,D). Higher values of SLR ranges meant greater extensibility of neural structures.

SLUMP test [17,18] was performed on a patient in a sitting position, with the neck and trunk bent forward and the sacral bone in a vertical position. The patient joined the upper limbs behind the back. A physiotherapist placed one hand on the back of the patient's neck and extended the patient's knee joint with the other hand until the first feeling of tension, at the same time maintaining the ankle joint in a neutral position. The measurement was made with a plurimeter placed at the lower leg below the tibial tuberosity. Verification of the affected structure was made based on the extended cervical segment of the spine (moving the chin away from the neck) (Figure 2E,F). Decreased symptoms meant disturbed NS slides. Lower values of the SLUMP ranges indicate greater neural tissue extensibility. Measurements with a plurimeter during SLR and SLUMP tests have been used in previous studies [12].

The ATR measurement in the thoracic and lumbar segments was performed with a scoliometer in a standing position, with the trunk bent forward. The reliability of this measurement has been assessed in the past. This test is widely used in screening for scoliosis and assessing the effects of treatment in patients with scoliosis [28,29].

The position of the spine in the sagittal plane was assessed with the Rippstein plurimeter zeroed vertically and placed at the cervical-thoracic junction (C), in the upper part of the thoracic spine (T1—spine segment Th1–Th3), at the thoracic–lumbar (T2—spine segment Th11–L1) and lumbosacral junction (LS—spine segment L5–S1). Moreover, the position of the sternum was measured by placing a plurimeter on the upper part of the sternum. In previous studies based on a similar methodology, the Rippstein plurimeter was used to assess the curvatures of the spine in the sagittal plane in children with scoliosis and healthy controls [30,31].

The ranges of hip flexion with knee extension and extension in the hip joint with knee flexion were measured in a supine position according to a widely applied methodology [32]. A plurimeter zeroed parallel to the floor was placed on the thigh above the patella when the hip joint was extended. In the past, the measurement of extension in hip joints made with the plurimeter proved to be a reliable test in children with neuromuscular disease [33]. Therefore, when measuring flexion in the hip joint with extension in the knee joint, the plurimeter was placed at the lower leg below the tibial tuberosity, similarly to the SLR and SLUMP tests.

The mobility of the lumbo-pelvic-hip complex was measured using the TPHA test using a plurimeter zeroed parallel to the floor. Values below the horizontal (greater ranges of movement) were designated as "+" in this study, and values above the level (movement restriction) were designated as "−". Previous studies have confirmed the good reliability of the TPHA test, which was used in adolescents with IS and their healthy peers [34,35].

Also, the FTF test has been used in previous studies in people with back pain. The good validity of this test has been demonstrated [13,36].

2.3. Statistical Analysis

Statistical analyses were performed using STATISTICA version 13. Normal distribution was assessed with the Shapiro–Wilk test. Due to the lack of a normal distribution, the Mann–Whitney U test was used to determine any differences between the tested parameters in both groups. Spearman's rank correlation coefficient was used to analyse the correlations between the parameters. Correlations were interpreted as: <0.3, —negligible correlation; 0.3–0.5, low correlation; 0.5–0.7, moderate correlation; 0.7–0.9, high correlation; and >0.9, very high correlation [37]. Quantitative variables were described as median ± quarter deviation; however, means ± SD were presented as additional information. The qualitative variables were analysed using the chi-square test. We adopted $p = 0.05$ as the level of significance.

3. Results

The study included 126 individuals: 69 patients with IS and 57 controls without scoliosis (C). The groups did not differ significantly in terms of age, body mass, or body height. In both groups, there were more girls than boys. There were definitely more adolescents with double-curve scoliosis in the IS group than with single-curve scoliosis. Within this group, the Cobb angle range was 11° to 69°. In total, 25 participants (36.3%) had low scoliosis at 11–20°, 41 were diagnosed with scoliosis at 21–50° (59.4%), and 3 participants (4.3%) had a Cobb angle greater than 50°. Most of the IS participants confirmed their participation in physiotherapy sessions. The pain was more common in adolescents with spinal deformities than in the control group. In both groups, the pain was most often located in the thoracic and lumbar segments of the spine. Detailed information on all of the participants is included in Table 1.

Table 1. Characteristics of adolescents with idiopathic scoliosis (IS) and the control group (C).

Characteristics	Idiopathic Scoliosis (n = 69)	Control Group (n = 57)	p
Age [years]			0.410
Median ± Q (range)	13.0 ± 1.5 (11.0–14.0)	12.0 ± 1.5 (11.0–14.0)	
Mean ± SD (range)	12.7 ± 1.7 (10.0–15.0)	12.4 ± 1.7 (10.0–15.0)	
Body mass [kg]			0.944
Median ± Q (range)	49.0 ± 5.0 (44.0–54.0)	48.0 ± 7.5 (40.0–55.0)	
Mean ± SD (range)	48.0 ± 10.2 (28.0–71.0)	47.9 ± 12.0 (29.0–75.0)	
Body height [cm]			0.815
Median ± Q (range)	160.0 ± 6.5 (154.0–167.0)	162.0 ± 10.0 (148.0–168.0)	
Mean ± SD (range)	159.3 ± 10.9 (132.0–181.0)	158.8 ± 12.5 (136.0–186.0)	
Gender n (%)			
Girls	57 (82.6%)	42 (73.7%)	
Boys	12 (17.4%)	15 (26.3%)	
Cobb angle [°]			
Double scoliosis Th	n = 54 (78.3%)		
Median ± Q (range)	22.5 ± 6.5 (20.0–33.0)		
Mean ± SD (range)	26.1 ± 12.6 (11.0–69.0)		
Double scoliosis L	n = 54 (78.3%)		
Median ± Q (range)	23.00 ± 7.50 (15.0–30.0)		
Mean ± SD (range)	24.8 ± 11.5 (11.0–68.0)		
Single scoliosis ThL	n = 15 (21.7%)		
Median ± Q (range)	16.0 ± 5.0 (15.0–25.0)		
Mean ± SD (range)	24.9 ± 11.5 (11.0–45.0)		
Physiotherapy (last year) n (%)	54 (78.3%)	18 (31.6%)	<0.001
Brace n (%)	25 (36.2%)	-	
Pain (last 3 months) n (%)	26 (37.7%)	7 (12.3%)	0.001
Head	3 (4.3%)	0 (0.0%)	
Back pain	20 (29.0%)	6 (10.5%)	
Cervical spine	5 (7.2%)	0 (0.0%)	
Thoracic spine	12 (17.4%)	4 (7.0%)	
Lumbar spine	15 (21.7%)	4 (7.0%)	
Upper limbs	1 (1.4%)	0 (0.0%)	
Lower limbs	4 (5.8%)	2 (3.5%)	
Several body parts	13 (18.8%)	3 (5.3%)	

Abbreviations: Q, quartiles; SD, standard deviation; n, number of participants; p, statistical significance.

3.1. Neurodynamic Tests, Postural Parameters, and Range of Motion

Significantly lower ranges of ULNT1 and SLUMP tests (lower extensibility) were observed on both sides of the body in participants with scoliosis compared to the control group. The SLR test values did not differ significantly (Figure 3, Table 2). Increased ULNT1left values (5° or more) were found in 36 adolescents with scoliosis (52.2%) and 12 (17.4%) healthy participants. Increased ULNT1right values occurred in 36 participants with scoliosis (52.2%) and 14 (20.3%) controls. The values of SLRleft and SLRright less than 60° (lower extensibility) were achieved by 36 participants with IS (52.2%) and 26 controls (45.6%). A group of 49 adolescents with IS (71.0%) and 23 participants without scoliosis (40.4%) achieved a SLUMPleft of more than 20° (higher neural tension). A SLUMPright greater than 20° was found in 53 participants with IS (76.8%) and 22 healthy (38.6%) participants.

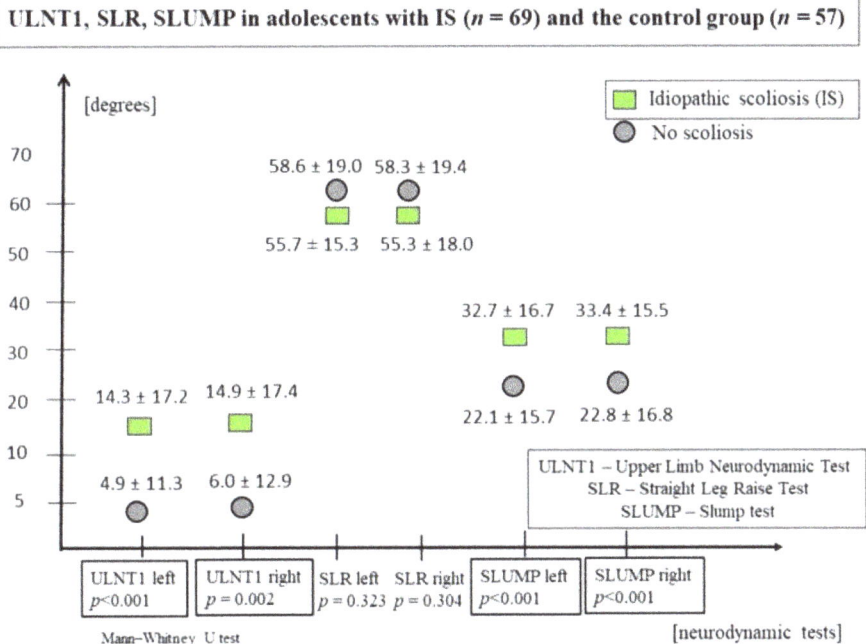

Figure 3. ULNT1, SLR and SLUMP values in adolescents with IS and in the control group.

During the analysis, we checked how many participants had unequal ranges of neurodynamic tests on the left and right sides of the body, assuming a 5° difference as asymmetry. In 31 (44.9%) individuals with scoliosis, there were differences between the ULNT1 ranges on the left and right sides, equal to or larger than 5°. In the control group, asymmetry was noted in only 10 (17.5%) out of 57 adolescents. The SLR test revealed a minimum 5° difference in 23 (33.3%) participants with scoliosis and 8 controls (14.0%). The SLUMP measurements were not equal (minimum 5°) in 23 (33.3%) adolescents with spine deformity and in 8 (14.0%) participants without scoliosis. The differences between the mean values of the neurodynamic tests (ULNT1, SLR, and SLUMP) on both sides of the body were not significant in the IS patients and the control group. Detailed analysis of left/right asymmetry in the neurodynamic tests showed that limitation of the range of motion occurs with a similar frequency of 40–60% on both the left and right sides of the body in participants with IS (limitations: ULNT1left 54.8%, ULNT1right 45.2%, SLRleft 43.5%, SLRright 56.5%, SLUMPleft 47.8%, SLUMPright 52.5%).

Table 2. The values of neurodynamic tests, postural parameters and ranges of motion in adolescents with idiopathic scoliosis (IS) and the control group (C).

Measurements	Idiopathic Scoliosis (n = 69)		Control Group (n = 57)		p
	Median ± Q	Mean ± SD	Median ± Q	Mean ± SD	
Neurodynamic tests (°)					
ULNT1left	5.0 ± 15.0 ***	14.3 ± 17.2	0.0 ± 0.0	4.9 ± 11.3	<0.001
ULNT1right	5.0 ± 15.0 **	14.9 ± 17.4	0.0 ± 0.0	6.0 ± 12.9	0.002
SLRleft	58.0 ± 15.0	55.7 ± 15.2	60.0 ± 17.5	58.6 ± 19.0	0.323
SLRright	58.0 ± 15.0	55.3 ± 18.00	60.0 ± 17.0	58.3 ± 19.4	0.304
SLUMPleft	35.0 ± 22.0 ***	32.7 ± 16.7	18.0 ± 12.0	22.1 ± 15.7	<0.001
SLUMPright	36.0 ± 21.5 ***	33.4 ± 15.5	17.0 ± 11.3	22.8 ± 16.8	<0.001
Postural parameters (°)					
ATRT	6.0 ± 3.5 ***	6.9 ± 4.9	2.0 ± 1.5	2.0 ± 1.9	<0.001
ATRL	4.0 ± 2.0 ***	4.2 ± 3.8	1.0 ± 1.0	1.4 ± 1.7	<0.001
Sternum	24.0 ± 2.5	25.3 ± 5.6	27.0 ± 3.5	26.7 ± 5.6	0.064
C	24.0 ± 5.0	24.7 ± 6.3	24.0 ± 3.0	25.7 ± 6.0	0.284
T1	13.0 ± 3.5 **	13.2 ± 6.1	16.0 ± 3.0	16.5 ± 5.0	0.001
T2	12.0 ± 4.0 **	12.3 ± 5.5	14.0 ± 3.0	14.8 ± 4.7	0.009
LS	20.0 ± 3.5	20.2 ± 5.2	20.0 ± 4.0	19.7 ± 5.8	0.331
Ranges of motion					
FTF (cm)	0.0 ± 6.5	6.5 ± 8.1	0.0 ± 5.5	5.9 ± 7.3	0.735
CRleft (°)	34.0 ± 4.0	32.9 ± 7.1	34.0 ± 3.0	32.7 ± 4.9	0.412
CRright (°)	30.0 ± 3.5	30.2 ±7.3	31.0 ± 3.0	30.1 ± 5.6	0.549
HEleft (°)	22.0 ± 2.0	23.4 ± 4.2	22.0 ± 2.0	22.05 ± 5.7	0.142
HEright (°)	22.0 ± 3.0	23.0 ± 5.6	22.0 ± 2.0	22.2 ± 5.6	0.205
HFleft (°)	68.0 ± 11.0	64.1 ± 14.8	66.0 ± 12.0	63.7 ± 16.2	0.943
HFright (°)	70.0 ± 11.0	65.0 ± 15.2	66.0 ± 12.0	63.8 ± 16.6	0.737
TPHAleft (°)	12.0 ± 2.0	11.9 ± 6.0	12.0 ± 2.0	12.1 ± 3.6	0.941
TPHAright (°)	10.0 ± 5.0	8.3 ± 9.4	10.0 ± 3.0	10.7 ± 5.8	0.165
JHM score	3.5 ± 1.5 **	3.5 ± 2.3	2.0 ± 1.5	2.3 ± 2.4	0.001

Abbreviations: ULNT1, upper limb neurodynamic test; SLR, straight leg raise test; SLUMP, slump test; ATRT, angle of trunk rotation in the thoracic spine; ATRL, angle of trunk rotation in the lumbar spine; Sternum, sternum inclination; C, inclination of the cervicothoracic junction; T1, inclination of the upper thoracic spine; T2, inclination of the thoracic-lumbar junction; LS, inclination of the lumbosacral junction; FTF, fingertip-to-floor test; CR, cervical rotation; HE, hip extension; HF, hip flexion with knee extension; TPHA, trunk-pelvis-hip angle; JHM, joint hypermobility; n, number of participants; p, statistical significance. Notes: Mann–Whitney U test; Significance of differences between IS and control group: (**)—at the level of $0.01 \geq p \geq 0.001$; (***)—at the level of $p < 0.001$.

The values of ATR in the thoracic and lumbar segments of the spine and Beighton score values were significantly higher in individuals with scoliosis. Measurements with the plurimeter revealed decreased values of T1 and T2 in the IS group compared to the control group, which indicates decreased kyphosis in patients with scoliosis. No significant differences were noted between the values of the measurements at the sternum, cervical-thoracic (C), and lumbosacral junction (LS). Further, the ranges of movement in the cervical spine, hip joints, and FTF test did not differ significantly (Table 2).

The analysis carried out in the subgroups of girls with scoliosis (n = 57) and without scoliosis (n = 42) revealed significant differences between the values of ULNT1left, ULNT1right, SLUMPleft and SLUMPright tests. The values of the SLR did not differ significantly. Girls with scoliosis demonstrated lower values of upper thoracic segment T1 inclination and higher values of ATRT, ATRL, and Beighton points (IS 3.73 ± 2.11; C 2.54 ± 2.47; p = 0.005) (Figure 4). No differences between the ranges of motion were found. Only a trend towards a lower range of TPHAright motion was observed in girls with scoliosis.

3.2. Correlations between Neurodynamic Tests and Postural Parameters

There was no significant relationship between the neurodynamic tests' values and the Cobb angle values in adolescents with IS. However, participants with deformation over 30° showed significantly lower ranges of motion in the SLUMPleft test ($p = 0.037$). The IS and control groups revealed medium and low correlations between the ULNT1, SLR, and SLUMP tests. The increase in nerve tension in one test was accompanied by increased tension in the others. With an increase in the ULNT1 values, the ranges of SLR decreased, while higher SLUMP values accompanied an increase in the ULNT1 values (Table 3).

Table 3. Correlations between neurodynamic tests, Cobb angle, age, body mass and height in adolescents with idiopathic scoliosis (IS) and the control group (C).

	ULNT1 Left	ULNT1 Right	SLR Left	SLR Right	SLUMP Left	SLUMP Right
Idiopathic Scoliosis ($n = 69$)						
ULNT1 right	0.665 ***	–	–	–	–	–
SLR left	−0.518 ***	−0.497 ***	–	–	–	–
SLR right	−0.506 ***	−0.529 ***	0.950 ***	–	–	–
SLUMP left	0.313 **	0.432 **	−0.575 ***	−0.524 ***	–	–
SLUMP right	0.383 **	0.462 **	−0.545 ***	−0.514 ***	0.900 ***	–
Cobb angle	0.016	−0.073	0.197	0.177	−0.176	−0.126
Age	0.370 **	0.215	−0.113	−0.112	−0.014	0.090
Body mass	0.226	0.115	−0.186	−0.176	0.030	0.102
Body height	0.325 **	0.217	−0.212	−0.184	0.118	0.189
Control Group ($n = 57$)						
ULNT1 right	0.928 ***	–	–	–	–	–
SLR left	−0.589 ***	−0.625 ***	–	–	–	–
SLR right	−0.601 ***	−0.622 ***	0.979 ***	–	–	–
SLUMP left	0.384 **	0.423 **	−0.650 ***	−0.644 ***	–	–
SLUMP right	0.373 **	0.426 **	−0.636 ***	−0.624 ***	0.976 ***	–
Age	0.140	0.147	−0.239	−0.218	0.190	0.184
Body mass	0.199	0.215	−0.321 *	−0.300 *	0.045	0.040
Body height	0.216	0.260	−0.316 *	−0.298 *	0.137	0.148

Abbreviations: ULNT1, upper limb neurodynamic test; SLR, straight leg raise test; SLUMP, slump test; n, number of participants; p, statistical significance. Notes: Significance of differences: (*)—at the level of $0.05 > p > 0.01$; (**)—at the level of $0.01 \geq p \geq 0.001$; (***)—at the level of $p < 0.001$.

In both girls with scoliosis and their healthy counterparts, a significantly low correlation was observed between the position of the C and T1 segments in the sagittal plane and the ULNT1 and SLR tests values. The increased angular inclination of the spine from the axis was accompanied by higher MNS. In the IS group, a low positive correlation was observed between ULNT1 and the position of the lumbosacral segment (LS). Higher values of pelvic inclination were associated with higher values of ULNT1 test (lower extensibility). A weak correlation between the pelvic position (LS) and SLR values was found in the control group. The increase in ATR was correlated with the increased range in the ULNT1 test in this group (Table 4).

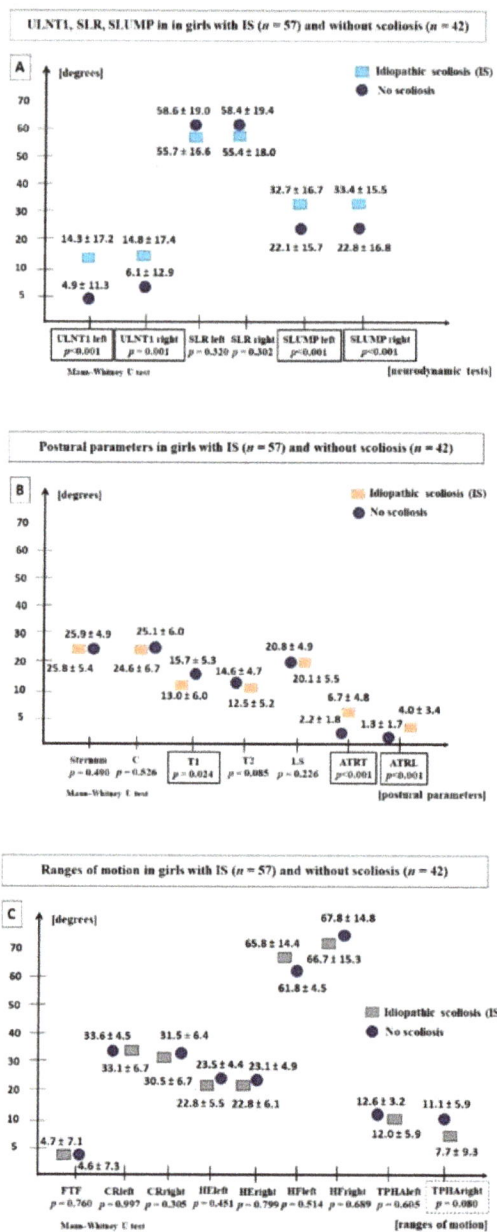

Figure 4. (**A**) ULNT1, SLR and SLUMP; (**B**) postural parameters; (**C**) ranges of motion in girls with IS (*n* = 57) and asymptomatic girls (*n* = 42). Abbreviations: ULNT1, Upper Limb Neurodynamic Test; SLR, Straight Leg Raise Test; SLUMP, Slump Test; ATRT, angle of trunk rotation in the thoracic spine; ATRL, angle of trunk rotation in the lumbar spine; Sternum, sternum inclination; C, inclination of the cervicothoracic junction; T1, inclination of the upper thoracic spine; T2, inclination of the thoracic-lumbar junction; LS, inclination of the lumbosacral junction; FTF, Fingertip-To-Floor test; CR, Cervical Rotation; HE, Hip Extension; HF, Hip Flexion with knee extension; TPHA, Trunk-Pelvis-Hip Angle; JHM, Joint Hypermobility; *p*, statistical significance (Mann–Whitney U test).

Table 4. Correlations between neurodynamic tests and postural parameters in adolescents with idiopathic scoliosis (IS) and the control group (C).

	Idiopathic Scoliosis (n = 69)					
	ULNT1 Left	ULNT1 Right	SLR Left	SLR Right	SLUMP Left	SLUMP Right
Sternum	0.067	−0.043	−0.010	−0.074	0.007	−0.002
C	0.425 ***	0.324 **	−0.377 **	−0.407 **	0.103	0.131
T1	0.487 ***	0.370 **	−0.450 ***	−0.432 ***	0.158	0.216
T2	0.294 *	0.175	−0.264 *	−0.281 *	0.118	0.164
LS	0.300 *	0.412 **	−0.135	−0.098	0.256 *	0.243 *
ATRT	−0.249 *	−0.282 *	0.160	0.169	−0.119	−0.198
ATRL	0.283 *	0.104	−0.124	−0.122	0.122	0.130
	Control Group (n = 57)					
	ULNT1 Left	ULNT1 Right	SLR Left	SLR Right	SLUMP Left	SLUMP Right
Sternum	0.023	−0.007	−0.122	−0.104	0.045	0.059
C	0.297 *	0.356 **	−0.526 ***	−0.544 ***	0.152	0.171
T1	0.352 **	0.265 *	−0.370 **	−0.383 **	0.173	0.125
T2	0.240	0.270 *	−0.253	−0.282 *	0.191	0.200
LS	0.190	0.272 *	−0.374 **	−0.346 **	0.292 *	0.301 *
ATRT	−0.429 **	−0.419 **	0.301 *	0.297 *	−0.021	−0.066
ATRL	−0.057	−0.109	0.141	0.174	−0.109	−0.136

Abbreviations: ULNT1, upper limb neurodynamic test; SLR, straight leg raise test; SLUMP, slump test; ATR, angle of trunk rotation; T, thoracic; L, lumbar; Sternum, sternum inclination; C, inclination of the cervicothoracic junction; T1, inclination of the upper thoracic spine; T2, inclination of the thoracic-lumbar junction; LS, inclination of the lumbosacral junction; n, number of participants; p, statistical significance. Notes: Significance of differences: (*)—at the level of $0.05 > p > 0.01$; (**)—at the level of $0.01 \geq p \geq 0.001$; (***)—at the level of $p < 0.001$.

The analysis showed several relationships between neurodynamic tests and range of motion. In both groups, a significant correlation was found between the ULNT1, SLR, and SLUMP tests and the range of flexion in the hip joint with the knee extended (HF). The grater HF ranges were accompanied by greater neural extensibility. The FLF test showed a low correlation with SLR in the IS group. A moderate correlation was found between FLF, SLR, and SLUMP in the control group. No significant relationship was found between JHM and neurodynamic tests in either group (Table 5).

In the IS group, the ranges of TPHAright were correlated with ULNT1 and SLR. Higher ULNT1 values (lower extensibility) were associated with greater ranges of motion in both TPHAright (better mobility), and SLR was correlated with lower values of the mobility of the lumbo-pelvic-hip complex (limited mobility) (Table 5).

3.3. Neurodynamic Tests and Pain

The values of neurodynamic tests obtained by adolescents with and without pain in both groups were compared to confirm or exclude the effect of pain on the measurements. In addition, the values were analysed in the group of participants with IS, considering a subgroup of adolescents with and without pain.

Significant differences were found between adolescents without pain with scoliosis (n = 43) and those without scoliosis (n = 50). In participants with IS there were reduced ranges of motion in the ULNT1left ($p < 0.001$), ULNT1right ($p < 0.001$), SLUMPleft ($p = 0.002$) and SLUMPright ($p = 0.001$) tests. Due to the insufficient number of adolescents in the control group with pain (n = 7), the differences between the groups of participants with pain are not discussed.

The analysis of adolescents with IS revealed that patients with pain (n = 26) showed increased mechanosensitivity in the SLRright ($p = 0.04$) and SLUMPright ($p = 0.006$) tests compared to participants without pain (n = 43).

Table 5. Correlations between neurodynamic tests and ranges of motion in adolescents with idiopathic scoliosis (IS) and the control group (C).

	ULNT1 Left	ULNT1 Right	SLR Left	SLR Right	SLUMP Left	SLUMP Right
Idiopathic Scoliosis (n = 69)						
FTF	−0.026	−0.141	−0.396 **	−0.370 **	0.189	0.201
CR left	−0.139	−0.015	0.096	0.058	−0.105	−0.125
CR right	−0.058	0.031	0.022	−0.020	−0.178	−0.168
HE left	0.120	0.049	0.268 *	0.211	−0.159	−0.120
HE right	0.213	−0.011	0.133	0.067	−0.124	−0.095
HF left	−0.447 **	−0.426 ***	0.941 ***	0.905 ***	−0.533 ***	−0.485 ***
HF right	−0.403 **	−0.347 **	0.895 ***	0.886 ***	−0.465 ***	−0.432 ***
TPHA left	0.206	0.202	−0.078	−0.101	−0.011	0.029
TPHA right	0.364 **	0.398 **	−0.350 **	−0.347 **	0.124	0.151
JHM	−0.136	−0.099	0.123	0.108	−0.082	−0.077
Control Group (n = 57)						
FTF	0.214	0.245	−0.543 ***	−0.504 ***	0.433 **	0.462 ***
CR left	0.025	−0.009	0.188	0.199	−0.275 *	−0.254
CR right	−0.097	−0.172	0.273 *	0.267 *	−0.477 ***	−0.462 ***
HE left	−0.045	−0.096	0.228	0.207	−0.026	−0.066
HE right	−0.192	−0.196	0.281 *	0.279 *	0.005	−0.030
HF left	−0.544 ***	−0.572 ***	0.965 ***	0.939 ***	−0.604 ***	−0.589 ***
HF right	−0.561 ***	−0.581 ***	0.952 ***	0.955 ***	−0.586 ***	−0.571 ***
TPHA left	0.350 **	0.353 **	−0.099	−0.113	0.208	0.215
TPHA right	0.303 *	0.250	0.180	−0.205	0.173	0.153
JHM	0.095	0.027	0.077	0.047	−0.017	−0.054

Abbreviations: ULNT1, upper limb neurodynamic test; SLR, straight leg raise test; SLUMP, slump test; ATR, angle of trunk rotation; Sternum, sternum inclination; C, inclination of the cervicothoracic junction; T1, inclination of the upper thoracic spine; T2, inclination of the thoracic-lumbar junction; LS, inclination of the lumbosacral junction; FTF, fingertip-to-floor test; CR, cervical rotation; HE, hip extension; HF, hip flexion with knee extension; TPHA, trunk-pelvis-hip angle; JHM, joint hypermobility; n, number of participants; p, statistical significance. Notes: Mann–Whitney U test; significance of differences between IS and control group: (*)—at the level of $0.05 > p > 0.01$; (**)—at the level of $0.01 \geq p \geq 0.001$; (***)—at the level of $p < 0.001$.

4. Discussion

The multivariant aetiology of IS, various health problems, and long-lasting treatment makes it necessary to conduct scientific studies aimed at a detailed description of this disease and the prevention of its symptoms in the musculoskeletal system. Unfortunately, current knowledge about the neurodynamic of the NS in patients with IS is limited. Therefore, this study aimed to evaluate MNS in adolescents with IS in comparison to a control group, which is an issue that has not previously been addressed in the literature.

The study included girls and boys with IS and asymptomatic adolescents aged 10–15 years. According to the World Health Organization, adolescents are defined as the period between childhood and adulthood, from ages 10 to 19 [38]. However, it is known that in this age, a rapid growth spurt and other puberty-related changes are observed [39,40]. Intensive changes related to maturation may affect posture and range of motion, and promote the development of scoliosis, making clinical reasoning difficult. The varied ages of the participants qualified for our study can therefore be considered factors that may affect the values of neurodynamic tests, postural parameters, and range of motion. It is worth conducting similar studies in different age categories among adolescents in the future.

For this study, three neurodynamic tests whose reliability had been previously confirmed in different groups of participants were selected: the ULNT1 [14–16], SLR [13,19,41], and SLUMP test [17,18]. In addition, we also applied other tests that have been used to assess patients with various dysfunctions, including scoliosis.

The results showed that MNS in adolescents with IS assessed using ULNT1 and SLUMP was larger than in the control group. No differences were noted in the ranges of SLR between the groups. These results indicate that adolescents with IS in puberty experience increased nerve sensitivity, but only in certain parts of NS. The upper part structures of the NS appeared to be more sensitive to stretching. The ULNT test used in this study was applied, inter alia, to assess the tension of the median nerve, that is, one of the nerves from the subclavicular part of the brachial plexus. During the SLUMP test, the structures of the spinal canal and intervertebral foramen in all segments of the spine were stretched. The SLR test assesses the extensibility of the nervous structures in the lower peripheral NS [3]. The study was conducted with a group of participants with various values of the Cobb angle. There was no correlation between the Cobb angle values and the parameters tested. However, participants with deformation over 30° showed a significantly lower range of motion in the SLUMPleft test than participants with less severe scoliosis, which may indicate some relationship between spine deformation and MNS.

Statistical analysis of painless participants showed increased mechanosensitivity in ULNT1 and SLUMP tests in adolescents with IS. At the same time, the increased range of motion in the SLRright and SLUMPright tests was observed in participants with IS and pain compared to their peers with IS, but without pain. These results indicate that both spinal deformities and the presence of pain may influence the MNS in adolescents.

Unfortunately, these results cannot be correlated with those of other studies since no similar studies have been conducted in adolescents with scoliosis to date. Further, no norms for neurodynamic functions have been defined in healthy children and youth groups. A few years ago, the reliability of the SLR test was assessed in a group of children with cerebral palsy [20]. Other studies have shown a higher intensity of the sensory response rate in the examination using the long sitting slump (LSS) test in children aged 6–12 years with a migraine or cervicogenic headaches than their healthy peers [21].

In our study, the analysis of the frequency of occurrence of differences between the ranges of motion on the left and right sides (equal to or larger than 5°) revealed that regardless of the type of neurodynamic test (ULNT1, SLR, SLUMP), such differences occurred more often in the IS group. These results suggest that scoliosis can lead to extensibility differences between the sides of the body.

In a study by Stalioraitis et al. [42] conducted on a group of asymptomatic individuals, no significant differences were noted in the range of motion in the ULNT1 test on the left and right sides of the body. Interestingly, our results revealed that differences between the mean values of neurodynamic tests (ULNT1, SLR, and SLUMP) on both sides of the body were not significant in either group, even though the frequency of asymmetry of measurements was higher in the IS group. It has also been observed that reduced range of motion in neurodynamic tests occurs in patients with IS at a similar frequency of 40–60% on both sides of the body. However, due to many variables such as Cobb angle, number and location of curvatures, the dominance of one of the curves in double-curve scoliosis, value of ATR, alignment in the sagittal plane, pain incidence, gender, hypermobility, the relationship between the left/right asymmetry and direction of the curvatures was not analysed in detail in this study. This phenomenon requires further analysis in a larger and more homogeneous group of adolescents with IS.

The limited range of motion in one neurodynamic test was accompanied by a significant decrease in other neurodynamic tests in both groups. This observation is valuable from a practical point of view. The finding of increased neural tension in one part of the nervous system may require therapy in other parts of the body, which is important because of the risk of irritation of the nerves and pain provocation [3–5].

The analysis of measurements in our study revealed decreased values of thoracic kyphosis in the IS group. This finding supports findings obtained by other authors who described changes in spinal curvature in the sagittal plane and suggested their influence on the development of scoliosis [43,44]. Numerous correlations were noted between the neurodynamic tests and the selected postural parameters. It appeared that the position of the C, T1, and LS segments in the sagittal plane was a significant factor affecting the values of the ULNT1 and SLR tests. This correlation could indicate that changes in the spine curvatures in the sagittal plane observed in patients with scoliosis affect MNS changes [43,44].

Our results also confirmed the theory that adolescents with IS experience a significantly higher JHM prevalence than their healthy peers [45]. In the study by Czaprowski et al. [45], JHM was observed in 51.4% of participants with IS and 19% in the control group, whereas in the present study, hypermobility was found in 33.3% of participants with IS and 14% of controls. No significant correlation was found between JHM and neurodynamic measurements in our study.

No differences were observed between the range of motion values in participants with IS and their control counterparts. The analysis showed that there are biomechanical connections between neurodynamic tests and range of motion. These correlations confirm that NS viscoelasticity is not only associated with the static position of the body, as mentioned above (sagittal alignment), but also with the mobility of the body. The HF test showed a significant relationship with all neurodynamic tests. The larger HF ranges were accompanied by lower NS tension in both groups. These results indicate that the HF test could be used to diagnose children in everyday clinical practice. However, this thesis requires confirmation in a larger group of children and adolescents with IS and those who are asymptomatic.

A comparison of the TPHA values achieved in both subgroups of girls showed that participants with IS tended to limit the range of rotational movement of the lumbo-pelvic-hip complex to the right (TPHAright). In a previous study by Stępień et al. [34] significant difference was observed between the TPHAright values in girls with IS and healthy peers. Further, a positive effect of rotational mobilisation on TPHA and ATR values was demonstrated in girls with double-curve scoliosis [35]. Earlier studies have also shown limitations in the range of rotation of the trunk and pelvis in adolescent girls with IS [46]. Rotational movement disorder was also recognised by Burwell et al. [47] as one of the factors in the development of scoliosis.

This study demonstrated a relationship between the TPHAright values and neurodynamic measurements in the IS group. As the TPHAright range increased, the mechanosensitivity increased in the ULNT1 and SLR tests. This relationship indicates a biomechanical relationship between neural tissues extensibility and rotational movements of the spine in individuals with scoliosis. Perhaps limiting the range of rotational movements of the spine leads to compensatory impairments of the NS. This theory, however, requires confirmation in future projects.

Increased NS irritation is often diagnosed in individuals experiencing pain. The literature reveals that pain occurs in adolescents with IS [22–26]. Prevention and reduction of pain are among the most important goals of conservative treatment for individuals with IS, although not the most important [2,26,27]. It is assumed that if Cobb's angle is above 30°, the risk of pain, health problems in adult life, and limitations in an everyday functioning increase [2].

Our results indicate that pain was observed significantly more often in adolescents with IS (37.7%) than in healthy controls (12.3%). A localised pain in different parts of the body occurred more often in participants with curvature angles higher than 30° (50.0%) than in patients with scoliosis below 30° (31.1%) or in healthy individuals (14%). This could indicate a relationship between three-dimensional spinal deformity and back pain, but in most studies, the pain has not shown a strong correlation with the Cobb angle [26]. The prevalence of back pain in our participants (29.0%) was less than in the population assessed by other authors. Teles et al. [25] showed that 90% of adolescents with IS reported back pain, mostly mild in intensity (37.5%). Sato et al. [22] conducted an epidemiological study among students aged 9–15 years. The authors showed a 58.8% prevalence of back pain in scoliotic patients, compared with 33% in non-scoliotic students. In a study by Théroux et al. [23], 47.3% of patients with IS aged 10–17 years had back pain, with the most severe pain in the lumbar region.

In studies by Wong et al. [24], depending on the analysed period (12 months, 30 days, 7 days), the prevalence of thoracic pain ranged from 6% (within 12 months) to 14% (within 7 days), whereas that in the lumbar region ranged from 6% to 29%. These results are similar to ours, where 17.4% of the IS adolescents complained the thoracic segment pain, and 21.7% had low back pain.

The frequency of occurrence of back pain in our project among children without scoliosis seems to be lower than in other studies, in which over 20% of healthy adolescents reported low back pain [48,49]. For example, studies conducted in Poland have shown that 12.2–61.5% of children aged 10–13 years and 14–65.7% aged 14–16 years report back pain, depending on the frequency of occurrence, location, intensity, and situations [50]. However, in our opinion, our results cannot be compared with others since our project did not consider the location and severity of pain, nor did we use reliable pain assessment methods.

SOSORT recommends that physiotherapeutic scoliosis-specific exercises (PSSEs) should be adapted to individual needs, including pain prevention or reduction in IS patients [2]. In our opinion, because pain occurred more often in adolescents with IS and the differences between neurodynamic tests in IS and healthy participants, impaired MNS should be treated as one of the factors predisposing to pain. Therefore, it is worth assessing neurodynamic functions during examinations to implement appropriate physiotherapeutic interventions and assess their effectiveness. Moreover, it provides valuable information in terms of clinical practice and the prevention of pain because non-treated tensions in one area of the body may, with time, generate broader dysfunctions of the nervous system.

The present study had certain limitations. Therapists were not blind to the existence of scoliosis. Blinding the researchers was difficult due to the symptoms of scoliosis visible during the body posture examination. A significant limitation was the lack of assessment of the reliability of the ULNT1, SLR, and SLUMP tests in a group of adolescents with IS. Our observations and conclusions in this study regarding the above-mentioned tests were based on previous studies. In the future, the reliability of neurodynamic tests should be verified in the population of children and youth with IS and healthy peers. Further, the age range of the participants was wide. The intense changes occurring at the age of 10–15 years during puberty and intensive growth could have impacted the values of the assessed parameters.

Incomplete analysis of pain among the participants was another limitation of the study. The participants only confirmed or denied that they had experienced pain in the last 3 months. However, the character and intensity of pain or provoking factors were not analysed, and the validated tool (questionnaire or scale) for pain assessment was not applied. In the future, the analysis should be carried out in a larger group, taking into account various types of spine deformity.

5. Conclusions

Our findings revealed increased MNS in adolescents with IS. Values of neurodynamic tests correlated with the sagittal profile of the spine and mobility of the spine and lower limb joints. Therefore, the examination of adolescents with IS should include an assessment of MNS. Future studies should extend the assessment of neurodynamic functions and explore this issue to improve the understanding of the mechanisms of IS.

Author Contributions: Conceptualization, A.S. and B.P.; Methodology, A.S. and B.P.; Formal Analysis, A.S.; Investigation, A.S. and B.P.; Resources, A.S. and B.P.; Data Curation, A.S.; Writing—Original Draft Preparation, A.S.; Writing—Review and Editing, B.P.; Visualization, A.S.; Supervision, A.S. All authors have read and agreed to the published version of the manuscript.

Funding: This research received no external funding.

Institutional Review Board Statement: The study was conducted according to the guidelines of the Declaration of Helsinki, and approved by the Institutional Ethics Committee at Józef Piłsudski University of Physical Education in Warsaw (SKE 01-30/2020, 19 January 2021).

Informed Consent Statement: Informed consent was obtained from all subjects involved in the study. Written informed consent was obtained from the patients to publish this paper.

Data Availability Statement: The data presented in this study are available on request from the corresponding author.

Acknowledgments: We would like to thank Witold Rekowski for professional support in statistical analysis.

Conflicts of Interest: The authors declare no conflict of interest.

References

1. Schlösser, T.P.C.; van der Heijden, G.J.M.G.; Versteeg, A.L.; Castelein, R.M. How 'Idiopathic' Is Adolescent Idiopathic Scoliosis? A Systematic Review on Associated Abnormalities. *PLoS ONE* **2014**, *9*, e97461. [CrossRef] [PubMed]
2. Negrini, S.; Donzelli, S.; Aulisa, A.G.; Czaprowski, D.; Schreiber, S.; de Mauroy, J.C.; Diers, H.; Grivas, T.B.; Knott, P.; Kotwicki, T.; et al. 2016 SOSORT Guidelines: Orthopaedic and Rehabilitation Treatment of Idiopathic Scoliosis during Growth. *Scoliosis Spinal Disord.* **2018**, *13*, 3. [CrossRef] [PubMed]
3. Shacklock, M. *Clinical Neurodynamics: A New System of Neuromusculoskeletal Treatment*, 1st ed.; Elsevier: Oxford, UK, 2005; ISBN 978-0-7506-5456-2.
4. Ellis, R.; Carta, G.; Andrade, R.J.; Coppieters, M.W. Neurodynamics: Is Tension Contentious? *J. Man. Manip. Ther.* **2022**, *30*, 3–12. [CrossRef] [PubMed]
5. Butler, D.S. *The Neurodynamic Techniques DVD and Handbook*; NOI Group Publications: Haarlem, The Netherlands, 2005.
6. Dwornik, M.; Kujawa, J.; Białoszewski, D.; Słupik, A.; Kiebzak, W. Electromyographic and Clinical Evaluation of the Efficacy of Neuromobilization in Patients with Low Back Pain. *Ortop. Traumatol. Rehabil.* **2009**, *11*, 164–176. [CrossRef] [PubMed]
7. Basson, A.; Olivier, B.; Ellis, R.; Coppieters, M.; Stewart, A.; Mudzi, W. The Effectiveness of Neural Mobilization for Neuromusculoskeletal Conditions: A Systematic Review and Meta-Analysis. *J. Orthop. Sports Phys. Ther.* **2017**, *47*, 593–615. [CrossRef] [PubMed]
8. Kleinrensink, G.J.; Stoeckart, R.; Mulder, P.G.; Hoek, G.; Broek, T.; Vleeming, A.; Snijders, C.J. Upper Limb Tension Tests as Tools in the Diagnosis of Nerve and Plexus Lesions. Anatomical and Biomechanical Aspects. *Clin. Biomech.* **2000**, *15*, 9–14. [CrossRef]
9. Van der Heide, B.; Allison, G.T.; Zusman, M. Pain and Muscular Responses to a Neural Tissue Provocation Test in the Upper Limb. *Man. Ther.* **2001**, *6*, 154–162. [CrossRef]
10. Majlesi, J.; Togay, H.; Unalan, H.; Toprak, S. The Sensitivity and Specificity of the Slump and the Straight Leg Raising Tests in Patients with Lumbar Disc Herniation. *J. Clin. Rheumatol.* **2008**, *14*, 87–91. [CrossRef]
11. Boyd, B.S.; Wanek, L.; Gray, A.T.; Topp, K.S. Mechanosensitivity of the Lower Extremity Nervous System during Straight-Leg Raise Neurodynamic Testing in Healthy Individuals. *J. Orthop. Sports Phys. Ther.* **2009**, *39*, 780–790. [CrossRef]
12. Walsh, J.; Hall, T. Agreement and Correlation between the Straight Leg Raise and Slump Tests in Subjects with Leg Pain. *J. Manip. Physiol. Ther.* **2009**, *32*, 184–192. [CrossRef]
13. Ekedahl, H.; Jönsson, B.; Frobell, R.B. Fingertip-to-Floor Test and Straight Leg Raising Test: Validity, Responsiveness, and Predictive Value in Patients with Acute/Subacute Low Back Pain. *Arch. Phys. Med. Rehabil.* **2012**, *93*, 2210–2215. [CrossRef]
14. Hines, T.; Noakes, R.; Manners, B. The Upper Limb Tension Test: Inter-Tester Reliability for Assessing the Onset of Passive Resistance R 1. *J. Man. Manip. Ther.* **1993**, *1*, 95–98. [CrossRef]
15. Vanti, C.; Conteddu, L.; Guccione, A.; Morsillo, F.; Parazza, S.; Viti, C.; Pillastrini, P. The Upper Limb Neurodynamic Test 1: Intra- and Intertester Reliability and the Effect of Several Repetitions on Pain and Resistance. *J. Manip. Physiol. Ther.* **2010**, *33*, 292–299. [CrossRef]
16. Oliver, G.S.; Rushton, A. A Study to Explore the Reliability and Precision of Intra and Inter-Rater Measures of ULNT1 on an Asymptomatic Population. *Man. Ther.* **2011**, *16*, 203–206. [CrossRef]
17. Philip, K.; Lew, P.; Matyas, T.A. The Inter-Therapist Reliability of the Slump Test. *Aust. J. Physiother.* **1989**, *35*, 89–94. [CrossRef]
18. Tucker, N.; Reid, D.; McNair, P. Reliability and Measurement Error of Active Knee Extension Range of Motion in a Modified Slump Test Position: A Pilot Study. *J. Man. Manip. Ther.* **2007**, *15*, E85–E91. [CrossRef]
19. Hunt, D.G.; Zuberbier, O.A.; Kozlowski, A.J.; Robinson, J.; Berkowitz, J.; Schultz, I.Z.; Milner, R.A.; Crook, J.M.; Turk, D.C. Reliability of the Lumbar Flexion, Lumbar Extension, and Passive Straight Leg Raise Test in Normal Populations Embedded within a Complete Physical Examination. *Spine* **2001**, *26*, 2714–2718. [CrossRef]
20. Marsico, P.; Tal-Akabi, A.; Van Hedel, H.J.A. Reliability and Practicability of the Straight Leg Raise Test in Children with Cerebral Palsy. *Dev. Med. Child. Neurol.* **2016**, *58*, 173–179. [CrossRef]
21. Von Piekartz, H.J.M.; Schouten, S.; Aufdemkampe, G. Neurodynamic Responses in Children with Migraine or Cervicogenic Headache versus a Control Group. A Comparative Study. *Man. Ther.* **2007**, *12*, 153–160. [CrossRef]

22. Sato, T.; Hirano, T.; Ito, T.; Morita, O.; Kikuchi, R.; Endo, N.; Tanabe, N. Back Pain in Adolescents with Idiopathic Scoliosis: Epidemiological Study for 43,630 Pupils in Niigata City, Japan. *Eur. Spine J.* **2011**, *20*, 274–279. [CrossRef]
23. Théroux, J.; Le May, S.; Fortin, C.; Labelle, H. Prevalence and Management of Back Pain in Adolescent Idiopathic Scoliosis Patients: A Retrospective Study. *Pain Res. Manag.* **2015**, *20*, 153–157. [CrossRef]
24. Wong, A.Y.L.; Samartzis, D.; Cheung, P.W.H.; Yin Cheung, J.P. How Common Is Back Pain and What Biopsychosocial Factors Are Associated With Back Pain in Patients With Adolescent Idiopathic Scoliosis? *Clin. Orthop. Relat. Res.* **2019**, *477*, 676–686. [CrossRef]
25. Teles, A.R.; St-Georges, M.; Abduljabbar, F.; Simões, L.; Jiang, F.; Saran, N.; Ouellet, J.A.; Ferland, C.E. Back Pain in Adolescents with Idiopathic Scoliosis: The Contribution of Morphological and Psychological Factors. *Eur. Spine J.* **2020**, *29*, 1959–1971. [CrossRef]
26. Balagué, F.; Pellisé, F. Adolescent Idiopathic Scoliosis and Back Pain. *Scoliosis Spinal Disord.* **2016**, *11*, 27. [CrossRef]
27. Negrini, S.; Grivas, T.B.; Kotwicki, T.; Maruyama, T.; Rigo, M.; Weiss, H.R.; Members of the Scientific society On Scoliosis Orthopaedic and Rehabilitation Treatment (SOSORT). Why Do We Treat Adolescent Idiopathic Scoliosis? What We Want to Obtain and to Avoid for Our Patients. SOSORT 2005 Consensus Paper. *Scoliosis* **2006**, *1*, 4. [CrossRef]
28. Côté, P.; Kreitz, B.G.; Cassidy, J.D.; Dzus, A.K.; Martel, J. A Study of the Diagnostic Accuracy and Reliability of the Scoliometer and Adam's Forward Bend Test. *Spine* **1998**, *23*, 796–802; discussion 803. [CrossRef]
29. Grivas, T.B.; Vasiliadis, E.S.; Koufopoulos, G.; Segos, D.; Triantafyllopoulos, G.; Mouzakis, V. Study of Trunk Asymmetry in Normal Children and Adolescents. *Scoliosis* **2006**, *1*, 19. [CrossRef]
30. Kluszczyński, M.; Czernicki, J.; Kubacki, J. The Plurimetric Assessment Of Spinal Curvature Changes In The Sagittal Plane In Children And Youths, Measured During 10 Years' Observation. *Adv. Rehabil.* **2013**, *27*, 1–8. [CrossRef]
31. Stolinski, L.; Kozinoga, M.; Czaprowski, D.; Tyrakowski, M.; Cerny, P.; Suzuki, N.; Kotwicki, T. Two-Dimensional Digital Photography for Child Body Posture Evaluation: Standardized Technique, Reliable Parameters and Normative Data for Age 7–10 Years. *Scoliosis Spinal Disord* **2017**, *12*, 38. [CrossRef]
32. Norkin, C.C.; White, D.J. *Measurement of Joint Motion: A Guide to Goniometry*, 5th ed.; F.A. Davis Company: Philadelphia, PA, USA, 2016; ISBN 978-0-8036-4566-0.
33. Stępień, A.; Jędrzejowska, M.; Guzek, K.; Rekowski, W.; Stępowska, J. Reliability of Four Tests to Assess Body Posture and the Range of Selected Movements in Individuals with Spinal Muscular Atrophy. *BMC Musculoskelet Disord.* **2019**, *20*, 54. [CrossRef]
34. Stępień, A.; Guzek, K.; Rekowski, W.; Radomska, I.; Stępowska, J. Assessment of the Lumbo-Pelvic-Hip Complex Mobility with the Trunk-Pelvis-Hip Angle Test: Intraobserver Reliability and Differences in Ranges of Motion between Girls with Idiopathic Scoliosis and Their Healthy Counterparts. *Adv. Rehabil.* **2020**, *30*, 27–39. [CrossRef]
35. Stępień, A.; Fabian, K.; Graff, K.; Podgurniak, M.; Wit, A. An Immediate Effect of PNF Specific Mobilization on the Angle of Trunk Rotation and the Trunk-Pelvis-Hip Angle Range of Motion in Adolescent Girls with Double Idiopathic Scoliosis-a Pilot Study. *Scoliosis Spinal Disord.* **2017**, *12*, 29. [CrossRef]
36. Perret, C.; Poiraudeau, S.; Fermanian, J.; Colau, M.M.; Benhamou, M.A.; Revel, M. Validity, Reliability, and Responsiveness of the Fingertip-to-Floor Test. *Arch. Phys. Med. Rehabil.* **2001**, *82*, 1566–1570. [CrossRef] [PubMed]
37. Mukaka, M.M. Statistics Corner: A Guide to Appropriate Use of Correlation Coefficient in Medical Research. *Malawi Med. J.* **2012**, *24*, 69–71. [PubMed]
38. World Health Organization. *Adolescent Health*; World Health Organization: Geneva, Switzerland, 2022.
39. Thakur, R.; Gautam, R. Differential Onset of Puberty and Adolescence among Girls and Boys of a Central Indian Town (Sagar). *Orient Anthropol.* **2017**, *17*, 137–147. [CrossRef]
40. Sawyer, S.M.; Azzopardi, P.S.; Wickremarathne, D.; Patton, G.C. The Age of Adolescence. *Lancet Child Adolesc. Health* **2018**, *2*, 223–228. [CrossRef]
41. Boyd, B.S. Measurement Properties of a Hand-Held Inclinometer during Straight Leg Raise Neurodynamic Testing. *Physiotherapy* **2012**, *98*, 174–179. [CrossRef]
42. Stalioraitis, V.; Robinson, K.; Hall, T. Side-to-Side Range of Movement Variability in Variants of the Median and Radial Neurodynamic Test Sequences in Asymptomatic People. *Man. Ther.* **2014**, *19*, 338–342. [CrossRef]
43. Burkus, M.; Schlégl, Á.T.; O'Sullivan, I.; Márkus, I.; Vermes, C.; Tunyogi-Csapó, M. Sagittal Plane Assessment of Spino-Pelvic Complex in a Central European Population with Adolescent Idiopathic Scoliosis: A Case Control Study. *Scoliosis Spinal Disord.* **2018**, *13*, 10. [CrossRef]
44. Schlösser, T.P.C.; Shah, S.A.; Reichard, S.J.; Rogers, K.; Vincken, K.L.; Castelein, R.M. Differences in Early Sagittal Plane Alignment between Thoracic and Lumbar Adolescent Idiopathic Scoliosis. *Spine J.* **2014**, *14*, 282–290. [CrossRef]
45. Czaprowski, D.; Kotwicki, T.; Pawłowska, P.; Stoliński, L. Joint Hypermobility in Children with Idiopathic Scoliosis: SOSORT Award 2011 Winner. *Scoliosis* **2011**, *6*, 22. [CrossRef]
46. Stępień, A. A Range of Rotation of the Trunk and Pelvis in Girls with Idiopathic Scoliosis. *Adv. Rehabil.* **2011**, *25*, 5–12. [CrossRef]
47. Burwell, R.G.; Cole, A.A.; Cook, T.A.; Grivas, T.B.; Kiel, A.W.; Moulton, A.; Thirlwall, A.S.; Upadhyay, S.S.; Webb, J.K.; Wemyss-Holden, S.A. Pathogenesis of Idiopathic Scoliosis. The Nottingham Concept. *Acta Orthop. Belg.* **1992**, *58* (Suppl. 1), 33–58.

48. Watson, K.D.; Papageorgiou, A.C.; Jones, G.T.; Taylor, S.; Symmons, D.P.M.; Silman, A.J.; Macfarlane, G.J. Low Back Pain in Schoolchildren: Occurrence and Characteristics. *Pain* **2002**, *97*, 87–92. [CrossRef]
49. Calvo-Muñoz, I.; Gómez-Conesa, A.; Sánchez-Meca, J. Prevalence of Low Back Pain in Children and Adolescents: A Meta-Analysis. *BMC Pediatr.* **2013**, *13*, 14. [CrossRef]
50. Kędra, A.; Czaprowski, D. Epidemiology of Back Pain in Children and Youth Aged 10–19 from the Area of the Southeast of Poland. *BioMed Res. Int.* **2013**, *2013*, 506823. [CrossRef]

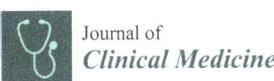

Article

Evolution of Early Onset Scoliosis under Treatment with a 3D-Brace Concept

Rebecca Sauvagnac and Manuel Rigo *

Rigo Quera Salvá S.L.P., 08021 Barcelona, Spain; rebecca.sauvagnac@gmail.com
* Correspondence: rigoquera@gmail.com; Tel.: +34-93-209-1330

Abstract: The objective of this study is to examine the evolution of all the braced patients diagnosed with early onset scoliosis in a private scoliosis center. All patients diagnosed with EOS and braced before the age of ten were retrospectively reviewed. The results have been defined in accordance with the Scoliosis Research Society (SRS) for bracing criteria, and with a minimum follow-up of one year. Improvement and stabilization were considered successful treatments, while failure was considered to be an unsuccessful treatment. Successful results were observed in 80% of patients (63% worst case). In the success group, the Cobb angle was reduced from 36.3° (21–68) to 25° (10–43), with 36% of patients being initially treated only with night-time bracing. Twenty percent of the patients failed, seven had more than 45° at the last control and five had undergone surgery. This study suggests that bracing, using a modern 3D-brace concept, could be an effective treatment option for early onset scoliosis and advocates exploring its effectiveness as an alternative to casting throughout studies of higher levels of evidence.

Keywords: early onset scoliosis; bracing; non-operative treatment

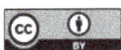

1. Introduction

Morphological scoliosis is a complex three-dimensional deformity of the trunk and spine that has multiple causes, which can appear during any period of life. When scoliosis has an unknown cause, it is called Idiopathic Scoliosis (IS). IS is the most common form of morphological scoliosis and appears in apparently healthy children during any growth period. The Scoliosis Research Society, in its revised glossary of terms [1], has established the chronological presentations of IS as: (1) infantile scoliosis: presenting from birth through age 2 + 11; (2) juvenile scoliosis: presenting from age 3 through age 9 + 11; (3) adolescent scoliosis: presenting from age 10 through age 17 + 11; (4) adult scoliosis: presenting from age 18 and beyond. Another common term is Early Onset Scoliosis (EOS). This term was used by Ponseti and Friedman to confirm a worse prognosis in scoliosis beginning before the age of 10 in comparison with scoliosis developing from aged 10 years and beyond, known as Late Onset Scoliosis (LOS) [2]. The term EOS was also used by Dickson as coinciding with infantile scoliosis [3], and later to define scoliosis present in children younger than 5 years of age [4]. Following some years of debate, the term EOS is now used globally and is defined by the SRS as a curvature of the spine ≥10 degrees in the frontal plane with onset before 10 years of age, including congenital, neuromuscular, syndromic and idiopathic. Thus, according to the SRS, EOS encompasses the two classical types: infantile and juvenile. In this paper, we will use this most-recently defined term for EOS, thus including infantile and juvenile.

EOS is a main priority for specialists due to its potential for early progression and, mainly in thoracic scoliosis, for its high risk of respiratory impairment. Currently, there are no treatment recommendations for these young patients. In 2007, Lenke [5] carried out a literature review and proposed brace treatment for scoliosis between 25° and 60°. The most widely used braces were the Milwaukee Brace (MB) and Thoraco-Lumbo-Sacral Orthosis

(TLSO) with eventual preliminary serial casting. Brace treatment should be abandoned in favor of surgical treatment by spinal fusion or with growing-rods with or without preliminary halo-gravity traction in curvatures of more than 60°. Early surgery can risk lessened spinal height, chest-wall and lung growth [6] and the crankshaft phenomenon [7].

Even if new surgery with growth-friendly instrumentation limits these complications, they often suppose multiple surgeries with the associated risk of cerebral neurodevelopmental due to repeated anesthesia [8,9].

In 2011, the Pediatric Orthopaedic Society of North America (POSNA) published a survey on EOS patients from 195 practitioners [10], showing that 89.1% braced their patients (albeit with no mention being made of the type of brace used), 62% cast them, 64.1% operated on them employing growing-rods, and 39.1% used chest wall expansion. In 2016, Yang et al. [11] conducted a review of patients exhibiting curves of more than 25° and with more than 10° documented progression. Yang et al. proposed bracing to maintain correction obtained from serial casting in order to delay surgery. Otherwise, most surgeons consider a scoliosis progression over 60° to indicate the need for distraction-based implants, as well as spinal fusion at the end [12].

It is now well known that bracing is effective in preventing progression to surgery in adolescent idiopathic scoliosis [13], but no consensus exists for infantile and juvenile idiopathic scoliosis. The most typically recommended braces for these patients are still the classic Milwaukee (MB) and TLSO braces. Harshavardhana and Lostein [14], in a retrospective study from 1956 to 1999 in 125 patients treated by the MB or TLSO braces before 10 years of age, showed an overall success rate of 45%. Khoshbin et al. [15] described around 88 patients with JIS treated by the MB, TLSO or Charleston braces between 1982 and 2011 and showed that 28% of the curves were improved or stabilized, 72% were progressing, and there was a 50% surgery rate. In comparison with these relatively poor results, in 2014 De Kleuver et al. [16] reported a 100% success rate with the Cobb angle decreasing in 42% of patients following brace treatment. However, this was in a cohort of only seven patients, three of whom had initially been treated by cast.

Although inspired by the old principles of correction from the 'Casting Era', some new braces do appear to be more effective in treating juvenile or infantile scoliosis. In 2014, Moreau et al. [17] studied the effect of a detorsion night-time brace pursuing Charleston principles, in 33 patients with brace onset at a mean age of 4 years and 2 months. They found a 67% success rate and a median Cobb angle reduction for success patients of 15° (3–27). More recently, Thometz et al. [18] have proposed an elongation-bending-derotation brace for infantile and juvenile scoliosis. This new brace system is made by using CAD/CAM in a corrective position and has been shown to achieve correction or stabilization in 75% of curves, with a progression incidence of only 25%.

The 3D brace used in this study is inspired by the so-called Chêneau brace and the French Casting Technique EDF. More than a type of brace identifiable with a specific curve pattern, it is a brace concept that can be recommended—using different techniques for design and construction—to treat most curve patterns in AIS and EOS. The principles of this brace have been described by its developer [19] and different authors have showed good results in treating AIS, but no data have been published on EOS [20–22]. We began using this brace concept for EOS in the late 1990s, introducing some modifications in the construction technique.

The main objective of our study is to evaluate the effect that rigid bracing (3D TLSO) has in EOS according to SRS criteria of success. The secondary aims are to study this effect on an EOS sub-group of patients with a known graver prognosis (younger than 5 years) and to evaluate factors that can influence treatment success.

2. Materials and Methods

Study design: This is a retrospective case series of all consecutive patients fulfilling inclusion criteria from 2007 to 2019.

Inclusion criteria were as follows: (1) Cobb angle of 25° or more; or Cobb angle of 20° to 24°, with documented progression; (2) starting brace treatment before 10 years of age; (3) minimum follow up of 1 year. We do not recommend bracing in all the cases with a Cobb angle of 25° or more as a single criterion for treatment, but rather we combine physical examination, Cobb angle degree, angle of vertebral rotation, costo-vertebral-angle difference, and factors such as positive family history. However, although these factors are taken into consideration when deciding on bracing or not, we did not collect these data for all the patients in a systematic way, which could have been used to discuss prognosis factors or report as outcomes. When considering the potential indications for bracing (25–60°), we try not to break the rules and, in most of the cases, we did not. Six patients with a Cobb angle between 21° and 24° were braced, all of them with a documented progression after an initial period of observation. Independent of the Cobb angle, they also presented some sign or signs of poor prognosis (e.g., high axial rotation, CVAD > 25°, high ATI value). Three patients with a Cobb angle over 60° were recommended bracing. Taking the Cobb angle as the only indication value is not always in accordance with the best clinical practice. For instance, we have rejected bracing for patients with curvatures less than 60°, or even less than 50°, due to the very high degree of rotation and rigidity, amount of lordotization and angular rib shape, making them poor candidates for any type of TLSO. As such, they were all referred to an orthopedic surgeon. The three cases with a Cobb angle over 60° who did undergo bracing still had curvatures flexible enough to accept a TLSO, although they were also visited by the orthopedic surgeon. However, following an interdisciplinary team approach, we decided by consensus to continue with bracing, for several reasons in relation with individual characteristics to try and buy time. Some patients diagnosed with EOS, however, were simply observed with no specific intervention other than regular medical controls, and radiographic controls only when indicated from clinical observation and exploration. Thus, not all the patients with a Cobb angle of 25 degrees or higher were directly recommended for bracing. Nevertheless, the patients included in this present study are those treated with a brace who fulfilled the inclusion criteria defined above. Where possible (i.e., a better prognosis) and after discussing the case with the parents, an initial recommendation for wearing time was 'night-time' (i.e., 6 to 12 H). In the cases with poorer initial prognoses, these were prescribed 'full time' wearing ($\geq$20 H) from the very beginning. That said, some parents would only accept 'partial time' (13–19 H), not full-time, for their children. We were not able to instigate in order to objectively report the real wearing time.

Exclusion criteria were pre-treated patients (casting or brace).

At each visit, patients had their brace checked and underwent a physical examination. Because we have a private practice and, in accordance with an evidence-based personalized approach model [23], we do not have a fixed protocol for radiographic control, an Out Of Brace (OOB) radiograph was ordered when (and only when) either a physical examination gave us a clear suspicion of curve deterioration, or we had to change the brace due to growth and development, or we suspected a change in the curve pattern necessitating a new brace design.

Before 2007, we had initiated treatment with the 3D brace concept in only four EOS cases without previous treatment (usually casting). Three of them were still under treatment when we started the informatics clinical files and data collection and were considered for inclusion in this study, albeit with initial data having to be added to the file retrospectively. The four patients were included, but one had incomplete data, and another was lost. Thus, this series includes all the EOS we have treated with a rigid TLS 3D brace, with no previous treatment; consequently, it is a series of consecutive treated cases.

The brace: The 3D brace according to Rigo principles can be either hand-made or built using CAD CAM. The basic idea is to design highly specific contact and expansion areas on a positive mould of the patient's trunk. The contact areas are designed into the brace's shape, orientation and level in order to produce the necessary combined detorsional forces. Thus, the brace follows, in most of cases, the simple general principle of correction defined from

Dubousset (1992) [24], 'reaching the best possible frontal and sagittal alignment by using detorsional forces', and some well-described specific principles of correction: (1) regional derotation plus cranial and caudal counter-rotation forces; (2) lateral as well as ventro-dorsal contacts for frontal and sagittal plane alignment guidance; (3) a special mechanism to fight against the structural lordotization of the thoracic region, which depends on the level, the shape and the orientation of the contact areas of the brace. As a whole, the objective is not the maximum correction in one single plane but rather reaching the best possible frontal and sagittal alignment while preventing any worsening of compensatory curvatures and/or imbalance (Figures 1 and 2). Thus, the level-orientation shape of where the detorsional forces are applied is of equal importance to the standard of the brace, as its implementation is in accordance with the clinical type and radiological curve pattern. The level of the main derotational force is the apical region of the main curve or curves, with counter-rotation forces acting at the proximal thoracic region and at the lumbo-pelvic or pelvic region. The design of the contact areas can then be made using CAD CAM or classical hand-made rectification of the pre-elongated mould. As a result, this is not a standardized orthopedic product but rather a treatment concept needing specific knowledge and experience from those prescribing, manufacturing and later controlling the brace. Once again, the knowledge and experience of the treatment team, as noted by the SOSORT guidelines for brace treatment [25], are essential areas of expertise.

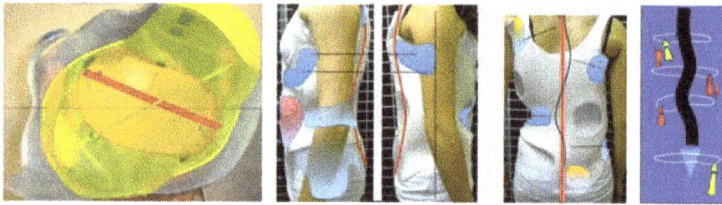

Figure 1. The brace design when treating a double structural scoliosis (Rigo B Type). Two mechanisms for regional derotation are applied, one at the main thoracic region and another at the lumbar/thoracolumbar region (red arrows). These two mechanisms for regional derotation work in combination with two counter-rotation forces (yellow arrows). Contact areas are provided, laterally, ventrally and dorsally, to guide the frontal as well as the sagittal plane alignment and balance. (The figures describe the brace design showing an adolescent. The brace design in EOS follows the same principles).

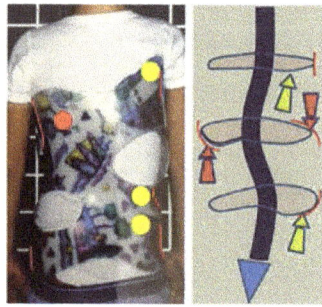

Figure 2. The brace design in a single thoracic scoliosis (Left convex in this EOS patient). One single mechanism of regional derotation (red arrows) works in combination with two counter-rotation forces (yellow arrows). Lateral, dorsal and ventral contacts are provided to guide frontal and sagittal plane alignment and balance.

Consistent with SRS criteria [26], we defined improvement to be a decrease of more than 5° of the Cobb angle between brace initiation and the final control, stabilization a Cobb angle variation ±5°, and failure an increase of more than 5°, Cobb > 45° at last control or at maturity, or a final need for surgery.

Improved and stabilized patients were all included in a simple success group. Thus, treatment could be defined as success or failure and patients as responders or not responders.

Because of its higher potential of progression, we also separately analyzed patients that could have originally been defined as EOS according to Dickson, i.e., those with a relevant spinal deformity before 5 years old.

Statistical analysis was performed using PSPP and GNU Software.

For quantitative variables, we analyzed means, standard deviations and ranges.

To evaluate the correlation between Cobb angles before and after treatment, we used a *t*-test for the paired sample, and to evaluate factors that could have influenced the success of the treatment we used a one-factor ANOVA.

3. Results

From a list of 280 patients younger than 10 years old coming for a consultation because of a suspicion of scoliosis and seen for at least a second time, we confirmed 84 EOS patients according to the SRS definition. Sixty-six patients fulfilled the inclusion criteria. Nine out of the sixty-six were excluded due to previous treatment (brace or cast). Twelve out of the fifty-seven patients finally included had incomplete (10) or lost data (2). Forty-five patients with complete data were fully analyzed and a worst-case analysis was then performed in terms of 'rate of success' considering the 12 patients, with lost or incomplete data, as failures (Figure 3).

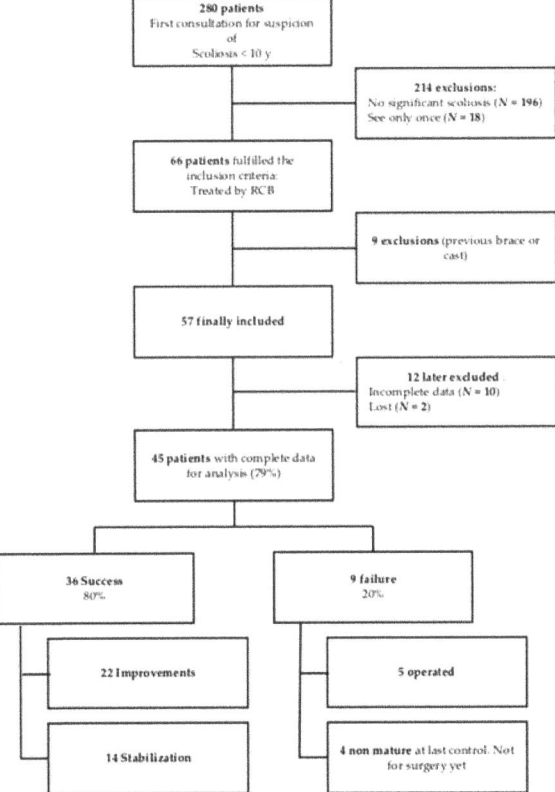

Figure 3. Flow chart. Worst case analysis = 63.2% success (36 success/57 finally included, presuming that cases lost to follow had failed).

Thus, 45 patients were finally analyzed, with a female–male ratio of 2:1.

Most of the patients (77%) had idiopathic scoliosis. Ten patients had a known cause: one congenital, five neurological, one Beals syndrome, one arthrogryposis, one Ehler Danlos syndrome, and one neurofibromatosis syndrome.

It was not possible using the Lenke classification to describe the radiological curve pattern of this present population. Using SRS terminology, however, 69% of the cases were single thoracic without lumbar, with functional lumbar or with a compensatory structural lumbar curve (Rigo clinical types A and C). Twenty-four percent of the cases were real double thoracic and lumbar or thoracolumbar (Rigo clinical type B), while only 4% were single lumbar or thoracolumbar (Rigo clinical type E). Figure 4 shows the distribution according to the Rigo classification [27].

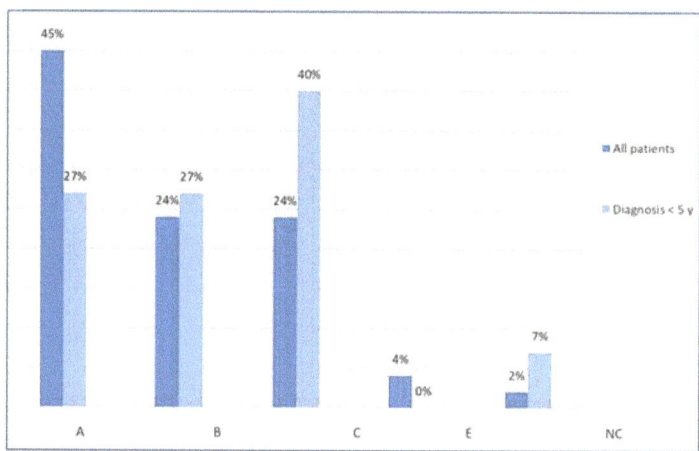

Figure 4. Distribution of clinical types according to Rigo Classification (A: Rigo type A; B: Rigo type B; C: Rigo Type C; E: Rigo Type E; NC: Not Classifiable).

The mean Cobb angle at brace initiation was 36.1 ± 11.6° (21.0–68.0). Age at first visit was 6.6 ± 2.0 years (2.5–9.8), age at last control was 13.2 ± 3.0 years (6.2–20.7). Mean years of follow-up was 6.5 ± 3.0 (1.0–15.6).

3.1. Treatment Success and Failure

Eighty percent of the patients met the success criteria at the last control: 49% improved and 31% stabilized their curves. Forty percent of all patients reached bone maturity (≥Risser 3 European Scale/≥4 American Scale) and 50% were still under a bracing regime at the last control.

In the success group (improved or stabilized), we observed a significant Cobb angle improvement from 36.3 ± 11.4° (21–68) to 25.0 ± 8.6° (10–43) when comparing initial values at the beginning, before starting brace treatment, and values at the last control ($p < 0.001$ by t-test Student). In the group of patients showing improvement (22 patients), the Cobb angle decreased by 17.1° ± 9.1 (7.0–37.0).

In the success group (improved or stabilized), 53% were treated initially using a full-time brace, 36% with a night-time brace and the remaining 11% with a part-time brace (Figure 5).

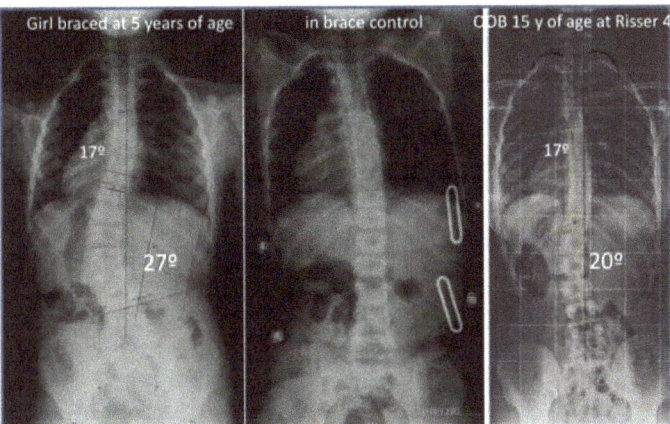

Figure 5. Example of success. Result of treatment in a girl braced at 5 years of age with a left lumbar scoliosis of 27°, completing treatment under night-time regimen until 15 years of age at Risser 4, stopping treatment with a left lumbar curvature of 20°.

Twenty percent (nine patients) failed, with a mean time of follow-up from the initiation of treatment to failure of 7.1 years ± 1.9 (5.2–10.1) and a mean progression of the Cobb angle of 22.7 ± 12.5° (10–46). Seven out of these nine patients had more than 45° at the last control (Figure 6). All the patients had been instructed to wear the brace full-time; however, we cannot report about the real compliance in these failed patients.

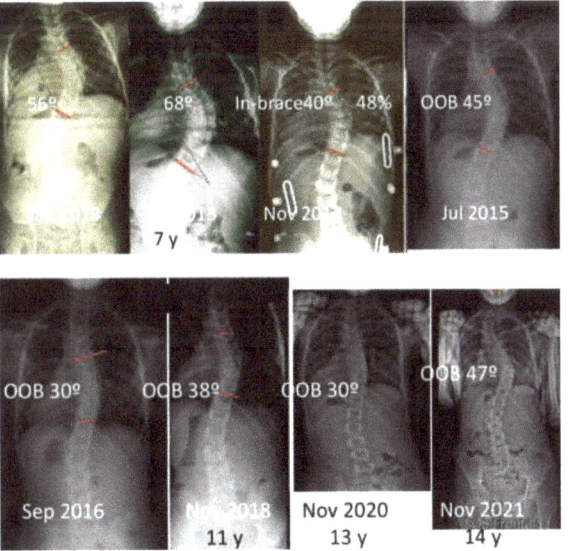

Figure 6. Girl treated with full-time brace, initiating the treatment at 7 years of age with a 68° thoracic scoliosis. With a 48% in-brace correction in her first brace she showed a good response until 10 years with a scoliosis of 30°. She was followed until 12 years of age still with a scoliosis of 30°. Next control at 13 years, she was still stable with 30°, but had developed a more relevant proximal curvature (after closing this present study). Between 2020 and 2021 (not registered in this present study), she showed a deterioration, with the development of a proximal curve of 43°, forcing us to stop bracing and recommending her to undergo surgery.

Treatment strategies for six out of the nine patients was changed when failure was detected: (1) increasing wearing time from night-time to full-time in four patients; and (2) two patients were recommended to undergo surgery. Three more patients had surgery sometime later, so, overall, five patients were finally operated on.

3.2. Prognosis Factors

When comparing the two groups showing success or failure, we did not find any significant difference in age (6.5 vs. 5.4 p 0.175), Cobb angle (36.3° vs. 35.6° p 0.875) at the initiation of brace treatment, and age at the last control (13.1 vs. 11.8 p 0.776) (Table 1).

Table 1. Cobb evolution in both successful and failure groups (significance $p < 0.05$).

	Successful Group (N36)		Failure Group (N9)		
	Mean	Range	Mean	Range	p
Age at brace onset (years)	6.5 ± 2.0	2.0–9.0	5.4 ± 2.5	1.0–8.0	0.175
Cobb angle at brace onset (°)	33.3 ± 11.4	21.0–68.0	35.6 ± 13.1	24.0–65.0	0.875
Age at last control (years)	13.1 ± 3.2	6.2–20.7	12.8 ± 2.7	7.0–16.0	0.776
Cobb angle at last control (°)	25.0 ± 8.9	10.0–43.0	58.2 ± 14.1	38.0–76.0	<0.001

3.3. Population under 5 Years of Age

Fifteen of the 47 patients were less than 5 years of age when they were diagnosed with EOS. As they are expected to have a poorer prognosis, we decided to analyze them separately. As expected, the female–male sex ratio was more balanced: 0.88:1 in this sub-group (vs. 2.13:1 in our total cohort).

Etiology was idiopathic scoliosis (73%), while others were congenital (1), neurological (2), and Beals syndrome (1).

Radiological curve patterns were mostly thoracic curves (67%) (A and C Rigo clinical type). Real double was observed in 27% of the cases (B Rigo clinical type). There were no single lumbar or thoracolumbar curves (Figure 2).

Follow-up time was not significantly different in this sub-group when compared with the whole cohort (Table 2).

Table 2. Baseline characteristics of study population (significance $p < 0.05$).

	All Patients	Diagnosis < 5 y	p
No. of patients	45	15	
Age at diagnosis, Mean ± SD (y)	5.3 ± 2.3	2.7 ± 1.2	<0.001
Sex			
Female	67% (30/45)	47% (7/15)	
Male	33% (15/45)	53% (8/15)	
Age at brace onset, Mean ± SD (y)	6.3 ± 2.1	4.6 ± 2.4	0.012
Age at last control, Mean ± SD (y)	13.1 ± 3.1	11.6 ± 2.9	0.106
Years of follow up, Mean ± SD (y)	6.5 ± 3.0	6.6 ± 2.3	0.865

Only six out of these 15 EOS patients started brace treatment before 5 years of age. Mean age at brace onset was 4.6 ± 2.3 years old (1.0–9.0).

Sixty-seven percent of the EOS patients from this sub-group showed treatment success. The 27.8° ± 7.4 (15–40) Cobb angle at the last brace control was significantly lower compared with the Cobb angle at the initiation of brace treatment 35.8° ± 10.0° (29–63) ($p = 0.027$, by t-test Student).

As in the total sample, age and Cobb angle at the initiation of brace treatment was not different in both groups showing success or failure in this sub-group (Table 3).

Table 3. Patients under 5 years at diagnosis. Cobb evolution in both successful and failure groups ($p < 0.05$).

	Successful Group (N10)		Failure Group (N5)		
	Mean	Range	Mean	Range	p
Age at brace onset (years)	4.8 ± 2.6	2.0–9.0	4.2 ± 2.8	1.0–8.0	0.667
Cobb angle at brace onset (°)	35.8 ± 10.0	29.0–63,0	40.4 ± 16.6	24.0–65.0	0.511
Age at last control (years)	11.1 ± 3.3	6.2–16.7	12.7 ± 1.6	10.9–14.8	0.378
Cobb angle at last control (°)	27.8 ± 7.4	15.0–40.0	66.2 ± 13.2	43.0–76.0	<0.001
Cobb evolution (°)	8.0 ± 9.6	−3.0–25.0	−25.8 ± 15.5	−46.0–−11.0	<0.001

4. Discussion

Comparison with previous studies. This is a cohort of 57 consecutive patients diagnosed with EOS (mostly Idiopathic) treated with a 3D-brace concept according to Rigo principles before the age of 10. Twelve patients were lost or presented incomplete data and were not included in the final analysis. We report an 80% success rate, defining success according to the SRS criteria of improvement or stabilization. In a worst-case analysis, the success rate was 63.2%. Our results are along the same lines as those reported by Moreau et al. [18] and Thometz et al. [19], both using new-generation 3D braces. Moreau et al. [18] had 67% of success with a mean Cobb angle reduction of 15°, a little bit lower than ours, but with all their patients receiving night-time bracing and being a little younger than ours. Notwithstanding this, a relevant proportion of our patients were instructed to wear their braces only at night, at least initially, and we did not find the age of the initiation of bracing to be different in our successful and unsuccessful patients. Moreau et al. used a detorsional night-time brace, only wearable at night due to its design. According to the description of the authors, the design of this brace was inspired by the Charleston bending brace and can be used only at night, but the horizontal plane action follows the Chêneau principles like our 3D brace. However, our brace does not have a different design when it is to be used only at night or to be worn full-time. We use a unique day/night design based on detorsional forces, which can be worn indistinctly at night or full-time, thus allowing us, when necessary and with greater flexibility, to increase the wearing time with no need to change the brace, yet still working well. Our results must be taken with precaution because, although 60% of our patients were scored Risser 3 (European), so able to be considered mature enough to stop bracing, our follow-up (6.5 years) was lower than the one reported by Moreau (10 y). Thometz et al. [19] reported around 75% of success (improvement or stabilization) in treating IS and JS with an Elongation Bending Derotation Brace. However, this report studies 38 patients followed only during their first year of treatment and must be considered as preliminary results.

What is important to mention is that, with all the limitations discussed below, our study, as well as the two previously discussed studies, suggests that new brace designs are superior to the classic Milwaukee and TLSO braces, as reported by Harshavardhana and Lonstein [15] and Khoshbin et al. [16], the two main papers about bracing in infantile and juvenile scoliosis. Harshavardhana and Lonstein report an overall success rate of 45%, defining success as 'not reaching a surgical value'. It is true that the sample size of these authors is greater (N = 125 patients); however, this sample comes from a long-term database and represents only 15% of the juvenile cases. From a database of 841 patients, 80% were excluded for different reasons and, although some of these patients were observed, many were undoubtedly treated with a brace. Our smaller series represents all the patients we have treated with this type of brace (some are still under treatment). The pre-brace age is, on the other hand, higher in the study from Harshavardhana and Lonstein [15] (8 years) in comparison with ours (6.6), while the initial mean Cobb angle is lower (30° vs. 36°). Moreover, 32 out of 125 patients in their study initiated brace treatment during adolescence. According to Donzelli et al. [28], patients diagnosed during the juvenile period but braced later, during adolescence, can be considered, in terms of prognosis, as adolescent scoliosis. It is true that, like us, they did not find age differences in successful and unsuccessful patients, but rather a higher pre-brace Cobb angle was observed in those failing. Thus, we can consider our population of having a poorer prognosis in comparison to those from Harshavardhana and Lonstein [15], as we did not include any patient braced at or after 10 years of age, and our patients also have a higher pre-brace Cobb angle. In contraposition, follow-up is longer in their study and some of our patients are still under treatment and have not yet reached their adolescent growth spurt. Patients needing surgery in the study of Harshavardhana and Lonstein [15] were stable during the juvenile period and did show progression during the adolescent growth spurt, so we could expect that some of our patients will fail and might finally need surgery. Notwithstanding this, the mean chronological age in our series, as well as the bone age (60% at Risser 3-European), indicates that a relevant number of patients already passed the peak of growth and are not far from becoming mature. On the other hand, reaching that period of growth with a successful result is remarkable, as one of the objectives of non-operative treatment in EOS is delaying early surgery, in other words, buying time. Thus, we must be prudent in affirming that our results, in correlation with those from Moreau et al. and Thometz et al., suggest that a new-generation brace might be more effective in preventing progression in EOS in comparison with the Milwaukee brace or the classic TLSO.

We cannot compare our study with the study from Khoshbin et al. [16]. In this last study, in a cohort of 88 patients diagnosed with JIS, the authors showed a 50% incidence of final surgery, with 28% of patients showing a minimal curve progression or improvement. On the other hand, they reported a low compliance (49% wore the brace full-time). Although this study is considered one of the main references in relationship with the effect of bracing on juvenile idiopathic scoliosis, the mean age at diagnosis was 8.4 years and the mean age at the initiation of bracing was 9.3 ± 1.5 years for the whole sample and 9.9 ± 1.4 for those not needing surgery. This clearly indicates that a highly relevant number of patients started wearing the brace at 10 years of age or older, coinciding with the ascending phase of growth in the adolescent period. The Cobb angle at baseline was 31° (20–71). According to Donzelli et al. [28], the response to bracing in patients diagnosed with JIS according to the SRS (from 3 years to 9 years and 11 months) but starting bracing at 10 years of age or later is not different to those diagnosed with AIS. Thus, we could expect a response similar to that of children with very early AIS in the Khoshbin et al. study (initiation of bracing and pre-brace curve magnitude), and, knowing that bracing is dose dependent in AIS [14], the high incidence of final surgery should be no surprise, considering a compliance under 50%.

Prognosis factors. In relationship with prognosis factors, we did not find any factor that could explain success or failure as a result of the treatment. Indeed, neither age at brace initiation, pre-brace cobb angle, nor initial wearing time are significantly different between those responding well and those failing. In the Moreau study [18], the unsuccessful group was older (58 months vs. 42 months) and had a higher main Cobb angle (35° vs. 28°) at the initial examination, compared with the success group. Our results could indicate that pre-brace age and Cobb angle are, contrary to the study from Moreau et al., not factors for a poorer treatment response, while having the chance to change from nigh- time to partial or full-time when necessary are. However, we must admit that with age and curve magnitude both being factors for prognosis when looking at the natural history of EOS, our results could be different with a bigger cohort and the exclusion of non-idiopathic cases. On the other hand, we did not look at compliance and in-brace correction as possible factors associated to brace response. We cannot report on real compliance as we did not use sensors. In any case, we have the impression that, once having discussed the proper wearing time with parents and accepting their final decision about this being full-time or partial night-time, compliance in EOS patients is good, as it depends mainly on parental care, at least before and during the ascending phase of growth in the adolescence or before menarche. We had very few cases where compliance was good during the pre-menarche period and failed afterwards. It looks to be easier for children wearing a brace before puberty to continue using the brace with good compliance during the more difficult time of adolescence in comparison with those starting bracing when they are already adolescents; this is, however, just a subjective impression. In-brace correction was not analyzed because, in accordance with our clinical protocols, we only look at in-brace correction in those patients that are recommended to wear the brace full-time, as in-brace correction as a prognosis factor is highly dependent on the wearing time [14]. Consequently, in most of our EOS patients, radiological controls are made out-of-brace.

The sub-group of patients younger than 5. Regarding the sub-group of EOS patients younger than 5 years of age with a relevant structural curvature at presentation, the 15 patients had the same characteristics as the whole cohort. As is known in the literature, we found a female–male ratio that tends to be towards boys (0.8:1) and a higher number of thoracic curves [29,30], and this could be interpreted as these patients being part of the real infantile scoliosis group, those going into progression during infantile and childhood periods before the properly defined juvenile period [31]. As in the entire cohort, we did not find any possible factors associated with success or unsuccessful results. It is noticeable that only six of this sub-group of 15 EOS patients diagnosed before the age of 5 years, were really braced at or before the age of 5 years. Two of these six patients failed and four succeeded ($p = 0.67$ by chi-2). However, the type of study and the number of cases analyzed in this particular sub-group do not allow us to draw any clear conclusion. The proportion of failures in this sub-group (5/15) in comparison with the whole sample (9/45) strongly suggest that this sub-group of patients has a poorer prognosis; consequently, we still believe it would of interest to analyze this sub-group of patients and those diagnosed at six years of age to 9 years and 11 months separately, as most probably there are two different conditions.

Good responders and night-time bracing. Looking at this present study, it is important to point out the apparently good response to night-time bracing. Early onset scoliosis with a Cobb angle over 25° is generally considered as having a poor prognosis. However, the Cobb angle by itself was found not to be the main factor associated with the risk of progression in EOS, but rather in combination with other more important factors, such as the amount of axial rotation [32] or the costovertebral angle difference [33]. Furthermore, independent of the initial Cobb angle, flexibility and the shape and magnitude of the rib hump could be determinant factors for a good response to treatment [34]. In our current clinical practice, we do not use a closed protocol based on a particular Cobb angle to initiate bracing, but we make a decision (in consensus with the family) based on a personalized approach and by taking into consideration values such as axial rotation, costovertebral angle difference, flexibility (tested only by clinical exploration) and the shape of the rib hump. We consider these factors to be important not only in brace indication but also in the prescribed wearing time. In AIS, there is consensus about recommending a wearing time of ≥ 18 h in scoliosis involving a high risk of surgery [34]. It is true that EOS is a population classically considered to be at high risk of needing surgery but, still, some patients with the diagnosis of EOS according to the SRS definition do not go into progression before the age of 10 but do so later during the adolescent period, showing the same behavior as classical AIS [28], while others do not progress or even regress. Thus, there was some data based on clinical experience and evidence supporting the expectation of good responders that might be treated with night-time bracing, and these results support the prescription of night-time bracing in some selected patients, i.e., basically those with relative degrees of rotation (<10° Perdriolle), Cobb angles under 35°, low costovertebral angle differences (<20°), with flexible curvatures and 'round versus angular rib humps'.

Limitations. Our study has important limitations. First, it comes from a unique center, showing results from a brace made by the main author of this article. Even if the main outcome was evaluated from a universal and reproducible measurement like the Cobb angle is, it would be necessary to investigate the effectiveness of this type of 3D brace when used by others. Notwithstanding this, the fact that our results are akin to those using similar brace principles minimizes this weak point. Second, a more important limitation is that this is a retrospective study with no control group, so conclusions will need to be in accordance with this low level of evidence. However, considering the very few studies of these characteristics and the general belief that casting is the main treatment option in EOS, we felt there is a strong need to report our experience to increase the amount of evidence in order to justify a prospective study with the highest possible methodology, comparing casting and bracing in EOS. After looking at our results and some parts of the previous discussion, we would suggest separately analyzing those EOS developing a relevant structural scoliosis before the age of 5, defining well what means 'relevant', with the need of bracing before the age of 5, rather than just taking the classic definitions of IIS and JIS. Idiopathic scoliosis and non-idiopathic should also be analyzed separately. Furthermore, it would be interesting to explore the possibility of 'serial bracing' in the youngest patients (i.e., younger than 3 years). This is something that we have already tried with a few patients when families rejected casting for various reasons, and after being informed about current evidence. The CAD CAM technology makes this easier, with no need to stress the child unnecessarily. Once the design has been made, the real cost of fabricating the plastic itself is not so high and, while it is necessary just to enlarge and elongate the brace for 'serial bracing', in general, it is not necessary to change the design significantly.

In retrospective studies, patients lost for the final analysis are always a problem. We had to exclude two lost patients and ten with incomplete data. Thus, we made a worst-case analysis (see Figure 3) by adding to the forty-five analyzed patients the ten with incomplete files and the two lost patients but, even so, we still obtained a final success percentage of 63.2% (36/57), with a percentage of unsuccessful cases of 36.2% (21/57). These numbers are still interesting, as they are closer to everyday clinical practice.

A further limitation is the fact that this series includes non-idiopathic scoliosis. First of all, we wanted to report on our experience in treating EOS with bracing, and the definition of EOS includes types of scoliosis other than idiopathic. On the other hand, the incidence of neurological anomalies in EOS was still a controversial issue at the time we started bracing in EOS. We were not routinely ordering MRIs at that time, but just in case we found some specific atypical features. In 2004, Morcuende et al. reported a relatively low probability of neurogenic lesions in EOS with atypical features other than severe curves or neurological abnormalities (3% probability) [35]. Thus, we ordered MRIs only in the cases where we found a severe curve or neurologic changes. We found three patients with an anomaly in the neuro axis (Chiari and Syrinx). Two of them had been operated on. One boy who had had surgery before the age of 3 did not show a regression of the curvature and he was consequently recommended to undergo bracing. The second patient was braced at the end of 7 years after observing a progression from 44° to 55° after neurosurgical decompression. The third patient was treated directly with bracing with no previous neurosurgical intervention, and she showed a spontaneous resolution of the syrinx. The latter two patients mentioned were presented in a double case report during the SOSORT meeting of 2012 in Milano [36]. All three patients showed a good response to bracing and did fall into the success group.

Other important outcomes that we were not able to report on in detail are breathing function, trunk shape, sagittal radiological values and quality of life. The first two, breathing function and trunk shape, especially the rib cage, are partially related. We believe that allowing the correct development of the rib cage and re-shaping the rib cage would be important factors for future breathing function and curve stability. It must be pointed out that, historically, many scoliosis specialists have advised against using TLSO in EOS due to the risk of worsening breath function and deforming the ribs. We must recognize that the type of brace used in this study, due to its sophisticated design, has an iatrogenic potential when used improperly and only looking at the Cobb angle correction. Sagittal radiological values are, nowadays, considered to be highly important from both clinical and scientific points of view. However, when these young patients started their treatment, the consensus about using initial radiographs in the lateral projection was not so clear, and we tried to use the fewest possible number of radiographs in this young population. Quality of life, from a biopsychosocial perspective, is another important aspect to consider. Although we routinely assess quality of life in adolescents and adults using validated instruments, we did not look at this data in this present study. We have the intention to look at all these important aspects (breathing function, trunk shape, sagittal alignment and balance and quality of life) in this same reported population once they have all finished their treatments with a minimum follow-up of two years. That said, we felt this was a good time to report on our experience with non-operative treatment in EOS.

5. Conclusions

This study suggests that bracing, using a modern 3D-brace concept, could be an effective treatment option for EOS and advocates exploring the effectiveness of bracing in EOS through studies of a higher level of evidence.

Author Contributions: R.S. and M.R. conceived and designed the study. R.S. collected and analyzed the data. All authors have read and agreed to the published version of the manuscript.

Funding: This research received no external funding.

Institutional Review Board Statement: Ethical review and approval were waived for this study, due to its retrospective case series design. This is not an experiment. We used already existing data collected from patients' clinical files retrospectively in a private clinic where patients sign a consent form for the use of their clinical data. Although there is low evidence, bracing in EOS is a common accepted practice. Data are related to a treatment which is in accordance with current good practice (POSNA survey reporting that 89.1% of practitioners braced their patients). The brace used in our institution is not a new or experimental brace but an accepted TLSO following well-known corrective principles since it was first introduced by Jacques Cheneau and Professor Mathias in 1979.

Informed Consent Statement: The authors used already existing data, so informed consent was not necessary. Written informed consent has been obtained from patients for the use of the radiographs used in the figures.

Data Availability Statement: The data presented in this study are available on request from the corresponding authors. The data are not publicly available due to privacy.

Acknowledgments: All the braces were designed and constructed in 'Ortopedia Grau Soler'. Beatriz Camos, owner of Grau Soler. Enric Alcolea, CPO Grau Soler.

Conflicts of Interest: R.S. declares no conflict of interest. M.R. declares: Honoraria for medical advice from Ortholutions (Germany) and from AlignClinic (California, USA). R.S. was an employee in the company Rigo Quera Salvá at the time the study was completed, working for the company until March 2020. Nowadays, R.S. is an employee of the French company UPNOS, working in the field of sleep disorders and also at Wandercraft, another French company, working in the field of exoskeletons. M.R. is an employer and director of the company Rigo Quera Salvá S.L.P., a private rehabilitation clinic for spinal deformities. All the braces were designed, manufactured and fitted in Ortopedia Grau Soler, Barcelona, Spain. M.R. personally designed all the braces. M.R. specifically declares that neither himself nor Rigo Quera Salvá S.L.P. have any type of commercial relationship, partnership, honoraria, direct or indirect incomes or benefits from Ortopedia Grau Soler.

References

1. Revised Glossary of Terms | Scoliosis Research Society. Available online: https://www.srs.org/professionals/online-education-and-resources/glossary/revised-glossary-of-terms (accessed on 2 July 2019).
2. Ponseti, I.V.; Friedman, B. Prognosis in idiopathic scoliosis. *J. Bone Jt. Surg. Am.* **1950**, *32A*, 381–395. [CrossRef]
3. Dickson, R. Conservative treatment for idiopathic scoliosis. *J. Bone Jt. Surg. Br.* **1985**, *67*, 176–181. [CrossRef] [PubMed]
4. Dickson, R.A. Idiopathic scoliosis. *BMJ* **1989**, *298*, 906–907. [CrossRef]
5. Lenke, L.G.; Dobbs, M.B. Management of Juvenile Idiopathic Scoliosis. *J. Bone Jt. Surg.* **2007**, *89*, 55–63. [CrossRef]
6. Winter, R. Scoliosis and spinal growth. *Orthop. Res.* **1977**, *6*, 17–20.
7. Dubousset, J.; Herring, J.A.; Shufflebarger, H. The Crankshaft Phenomenon. *J. Pediatr. Orthop.* **1989**, *9*, 541–550. [CrossRef]
8. Flick, R.P.; Katusic, S.K.; Colligan, R.C.; Wilder, R.T.; Voigt, R.G.; Olson, M.D.; Sprung, J.; Weaver, A.L.; Schroeder, D.R.; Warner, D.O. Cognitive and Behavioral Outcomes After Early Exposure to Anesthesia and Surgery. *Pediatrics* **2011**, *128*, e1053–e1061. [CrossRef]

9. Hu, D.; Flick, R.P.; Zaccariello, M.J.; Colligan, R.C.; Katusic, S.K.; Schroeder, D.R.; Hanson, A.C.; Buenvenida, S.L.; Gleich, S.J.; Wilder, R.T.; et al. Association between Exposure of Young Children to Procedures Requiring General Anesthesia and Learning and Behavioral Outcomes in a Population-based Birth Cohort. *Anesthesiology* **2017**, *127*, 227–240. [CrossRef]
10. Fletcher, N.D.; Larson, A.N.; Richards, B.S.; Johnston, C.E. Current treatment preferences for early onset scoliosis: A survey of POSNA members. *J. Pediatr. Orthop.* **2011**, *31*, 326–330. [CrossRef]
11. Yang, S.; Andras, L.M.; Redding, G.J.; Skaggs, D.L. Early-Onset Scoliosis: A Review of History, Current Treatment, and Future Directions. *Pediatrics* **2016**, *137*, e20150709. [CrossRef]
12. Corona, J.; Miller, D.J.; Downs, J.; Akbarnia, A.B.; Betz, R.R.; Blakemore, L.C.; Campbell, R.M.; Flynn, J.M.; Johnston, E.C.; McCarthy, E.R.; et al. Evaluating the Extent of Clinical Uncertainty Among Treatment Options for Patients with Early-Onset Scoliosis. *J. Bone Jt. Surg.* **2013**, *95*, e67. [CrossRef] [PubMed]
13. Weinstein, S.L.; Dolan, L.; Wright, J.G.; Dobbs, M.B. Effects of Bracing in Adolescents with Idiopathic Scoliosis. *N. Engl. J. Med.* **2013**, *369*, 1512–1521. [CrossRef]
14. Harshavardhana, N.S.; Lonstein, J.E. Results of Bracing for Juvenile Idiopathic Scoliosis. *Spine Deform.* **2018**, *6*, 201–206. [CrossRef] [PubMed]
15. Khoshbin, A.; Caspi, L.; Law, P.W.; Donaldson, S.; Stephens, D.; Da Silva, T.; Bradley, C.S.; Wright, J.G. Outcomes of Bracing in Juvenile Idiopathic Scoliosis Until Skeletal Maturity or Surgery. *Spine* **2015**, *40*, 50–55. [CrossRef]
16. Van Hessem, L.; Schimmel, J.J.; Graat, H.C.; de Kleuver, M. Effective nonoperative treatment in juvenile idiopathic scoliosis. *J. Pediatr. Orthop. B* **2014**, *23*, 454–460. [CrossRef] [PubMed]
17. Moreau, S.; Lonjon, G.; Mazda, K.; Ilharreborde, B. Detorsion night-time bracing for the treatment of early onset idiopathic scoliosis. *Orthop. Traumatol. Surg. Res.* **2014**, *100*, 935–939. [CrossRef] [PubMed]
18. Thometz, J.; Liu, X.; Rizza, R.; English, I.; Tarima, S. Effect of an elongation bending derotation brace on the infantile or juvenile scoliosis. *Scoliosis Spinal Disord.* **2018**, *13*, 13. [CrossRef] [PubMed]
19. Rigo, M.; Jelačić, M. Brace technology thematic series: The 3D Rigo Chêneau-type brace. *Scoliosis Spinal Disord.* **2017**, *12*, 1–46. [CrossRef] [PubMed]
20. Ovadia, D.; Eylon, S.; Mashiah, A.; Wientroub, S.; Lebel, E.D. Factors associated with the success of the Rigo System Chêneau brace in treating mild to moderate adolescent idiopathic scoliosis. *J. Child. Orthop.* **2012**, *6*, 327–331. [CrossRef]
21. Rivett, L.; Stewart, A.; Potterton, J. The effect of compliance to a Rigo System Cheneau brace and a specific exercise programme on idiopathic scoliosis curvature: A comparative study: SOSORT 2014 award winner. *Scoliosis* **2014**, *9*, 5. [CrossRef]
22. Minsk, M.K.; Venuti, K.D.; Daumit, G.L.; Sponseller, P.D. Effectiveness of the Rigo Chêneau versus Boston-style orthoses for adolescent idiopathic scoliosis: A retrospective study. *Scoliosis Spinal Disord.* **2017**, *12*, 7. [CrossRef] [PubMed]
23. Negrini, S.; Donzelli, S.; Negrini, F.; Arienti, C.; Zaina, F.; Peers, K. A Pragmatic Benchmarking Study of an Evidence-Based Personalised Approach in 1938 Adolescents with High-Risk Idiopathic Scoliosis. *J. Clin. Med.* **2021**, *10*, 5020. [CrossRef] [PubMed]
24. Dubousset, J. Importance of the three-dimensional concept in the treatment of scoliotic deformities. In *International Symposium on 3D Scoliotic Deformities Joined with the VIIth International Symposium on Spinal Deformity and Surface Topography*; Éditions de l'École Polytechnique de Montréal; Gustav Fischer Verlag: Stuttgart, Germany, 1992; pp. 302–311.
25. Negrini, S.; Donzelli, S.; Aulisa, A.G.; Czaprowski, D.; Schreiber, S.; De Mauroy, J.C.; Diers, H.; Grivas, T.B.; Knott, P.; Kotwicki, T.; et al. 2016 SOSORT guidelines: Orthopaedic and rehabilitation treatment of idiopathic scoliosis during growth. *Scoliosis Spinal Disord.* **2018**, *13*, 3. [CrossRef] [PubMed]
26. Richards, B.S.; Bernstein, R.M.; D'Amato, C.R.; Thompson, G.H. Standardization of criteria for adolescent idiopathic scoliosis brace studies: SRS Committee on Bracing and Nonoperative Management. *Spine* **2005**, *30*, 2068–2075, discussion 2076. [CrossRef]
27. Rigo, M.D.; Villagrasa, M.; Gallo, D. A specific scoliosis classification correlating with brace treatment: Description and reliability. *Scoliosis* **2010**, *5*, 1. [CrossRef]
28. Donzelli, S.; Zaina, F.; Lusini, M.; Minnella, S.; Negrini, S. In favour of the definition "adolescents with idiopathic scoliosis": Juvenile and adolescent idiopathic scoliosis braced after ten years of age, do not show different end results. SOSORT award winner 2014. *Scoliosis* **2014**, *9*, 7. [CrossRef] [PubMed]
29. James, J.I. Two Curve Patterns in Idiopathic Structural Scoliosis. *J. Bone Jt. Surg. Br.* **1951**, *33*, 399–406. [CrossRef]
30. Wynne-Davies, R. Infantile idiopathic scoliosis: Causative factors, particularly in the first six months of life. *J. Bone Jt. Surg. Br.* **1975**, *57*, 138–141. [CrossRef]
31. Ulijaszek, S.; Johnston, F.; Preece, M.; Heinig, M. The Cambridge encyclopedia of human growth and development. *Am. J. Clin. Nutr.* **1999**, *70*, 1114.
32. Perdriolle, R.; Vidal, J. Thoracic Idiopathic Scoliosis Curve Evolution and Prognosis. *Spine* **1985**, *10*, 785–791. [CrossRef]
33. Mehta, M.H. The rib-vertebra angle in the early diagnosis between resolving and progressive infantile scoliosis. *J. Bone Jt. Surg. Br.* **1972**, *54*, 230–243. [CrossRef]
34. Roye, B.D.; Simhon, M.E.; Matsumoto, H.; Bakarania, P.; Berdishevsky, H.; Dolan, L.A.; Grimes, K.; Grivas, T.; Hresko, M.T.; Karol, L.A.; et al. Establishing consensus on the best practice guidelines for the use of bracing in adolescent idiopathic scoliosis. *Spine Deform.* **2020**, *8*, 597–604. [CrossRef] [PubMed]

35. Morcuende, J.A.; Dolan, L.A.; Vazquez, J.D.; Jirasirakul, A.; Weinstein, S.L. A prognostic model for the presence of neurogenic lesions in atypical idiopathic scoliosis. *Spine* **2004**, *29*, 51–58. [CrossRef] [PubMed]
36. Rigo, M.; Janssen, B.; Campo, R.; Tremonti, L. Conservative treatment of juvenile with Chiari I malformation, syringomyelia and scoliosis. Two case reports. *Scoliosis* **2013**, *8*, O52. [CrossRef]

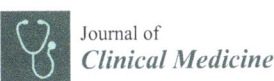

Article

Regular School Sport versus Dedicated Physical Activities for Body Posture—A Prospective Controlled Study Assessing the Sagittal Plane in 7–10-Year-Old Children

Mateusz Kozinoga [1,*], Łukasz Stoliński [2], Krzysztof Korbel [3], Katarzyna Politarczyk [1], Piotr Janusz [1] and Tomasz Kotwicki [1]

1. Department of Spine Disorders and Pediatric Orthopedics, University of Medical Sciences, 61-545 Poznan, Poland; k.politarczyk@gmail.com (K.P.); mdpjanusz@gmail.com (P.J.); kotwicki@ump.edu.pl (T.K.)
2. Spine Disorders Center, 96-100 Skierniewice, Poland; stolinskilukasz@op.pl
3. Department of Physiotherapy, University of Medical Sciences, 61-545 Poznan, Poland; kkorbel@ump.edu.pl
* Correspondence: mkozinoga@hotmail.com

Abstract: Body posture develops during the growing period and can be documented using trunk photography. The study aims to evaluate the body posture in children aged 7–10 years undergoing a dedicated physical activities program versus regular school sport. A total of 400 children, randomly chosen from a cohort of 9300 participating in a local scoliosis screening program, were evaluated twice at a one-year interval. A total of 167 children were involved in regular school sport (control group), while 233 received both school sport and a dedicated physical activities program (intervention group). Standardized photographic habitual body posture examination was performed at enrollment (T0) and one-year after (T1). Sacral slope (SS), lumbar lordosis (LL), thoracic kyphosis (TK), chest inclination (CI), and head protraction (HP) were measured. At T0, the body posture parameters did not differ between groups. At T1 in the controls, all five parameters tended to deteriorate (insignificant): SS $p = 0.758$, LL $p = 0.38$, TK $p = 0.328$, CI $p = 0.081$, and HP $p = 0.106$. At T1 in the intervention group, the SS decreased ($p = 0.001$), the LL tended to decrease ($p = 0.0602$), and the TK, CI, and HP remained unaltered. At T1, the SS and LL parameter differed between groups statistically ($p = 0.0002$ and $p = 0.0064$, respectively) and clinically (2.52° and 2.58°, respectively). In 7–10-year-old children, participation in dedicated physical activities tends to improve their body posture compared to regular school sport.

Keywords: body posture; sports activity; corrective exercises; digital photography

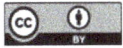

1. Introduction

Harmonious arches characterize the shape of sagittal curvatures in a normal spine, which provides both mobility and stability [1]. Body posture develops throughout childhood and adolescence [2]. Increased sagittal spine curvatures (thoracic kyphosis or lumbar lordosis) combined with increased chest inclination and head protraction are observed in children with weak postural muscles [3] and in adults with myofascial pattern back pain [4]. The standardized photographic assessment of lateral trunk view can reliably quantify body posture and was validated for 7–10-year-old children [5]. The influence of physical activity on a child's body posture has not been extensively studied so far. The study aims to assess the impact of dedicated physical activities versus regular school sports on a child's body posture in a cohort of 7–10-year-old children.

2. Materials and Methods

2.1. Study Population

An observational, prospective controlled study was undertaken within the frame of a scoliosis screening program addressed to primary school children, inhabitants of a half million city. A total of 400 children, 200 girls and 200 boys, aged 7–10 years, were randomly selected from a base consisting of 9300 children, including all primary schools' pupils of the city, previously negatively screened for idiopathic scoliosis or Scheuermann kyphosis. The technique of cluster randomization [6] was applied, assigning schools to districts first, then using a computer-generated sequence to select the order of districts randomly, and then the order of schools in individual districts. Inclusion criteria were age 7–10 years old, no structural deformation of the spine (i.e., idiopathic scoliosis or Scheuermann kyphosis), and availability of a full set of digital photographs. During school screening, the body posture assessment consisted of an inspection of spinal curvatures and position of the head. The assessments were performed by physiotherapists experienced in body posture examination. The examination was carried out according to a structured protocol. Physiotherapists received training before the procedure. Children were assigned into two groups: (1) the control group without any posture misalignment, who performed regular school sport and was considered natural history (N = 167), and (2) the intervention group of children presenting any posture misalignment, who received both school sport and dedicated physical activities (N = 233). The study was performed before the COVID-19 pandemic. The screening program was supported with a grant from the EEA Financial Mechanism. The study was approved by the local Institutional Review Board of the Poznan University of Medical Sciences, No. 283/16.

2.2. Intervention

The program for the prevention of postural misalignments (city of Poznan scoliosis screening program) comprised the participation of children in a system of organized dedicated physical activities. The group sessions, once per week, were organized and supervised by a physiotherapist. Several physiotherapists were engaged in the intervention, which could decrease the homogeneity of the intervention itself (study limitation). However, all of them received training and the dosage stayed fixed.

Children with postural misalignments (N = 233) entered in a weekly, one hour long, dedicated physical activities program, lasting ten months (September–June). Two major groups of activities were applied: either movement games and dance or swimming. All activities were supervised by a physiotherapist.

All children (N = 400) participated in regular 45 min long school sport activities (such as running, athletics, volleyball, basketball, handball, and football) four times per week, which is a standard frequency of school sport in primary schools in Poland.

2.3. Assessment

Each child underwent photographic registration of the body posture from the front (A), back (B), right lateral (C), and left lateral (D). The posture images were captured with a Canon® (Tokyo, Japan) Power shot A590 IS digital camera (matrix CCD 1/2.5, 8.3 M pixels, focal length 35–140 mm). The camera was mounted on a tripod at the height of 90 cm and paralleled to the floor, 300 cm from the examined person. The photographic technique was standardized and consistent with the methodology published by Stolinski et al. [5].

The habitual standing posture of both groups was compared before (T0) and after one year (T1), at the end of the postural school program.

Five postural parameters were measured on digital photographs using a dedicated semiautomatic software SCODIAC v. 2.0 (Pavel Cerny, Prague, Czech Republic) [7] (Figure 1): (1) sacral slope angle (SS), (2) lumbar lordosis angle (LL), (3) thoracic kyphosis angle (TK), (4) chest inclination angle (CI), and (5) head protraction angle (HP). The increase of postural angular parameter was interpreted as a posture worsening, while decrease of postural angular parameter was interpreted as an improvement of body posture.

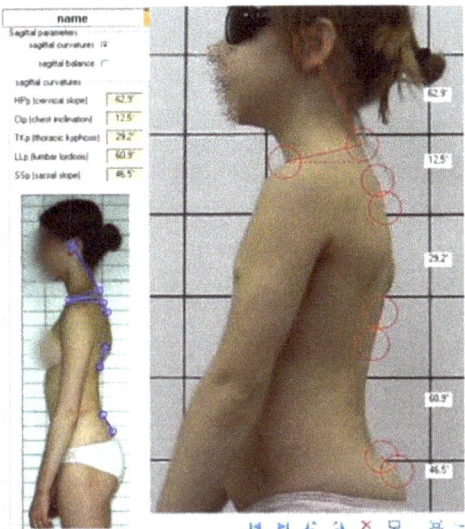

Figure 1. SCODIAC software v 2.0: top left—values of parameters; bottom left—instruction for use; right—measurement.

Clinically relevant differences were fixed as doubled SEM and revealed: SS 2.01°, LL 2.45°, TK 2.34°, CI 1.8°, and HP 0.89°.

2.4. Intra- and Inter-Rater Reliability

To determine the repeatability (intra-observer reliability), 40 digital photographs were evaluated three times in a one-week interval. Intraclass Correlation Coefficient (ICC), Confidence Interval (C.I.), Standard Error of Measurement (SEM), and Standard Deviation (SD) were calculated.

To determine reproducibility (inter-observer reliability), 30 digital photographs were evaluated by three observers three times each.

2.5. Statistical Analysis

GraphPad, MEDCALC, and Microsoft Excel were used. ICC values 0.81–1.00 were considered as excellent [8]. C.I. of 95% probability was taken. The normality of distribution was assessed using the Kolmogorov–Smirnov test. To assess the significant differences in average values, a t–Student test was used. The significance level was defined as $p = 0.05$.

3. Results

The repeatability (intra-observer reliability) for all five postural parameters was excellent (ICC 0.975 to 0.995), with SEM from 0.447° for HP to 1.225° for LL (Table 1).

Table 1. Repeatability of photographic parameters measurements (Intra-observer).

Parameter	ICC	95% C.I.	SEM [°]	SD [°]
Sacral slope	0.975	0.884–0.986	1.007	6.4
Lumbar lordosis	0.981	0.968–0.989	1.225	8.88
Thoracic kyphosis	0.987	0.977–0.992	1.170	10.14
Chest inclination	0.981	0.968–0.989	0.901	6.55
Head protraction	0.995	0.991–0.997	0.447	6.32

ICC—Intraclass correlation coefficient, C.I.—Confidence Interval, SEM—Standard Error of Measurement, SD—standard deviation.

The reproducibility (inter-observer reliability) was also excellent (ICC 0.885 to 0.975), with SEM from 0.888° for LL to 0.949° for HP (Appendix A, Table A1).

At study enrolment (T0), the habitual posture parameters SS, LL, TK, CI, and HP were not significantly different between both groups; the p level was 0.210, 0.366, 0.524, 0.757, and 0.611, respectively (Table 2).

Table 2. Comparison of habitual posture between the control and the intervention group at T0 time.

Posture Parameter	Control N = 167	Intervention N = 233	p
Sacral slope [°]	29.58 ± 7.23	28.63 ± 7.6	0.210
Lumbar lordosis [°]	46.94 ± 8.96	46.08 ± 9.78	0.366
Thoracic kyphosis [°]	41.63 ± 9.55	42.23 ± 9.11	0.523
Chest inclination [°]	15.9 ± 7	16.1 ± 5.64	0.757
Head protraction [°]	31.65 ± 5.16	31.96 ± 6.44	0.611

Mean value ± standard deviation is presented. N—group size, p—significance.

The habitual posture assessment at one-year (T1 vs. T0) revealed differences in the control versus the intervention group. In the control group, small (from 0.17° to 0.96°), and statistically nonsignificant differences were found for all parameters (SS p = 0.758, LL p = 0.38, TK p = 0.328, CI p = 0.081, and HP p = 0.106, respectively). The values of all parameters tended to increase (Table 3).

Table 3. Comparison of habitual posture between T0 and T1 in the control group (N = 167).

Posture Parameter	H_0	H_1	p
Sacral slope [°]	29.58 ± 7.23	29.75 ± 6.79	0.758
Lumbar lordosis [°]	46.94 ± 8.96	47.50 ± 9.19	0.38
Thoracic kyphosis [°]	41.63 ± 9.55	42.38 ± 9.39	0.328
Chest inclination [°]	15.9 ± 7	16.86 ± 6.32	0.081
Head protraction [°]	31.65 ± 5.16	32.45 ± 6.08	0.106

Mean value ± standard deviation is presented. H_0—habitual posture at T0, H_1—habitual posture at T1, N—group size, p—significance.

In the intervention group, the SS significantly decreased (1.4°, p = 0.001), LL tended to decrease (1.59°, p = 0.062), and no significant change for the TK, CI, and HP was found (Table 4).

Table 4. Comparison of habitual posture between T0 and T1 time in the intervention group (N = 233).

Posture Parameter	H_0	H_1	p
Sacral slope [°]	28.63 ± 7.6	27.23 ± 6.68	0.001
Lumbar lordosis [°]	46.08 ± 9.78	44.49 ± 9.34	0.062
Thoracic kyphosis [°]	42.23 ± 9.11	42.79 ± 9.98	0.404
Chest inclination [°]	16.1 ± 5.64	16.37 ± 5.95	0.547
Head protraction [°]	31.96 ± 6.44	32.80 ± 6.07	0.058

Mean value ± standard deviation is presented. H_0—habitual posture at T0, H_1—habitual posture at T1, N—group size, p—significance.

The habitual posture assessment at one-year (T1 intervention vs. T1 control) revealed statistically and clinically significant lower values of the SS and LL parameter (p = 0.0002, 2.52°; p = 0.0064, 2.58°, respectively) in the intervention group. The three other parameters did not differ between groups (Table 5).

Table 5. Comparison of habitual posture between the control and the intervention group at T1 time.

Parameter	Posture	Control N = 167	Intervention N = 233	p
Sacral slope [°]		29.747 ± 6.79	27.23 ± 6.68	0.0002
Lumbar lordosis [°]		47.50 ± 9.19	44.92 ± 9.34	0.0064
Thoracic kyphosis [°]		42.38 ± 9.38	42.79 ± 9.98	0.674
Chest inclination [°]		16.86 ± 6.32	16.37 ± 5.95	0.427
Head protraction [°]		32.45 ± 6.08	32.80 ± 6.07	0.57

Mean value ± standard deviation is presented. N—group size, p—significance.

4. Discussion

4.1. Body Posture Evaluation Technique

The photographic technique of the body posture evaluation presents an advantage to be non-invasive, objective, and easy to use (does not require the use of external skin markers). The terms of thoracic kyphosis, lumbar lordosis, or sacral slope denote the surface shape of the trunk but not the radiographic imaging. The methodology of photographic posture evaluation has been published [5,9–11], and the repeatability and reproducibility have been verified [5,9,12–15]. The previous study confirms excellent intra- and inter-reliability [5,9–15] and reflects the results by Stolinski et al. [5,15]. The ICC coefficient varied from 0.885 for the HP, up to 0.975 for the LL.

Archiving digital photography provides easy storage and reproduction of images, while respecting the patient's anonymity. Canales et al. [16] used photographs of patients with mental disorders (depression) to document their postures. The technique allows for a combined photographic and clinical analysis of body posture, thus enhancing a child's understanding of posture defect, which improves their cooperation during exercising.

4.2. Sample Selection

According to studies by McEvoy (U.S. population) and Shumway-Cook (Australian population) [13,17], the peri-pubertal growth spurt occurs at the age of 9–12 years (sooner for girls, later for boys). The study by Kułaga (Polish population) [18] in 2007–2012 on 22,000 children, aged 3–18 years, confirmed that the growth acceleration began at 9 years and 6 months for girls, and at 10 years and 3 months for boys. The Peak Height Velocity [19]—the most significant 12-month body height increase—equals 6.8 cm in girls and falls between 10 years and 8 months and 11 years and 8 months, while it equals 7.5 cm for boys and falls between 12 years and 6 months and 13 years and 6 months [18]. The rapid growth period corresponds to a period of deterioration of both structural spine deformities (idiopathic scoliosis) and non-structural ones (postural spine misalignments). Concerning the sample studied, the children presenting relevant trunk rotation during scoliometer examination had been previously identified and adequately managed. The remaining children were examined by physiotherapists and postural defects were noticed with inspection in about 40% of them. These children entered the dedicated program of physical activity in order to prevent further posture deterioration, improve motor skills, and enhance postural muscles force.

In this study, we examined the posture immediately before the critical period of the pubertal growth spurt. Comparing the values of the five postural photographic parameters between the two groups, no significant difference in the habitual posture at T0 was revealed.

4.3. Impact of Physical Activities on the Body Posture

In the control group (Table 3), no significant differences were noticed between the initial examination (T0) and the one-year examination (T1) for all parameters. All the values presented tendency to slightly increase. It can be supposed that in natural history (without the intervention of additional physical activities), postural parameters slightly deteriorate during the growing phase. Still, this change did not reach neither statistical nor clinically relevant values.

Among children from the intervention group (Table 4), examined in the habitual posture, between the initial examination (T0) and the one-year examination (T1), a significant ($p = 0.001$, Type II risk error 0.188) SS decrease of 1.40° was found, which should be interpreted as improved posture. The LL and HP parameter change was at the limit of significance ($p = 0.062$, Type II risk error 0.648; $p = 0.058$, Type II risk error 0.64, respectively). Other parameters did not change significantly, which can be interpreted as stabilization of postural photographic parameters in children from the intervention group.

Comparison of the habitual posture between both groups after one year (T1) has shown lower values of SS ($p = 0.0002$) and LL ($p = 0.0064$) in the intervention group, which signifies posture improvement. What is more, both differences were clinically significant (for SS: 2.52° (doubled SEM = 2.01°) and for LL: 2.58° (doubled SEM = 2.45°)) (Table 5).

The overall results indicate a positive effect of additional physical activities on a child's body posture. The hypothetic cause could be a higher unconscious tension and activity of the abdominal muscles while standing.

4.4. Impact of Corrective Activities on Body Posture in the Literature

Dutkiewicz [20] examined the impact of 10-month corrective exercises among 370 children (190 study, 180 control) aged 6–17 years. The surface topography and Kasperczyk scoring method were used. Both groups at T0 did not differ. The highest reduction of posture defects was noted for the head position in the age group 6–9 years (from 23.6% to 13.9%) and 10–14 years (from 33.4% to 23.6% of prevalence). For children 6–9 years, the reduction of excessive thoracic kyphosis occurrence was significant (from 24.1% to 15.7%), as well as the reduction of excessive lumbar lordosis (from 23.8% to 18.8%).

The results of our study, similar to Dutkiewicz's results, indicate an improvement in the thoracic kyphosis, however, we do not confirm the positive change in the head position and in lumbar lordosis angle.

Cosma et al. [21] reported on the influence of corrective exercises (static, dynamic, breathing, correcting, and hyper-correcting specific misalignments) on the body posture of 20 children aged 6–9 years. Body posture was assessed using the "PostureScreen Mobile" mobile application. The measurements were taken at the beginning of the study and after six months of physical exercises. The position of the head (protraction) and hip in the sagittal plane were assessed. A significant improvement of all measured postural parameters was noted. The study limitation, apart from a small study group, may be the fact that children were photographed in clothes, which makes it difficult to identify reference points on the body (such as sternum incision, acromions, waist, anterior superior iliac spines, greater trochanters, or external malleolus).

Torlaković et al. [22] published a study on the impact of physical exercises at the pool (swimming in combination with aquaerobics and corrective exercises) on the posture of 50 boys aged 5.2 ± 0.6 years in Sarajevo (Bosnia and Herzegovina). The posture was assessed by the Wolański visual method, assessing the position of the head, shoulders, shoulder blades, chest shape, spine, abdomen shape, knees, feet, and overall body posture. The program consisted of two weekly meetings of 60 min each for 16 weeks. Significant improvement in all parameters was noted, except for the chest shape and the head position. The limitation of the study is the use of a subjective method of assessing the children's body posture.

4.5. Impact of Physical Activities on the General Health of the Child

The positive impact on body posture is not the only benefit coming from regular physical activities performed by children. The U.S. Department of Health and Human Services, in their Physical Activity Guidelines Advisory Committee Report, 2008 [23], stated that children and adolescents who maintain regular physical activity demonstrate a higher level of physical fitness (cardiorespiratory endurance and muscle strength), reduced body fat, favorable cardiovascular and metabolic disease risk profiles, enhanced bone health, and reduced psychological symptoms such as depression or anxiety. The positive impact of physical activities on bone mass was confirmed by Sundberg et al. [24], Welten et al. [25], and Bielemann et al. in the systematic review [26].

4.6. Practical Implications

We observe that regular school sport, even if extremely beneficial for physical development of children, may be insufficient to ensure a normal posture development due to the modern model of sedentary life. There is an important practical issue whether it could be enriched by out-of-school sport activities. Numerous initiatives of supporting children's physical development are observed at the local, municipal, or regional level. Additionally, while strongly supporting children's additional physical activities, we would like to emphasize the advantage of using objective tools (such as photographic posture assessment) for evaluating various programs raised throughout the country, especially while based on public funding.

5. Conclusions

(1) Participation in additional physical activities performed as a part of a dedicated program tended to improve body posture in 7–10-year-old children.

(2) Regular school sport activity may be insufficient as a compensation of the contemporary model of sedentary lifestyle in children and could be enriched by after-school sports activities.

Author Contributions: Conceptualization M.K. and T.K.; methodology M.K., T.K., Ł.S. and K.P.; software, Ł.S. and P.J.; validation, M.K., Ł.S. and K.K.; formal analysis, M.K., T.K., K.K. and K.P.; investigation, M.K..; resources, M.K. and K.K.; data curation, M.K. and Ł.S.; writing—original draft preparation, M.K. and K.P.; writing—review and editing, T.K.; visualization, M.K.; supervision, T.K.; project administration, M.K.; funding acquisition, K.K. All authors have read and agreed to the published version of the manuscript.

Funding: This study was supported by the Poznan University of Medical Sciences (Young Medical Scientist grant number 502-14-01115157-41181). The activities program was supported with a grant from Iceland, Liechtenstein, and Norway through the EEA Financial Mechanism.

Institutional Review Board Statement: The study was conducted according to the guidelines of the Declaration of Helsinki and approved by the Institutional Review Board of the Poznan University of Medical Sciences, Poznan, Poland, No. 283/16.

Informed Consent Statement: Informed consent was obtained from the parents and the children involved in the study.

Data Availability Statement: The data presented in this study are available on request from the corresponding author.

Conflicts of Interest: The authors declare no conflict of interest.

Appendix A

Table A1. Reliability of photographic parameters measurements (Inter-observer).

Parameter	ICC	95% C.I.	SEM [°]	SD [°]
Sacral slope	0.940	0.892–0.969	0.910	6.5
Lumbar lordosis	0.975	0.954–0.987	0.888	9.82
Thoracic kyphosis	0.920	0.856–0.959	0.913	7.10
Chest inclination	0.916	0.842–0.958	0.913	5.76
Head protraction	0.885	0.802–0.939	0.949	4.59

ICC—Intraclass correlation coefficient, C.I.—Confidence Interval, SEM—Standard Error of Measurement, SD—standard deviation.

References

1. Claus, A.P.; Hides, J.A.; Moseley, G.L.; Hodges, P.W. Is 'ideal' sitting posture real? Measurement of spinal curves in four sitting postures. *Man Ther.* **2009**, *14*, 404–408. [CrossRef] [PubMed]
2. Angelakopoulos, G.; Savelsbergh, G.J.; Bennett, S.; Davids, K.; Haralambos, T.; George, G. Systematic review regarding posture development from infancy to adulthood. *Hell. J. Phys. Educ. Sport Sci.* **2008**, *68*, 35–43.
3. Czaprowski, D.; Stoliński, Ł.; Tyrakowski, M.; Kozinoga, M.; Kotwicki, T. Non-structural misalignments of body posture in the sagittal plane. *Scoliosis Spinal Disord.* **2018**, *13*, 6. [CrossRef] [PubMed]
4. Dewitte, V.; De Pauw, R.; De Meulemeester, K.; Peersman, W.; Danneels, L.; Bouche, K.; Roets, A.; Cagnie, B. Clinical classification criteria for nonspecific low back pain: A Delphi-survey of clinical experts. *Musculoskelet. Sci. Pract.* **2018**, *34*, 66–76. [CrossRef]
5. Stolinski, L.; Kozinoga, M.; Czaprowski, D.; Tyrakowski, M.; Cerny, P.; Suzuki, N.; Kotwicki, T. Two-dimensional digital photography for child body posture evaluation: Standardized technique, reliable parameters and normative data for age 7–10 years. *Scoliosis Spinal Disord.* **2017**, *12*, 38. [CrossRef] [PubMed]
6. Hemming, K.; Eldridge, S.; Forbes, G.; Weijer, C.; Taljaard, M. How to design efficient cluster randomized trials. *BMJ* **2017**, *358*, 3064. [CrossRef]
7. Cerny, P.; Stolinski, L.; Drnkova, J.; Czaprowski, D.; Kosteas, A.; Marik, I. Skeletal deformities measurements of X-ray images and photos on the computer. *Locomot. Syst. J.* **2016**, *23*, 32–36.
8. Weir, J.P. Quantifying test-retest reliability using the intraclass correlation coefficient and the SEM. *J. Strength Cond. Res.* **2005**, *19*, 231–240.
9. Stoliński, Ł.; Czaprowski, D.; Kozinoga, M.; Kotwicki, T. Clinical measurement of sagittal trunk curvatures: Photographic angles versus Rippstein plurimeter angles in healthy school children. *Scoliosis* **2014**, *9*, 15. [CrossRef]
10. Stolinski, L.; Kotwicki, T.; Czaprowski, D.; Chowanska, J.; Suzuki, N. Analysis of the Anterior Trunk Symmetry Index (ATSI). Preliminary report. *Stud. Health Technol. Inf.* **2012**, *176*, 242–246. [CrossRef]
11. Young, S. Research for medical photographers: Photographic measurement. *J. Audiov. Media Med.* **2002**, *25*, 94–98. [CrossRef] [PubMed]
12. Dunk, N.M.; Lalonde, J.; Callaghan, J.P. Implications for the use of postural analysis as a clinical diagnostic tool: Reliability of quantifying upright standing spinal postures from photographic images. *J. Manip. Physiol.* **2005**, *28*, 386–392. [CrossRef] [PubMed]
13. Van Niekerk, S.M.; Louw, Q.; Vaughan, C.; Grimmer-Somers, K.; Schreve, K. Photographic measurement of upper-body sitting posture of high school students: A reliability and validity study. *BMC Musculoskelet. Disord.* **2008**, *9*, 113–123. [CrossRef] [PubMed]
14. McEvoy, M.P.; Grimmer, K. Reliability of upright posture measurements in primary school children. *BMC Musculoskelet. Disord* **2005**, *6*, 35. [CrossRef]
15. Stoliński, Ł. Ocena Postawy Ciała z Wykorzystaniem Fotografii Cyfrowej: Opracowanie Metody Wraz z Normami Dla Wieku 8–11 lat. Ph.D. Thesis, Poznan University of Medical Sciences, Poznan, Poland, 2015. (In Polish)
16. Canales, J.Z.; Cordás, T.A.; Fiquer, J.T.; Cavalcante, A.F.; Moreno, R.A. Posture and body image in individuals with major depressive disorder: A controlled study. *Rev. Bras. Psiquiatr.* **2010**, *32*, 375–380. [CrossRef] [PubMed]
17. Shumway-Cook, A.; Woollacott, M.H. *Motor Control: Theory and Practical Applications*; Lippincott Williams & Wilkins: Baltimore, MD, USA, 2001.
18. Kułaga, Z.; Różdżyńska-Świątkowska, A.; Grajda, A.; Gurzkowska, B.; Wojtyło, M.; Góźdź, M.; Świąder-Leśniak, A.; Litwin, M. Siatki centylowe dla oceny wzrastania i stanu odżywienia polskich dzieci i młodzieży od urodzenia do 18 roku życia. *Stand. Med. Pediatr.* **2015**, *12*, 119–135. (In Polish)
19. Neinstein, L.S.; Kaufman, F.R. Chapter 1: Normal Physical Growth and Development. In *Adolescent Health Care: A Practical Guide*, 4th ed.; Neinstein, L.S., Ed.; Lippincott Williams & Wilkins: Baltimore, MD, USA, 2002.
20. Dutkiewicz, R. *Skuteczność Zajęć Korekcyjno-Wyrównawczych w Zniekształceniach Statycznych Ciała u Dzieci w Wieku Szkolnym*; Wydawnictwo Uniwersytetu Humanistyczno-Przyrodniczego Jana Kochanowskiego: Kielce, Poland, 2010. (In Polish)
21. Cosma, G.; Ilinca, I.; Rusu, L.; Nanu, C.; Burileanu, A. Physical exercise and its role in a correct postural alignment. *Phys. Edu. Sport Kinetotherapy J.* **2015**, *11*, 39.
22. Torlaković, A.; Muftić, M.; Avdić, D.; Kebata, R. Effects of the combined swimming, corrective and aqua gymnastics programme on body posture of preschool age children. *J. Health Sci.* **2013**, *3*, 103–108.
23. US Department of Health and Human Services. Physical Activity Guidelines Advisory Committee Report. 2008. Available online: https://health.gov/sites/default/files/2019-10/CommitteeReport_7.pdf (accessed on 11 November 2021).
24. Sundberg, M.; Gärdsell, P.; Johnell, O.; Karlsson, M.K.; Ornstein, E.; Sandstedt, B.; Sernbo, I. Physical Activity Increases Bone Size in Prepubertal Boys and Bone Mass in Prepubertal Girls: A Combined Cross-Sectional and 3-Year Longitudinal Study. *Calcif. Tissue Int.* **2002**, *71*, 406–415. [CrossRef]
25. Welten, D.C.; Kemper, H.C.; Post, G.B.; Van Mechelen, W.; Twisk, J.; Lips, P.; Teule, G.J. Weight-bearing activity during youth is a more important factor for peak bone mass than calcium intake. *J. Bone Min. Res.* **1994**, *9*, 1089–1096. [CrossRef] [PubMed]
26. Bielemann, R.M.; Martinez-Mesa, J.; Gigante, D.P. Physical activity during life course and bone mass: A systematic review of methods and findings from cohort studies with young adults. *BMC Musculoskelet. Disord.* **2013**, *14*, 77. [CrossRef] [PubMed]

MDPI
St. Alban-Anlage 66
4052 Basel
Switzerland
Tel. +41 61 683 77 34
Fax +41 61 302 89 18
www.mdpi.com

Journal of Clinical Medicine Editorial Office
E-mail: jcm@mdpi.com
www.mdpi.com/journal/jcm

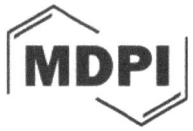

www.ingramcontent.com/pod-product-compliance
Lightning Source LLC
LaVergne TN
LVHW070456100526
838202LV00014B/1735